Nursing Health Assessment:

Assessment:

Clinical Pocket Guide

Nursing Health Assessment:
Clinical Pocket Guide

Patricia M. Dillon, DNSc, RN

Adjunct Faculty
Temple University
College of Allied Health Professions
Department of Nursing
Philadelphia, Pennsylvania

F.A. Davis Company/Publishers • Philadelphia

F. A. Davis Company
1915 Arch Street
Philadelphia, PA 19103
www.fadavis.com

Printed in the United States of America

Last digit indicates print number: 10 9 8 7 6 5 4 3 2 1

Acquisitions Editor: Lisa B. Deitch
Developmental Editor: Alan Sorkowitz
Production Editor: Jessica Howie Martin
Cover Designer: Louis J. Forgione

As new scientific information becomes available through basic and clinical
research, recommended treatments and drug therapies undergo changes.
The author and publisher have done everything possible to make this book
accurate, up to date, and in accord with accepted standards at the time of
publication. The author, editors, and publisher are not responsible for
errors or ommisions or for consequences from application of the book, and
make no warranty, expressed or implied, in regard to the contents of the
book. Any practice described in this book should be applied by the reader
in each situation. The reader is advised always to check product information (package inserts) for changes and new information regarding dose and
contraindications before administering any drug. Caution is especially urged
when using new or infrequently ordered drugs.

Library of Congress Cataloging-in-Publication Data

Dillon, Patricia M.
     Nursing health assessment : clinical pocket guide / Patricia M. Dillon.
         p. ; cm.
     Includes index.
     ISBN 0-8036-0881-0 (soft cover)
         1. Nursing assessment—Handbooks, manuals, etc. I. Title.
     [DNLM: 1. Nursing Assessment—Case Report. 2. Nursing Assessment—
     Handbooks. 3. Medical History Taking—methods—Case Report.
     4. Medical History Taking—methods—Handbooks. 5. Physical
     Examination—methods—Case Report. 6. Physical Examination—
     methods—Handbooks. WY 49 D579n 2004]
RT48.D544 2004
616′.075—dc21   2003051623

DEDICATION

To my patients and students

ACKNOWLEDGMENTS

I would like to acknowledge the staff of F. A. Davis, especially Lisa Deitch, for their support and expertise throughout this project. I would also like to thank Alan Sorkowitz for his editorial acumen and "good eyes."

PREFACE

■ ■ ■

Dear Students,

Now that you have learned the theory behind assessment in class, you need to apply that theory when assessing your patients. *Nursing Health Assessment: Clinical Pocket Guide* will help you to bridge the gap from the classroom to the clinical area.

The *Clinical Pocket Guide* contains:
• Primary function of every system
• Developmental and cultural considerations
• Key history questions for specific symptoms
• Integration with other systems
• The physical assessment, which includes:
     • Anatomical landmarks
     • Approach
     • Position for exam
     • Tools needed for exam
     • Assessment procedure and normal and abnormal findings with **helpful hints** in bold type and ***alerts*** in bold italic type

Think of this pocket guide as another valuable assessment tool that will help you to assess your patients. Take this guide with you wherever you are practicing nursing: the hospital, the home, the community, schools, long-term care facilities. Use the *Clinical Pocket Guide* to help you:
• Perfect your assessment skills
• Differentiate normal from abnormal findings
• Validate your assessment findings

Never forget that you learn much from your patients, so view your encounters with them as a means to learn assessment and develop your skills. And practice, practice, practice!

Patricia Dillon, DNSc, RN

CONTENTS

CHAPTER 24

THE COMPLETE HEALTH ASSESSMENT

A complete health assessment includes a comprehensive history and a complete physical assessment.

Complete Health History

Biographical Data

Includes name, address, phone number, contact person, age, birth date, place of birth, gender, race/ethnicity/nationality, religion, marital status, number of dependents, educational level, occupation, social security number/health insurance, source of history/reliability, referral, advance directive.

Current Health Status

Includes symptom analysis for chief complaint and current medications.

Past Health History

Includes childhood illnesses, surgeries, hospitalizations, serious injuries, medical problems, medications, allergies, immunizations, and recent travel or military service.

Family History

Includes client, spouse, children, siblings, parents, aunts, uncles, and grandparents' health status or, if deceased, age and cause of death.

Review of Systems

Includes questions specific to each body system and analysis of any positive symptoms.

Psychosocial Profile

Includes health practices and beliefs, typical day, nutritional patterns, activity/exercise patterns, recreation, pets/hobbies, sleep/rest patterns, personal habits, occupational health patterns, socioeconomic status, environmental health patterns, roles/relationships, sexuality patterns, social supports, and stress/coping patterns.

Complete Physical Assessment

Approach

Two methods are used for completing a total physical assessment: a systems approach and a head-to-toe approach.

- A systems approach allows for a thorough assessment of each system, doing all assessments related to one system before moving on to the next. Better for a focused assessment.
- A head-to-toe assessment includes the same examinations as a systems assessment, but you assess each region of the body before moving on to the next. Better for a complete assessment.

No matter which approach you use, be systematic and consistent.

All four assessment techniques—inspection, percussion, palpation, and auscultation—are used to perform a complete assessment. Remember:

- Inspect for abnormalities and normal variations of visible body parts.
- Palpate to identify surface characteristics, areas of pain or tenderness, organs, and abnormalities, including masses and fremitus.
- Percuss to determine the density of underlying tissues and to detect abnormalities in underlying organs.
- Auscultate for sounds made by body organs, including the heart, lungs, intestines, and vascular structures.

Assessment data are usually charted by systems (e.g., respiratory or neurological) and by regions to a limited extent

Percussion sounds

Percussion produces sounds that vary according to the tissue being percussed. This chart shows important percussion sounds along with their characteristics and typical locations.

Sound	Intensity	Pitch	Duration	Quality	Source
Resonance	Moderate to loud	Low	Long	Hollow	Normal lung
Tympany	Loud	High	Moderate	Drumlike	Gastric air bubble; intestinal air
Dullness	Soft to moderate	High	Moderate	Thudlike	Liver; full bladder; pregnant uterus
Hyperresonance	Very loud	Very low	Long	Booming	Hyperinflated lung (as in emphysema)
Flatness	Soft	High	Short	Flat	Muscle

(e.g., head/neck). Your documentation can focus only on positive findings or on both positive and negative findings. No matter which format you use, always be brief and to the point and avoid generalizations.

TOOLBOX
You will need all of the tools of assessment identified in the other chapters of this book.

Performing a Head-to-Toe Physical Assessment

Here are some helpful hints to keep in mind as you conduct the assessment:

- Wash your hands before you begin!
- Listen to your client!
- Provide a warm environment.
- If your client has a problem, start at that point.
- Work from head to toe.
- Compare side to side.
- Let your client know your findings.
- Use your time not only to assess but also to teach your client.
- Leave sensitive or painful areas until the end of the examination.

GENERAL SURVEY
Get anthropometric data and vital signs, and evaluate client's clothing, hygiene, state of well-being, nutritional status, emotional status, speech patterns, level of consciousness, affect, posture, gait, coordination and balance, and gross deformities.

SKIN/HAIR/NAILS
- Inspect and palpate client's visible skin for color, lesions, texture, and warmth. Continue observation throughout the examination.
- Note hair color, texture, and distribution over body.
- Observe hands and nails for clubbing or other abnormalities.

HEAD/FACE
- Note head size, shape, and position.
- Note scalp tenderness, lesions, or masses.

The effect of age on vital signs

Normal vital sign ranges vary with age, as this chart shows.

Age	Temperature		Pulse Rate	Respiratory Rate	Blood Pressure
	° Fahrenheit	° Celsius			
Newborn	98.6 to 99.8	37 to 37.7	70 to 190	30 to 80	systolic: 50 to 52 diastolic: 25 to 30 mean: 35 to 40
3 years	98.5 to 99.5	36.9 to 37.5	80 to 125	20 to 30	systolic: 78 to 114 diastolic: 46 to 78
10 years	97.5 to 98.6	36.3 to 37	70 to 110	16 to 22	systolic: 90 to 132 diastolic: 56 to 86
16 years	97.6 to 98.8	36.4 to 37.1	55 to 100	15 to 20	systolic: 104 to 108 diastolic: 60 to 92
Adult	96.8 to 99.5	36 to 37.5	60 to 100	15 to 20	systolic: 95 to 140 diastolic: 60 to 90
Older adult	96.5 to 97.5	35.9 to 36.3	60 to 100	15 to 25	systolic: 140 to 160 diastolic: 70 to 90

- Observe for facial symmetry and note facial expressions (cranial nerve [CN] VII).
- Test sensation on face (CN V).
- Palpate temporomandibular joint for popping or tenderness.
- Test range of motion (ROM) of neck and assess muscle strength.

EYES
- Test visual acuity (CN I) with Snellen test or pocket vision screener.
- Perform test of extraocular movements (CN III, IV, VI).
- Perform cover test and corneal light reflex test.
- Test visual fields by confrontation.
- Inspect general appearance and eyelids.
- Inspect cornea, iris, and lens with oblique lighting.
- Observe sclera and conjunctivae.
- Perform pupillary reaction to light and accommodation.
- Perform fundoscopic examination to test for red reflex and to observe disks and retinal vessels.

EARS
- Inspect external ear and canal.
- Inspect position and angle of attachment.
- Palpate tragus, mastoid, and helix for tenderness.
- Perform Weber test for lateralization, Rinne test for bone and air conduction, and whisper test for low-pitch or low-tone hearing loss (CN VIII).
- Perform otoscopic examination of canal and tympanic membrane.

NOSE
- Test for patency of each nostril.
- Test sense of smell (CN I).
- Palpate for sinus tenderness.
- Observe nasal mucosa, septum, and turbinates with speculum.

MOUTH/PHARYNX
- Inspect and palpate lips and oral mucosa.
- Inspect teeth, gingiva, and palate.
- Inspect pharynx and tonsils.

- Test gag and swallow reflexes, and have client say "ah" (CN IX, X).
- Test taste on anterior and posterior tongue (CN VII, IX).
- Inspect tongue for abnormalities, and check ROM of tongue by having client say "d, l, n, t" (CN XII).

NECK
- Inspect and palpate thyroid gland.
- Inspect for masses, abnormal pulsations, or tracheal deviation.
- Palpate carotid pulse and listen for bruits.
- Inspect jugular veins.
- Measure jugular venous pressure.
- Palpate lymph nodes in head, neck, and clavicular areas.
- Test ROM of neck.
- Test muscle strength of neck and shoulder muscles (CN XI).

UPPER EXTREMITIES
- Test for ROM and muscle strength.
- Inspect joints for swelling, redness, and deformities.
- Test hand grip.
- Test superficial and deep sensations.
- Palpate radial, ulnar, and brachial pulses.
- Test for deep tendon reflexes of biceps, triceps, and brachioradialis.
- Test coordination, rapid alternating movements, and finger-thumb opposition.
- Inspect and palpate nails, checking capillary refill and angle of attachment.
- Test for pronator drift.
- Test for accuracy of movements with point-to-point movements.

POSTERIOR THORAX/BACK
- Palpate thyroid from behind (if not done previously).
- Inspect spine and palpate muscles along spine.
- Percuss and auscultate lung fields.
- Fist/blunt percuss costovertebral angle tenderness.
- Palpate and percuss chest excursion.
- Palpate tactile fremitus.
- Note normal curvatures of spine.

- Test for kyphosis, scoliosis, and lordosis.
- Check ROM of spine.

ANTERIOR THORAX
- Inspect, palpate, percuss, and auscultate lungs.
- Inspect and palpate precordium for pulsations, point of maximal impulse, and thrills.
- Auscultate heart.
- Inspect and palpate breasts.
- Palpate axillary and epitrochlear lymph nodes.

ABDOMEN
- Inspect for shape, scars, movements, and abnormalities.
- Auscultate for bowel sounds and vascular sounds.
- Percuss abdomen and organs for size.
- Obtain a liver measurement.
- Palpate lightly for tenderness.
- Palpate deeply for masses and enlarged liver, spleen, kidneys, and aorta.
- Palpate femoral arteries and inguinal lymph nodes.
- If ascites suspected, percuss for shifting dullness.

LOWER EXTREMITIES
- Inspect for skin color, hair distribution, temperature, edema, and varicose veins.
- Test for ROM, muscle strength, and superficial and deep sensations.
- Palpate pulses.
- Test deep tendon reflexes and plantar reflex.
- Observe gait, toe walk, heel walk, heel-to-toe walk, and deep knee bend.
- Perform Romberg's test and proprioception test.
- Test coordination with toe tapping and heel down shin.
- Test superficial and deep sensations.
- If indicated, test knees for fluid with bulge sign or patellar tap.
- If indicated, test for torn meniscus with Apley's or McMurray's test.
- Observe ROM of lower extremities.
- Test muscle strength of lower extremities.

FEMALE GENITALIA/RECTUM
- Inspect and palpate external genitalia and inguinal lymph nodes.
- Perform internal examination: Inspect vagina and cervix, collect Pap smear and cultures.
- Palpate uterus and adnexa.
- Inspect perianal area and palpate anal canal and rectum.
- Test stool for occult blood.

MALE GENITALIA/RECTUM
- Inspect and palpate external genitalia.
- Palpate for hernias.
- Inspect perianal area for hemorrhoids or abnormalities.
- Palpate anal canal, rectum, and prostate.
- Test stool on glove for occult blood.

Documenting Physical Assessment Findings

Document physical assessment findings by system, using the following sequence:

- General survey, including anthropometric measurements and vital signs
- Integumentary
- Head, face, and neck
- Eyes
- Ears, nose, and throat
- Respiratory
- Cardiovascular
- Breasts
- Abdomen
- Male/female genitourinary
- Musculoskeletal
- Neurological

Focused Physical Assessments

- Focused assessments are only partial ones, dealing only with systems that relate to the client's problem, so less data are collected.
- Focused assessments are used when the client's condition or time restraints preclude a comprehensive assessment.
- A focused physical assessment should include the following:

- A general survey with vital signs and weight
- Assessment of level of consciousness
- Assessment of skin color, temperature, and texture
- Testing of gross motor balance and coordination
- Testing of extraocular movements
- Testing of pupillary reaction
- Testing of gross vision and hearing
- Inspection of oral mucosa as client says "ah"
- Auscultation of anterior and posterior breath sounds
- Palpation of apical impulse, point of maximal impulse
- Auscultation of heart sounds
- Auscultation of abdomen
- Percussion of abdomen
- Palpation of abdomen
- Palpation of peripheral pulses
- Testing sensation to touch on extremities
- Palpation of muscle strength of upper and lower extremities

CHAPTER 2

ASSESSING THE INTEGUMENTARY SYSTEM

Primary Functions

- Body's first line of defense
- Protects against trauma
- Protects against ultraviolet radiation
- Supports nerve tissue, blood vessels, sweat and sebum glands, and hair follicles
- Helps maintain body temperature
- Helps maintain fluid balance
- Provides sensation with external environment
- Involved in absorption and excretion
- Involved with immunity
- Synthesizes vitamin D

Developmental Considerations

Infants

- Skin is smooth, with little subcutaneous tissue.
- Color changes can be seen readily. Newborns often appear pinker/redder because of the lack of subcutaneous tissue.
- Physiologic jaundice may occur 2 to 3 days after birth.
- Newborns have little or no coarse terminal hair; hair is shed at approximately 3 months and then is soon replaced.

- Eccrine sweat glands begin to function within a month after birth.
- Immature sweat glands lead to poor thermoregulation.
- Because there are no functioning apocrine sweat glands, babies' skin is less oily than adults' and lacks offensive odor.
- Secretion of sebum by the sebaceous glands can result in cradle cap.
- Numerous skin lesions may be seen on the newborn, such as mongolian spots, nevus flammeus (port-wine stains), capillary hemangiomas (stork bites), hemangioma simplex (strawberry marks), milia, and erythema toxicum neonatorum.

Adolescents

- Apocrine glands begin to enlarge and function.
- Axillary sweating increases, with the potential for a more pronounced body odor.
- Sebum production increases and the skin becomes more oily, leading to acne.
- Pubic and axillary hair appear, and male and female body hair patterns become apparent.

Pregnant Clients

- Increased blood flow to the skin, particularly to the hands and feet, occurs as vessels dilate and the number of capillaries increases to dissipate heat.
- Sweating and sebaceous activity increase.
- Skin thickens and separates with stretching, with the appearance of striae.
- Hormonal changes result in hyperpigmentation. Pigmentary changes occur on the face (resulting in chloasma); on abdominal midline (the linea alba becomes the linea nigra); and on the nipples, areolae, axillae, and vulva.

Menopausal Women

- Hormonal fluctuations result in hot flashes, often accompanied by flushing of the skin and increased pigmentation.
- Facial hair increases, and there is some degree of scalp hair loss.
- Incidence of skin tags increases at menopause.

Older Adults

- Skin atrophies.
- Sebum and sweat production decreases.
- Skin becomes drier and flattens, often becoming paper-like.
- Elasticity decreases and wrinkles develop.
- Decreased melanocyte function causes gray hair and pale skin. Target areas of increased melanocyte function result in "age spots."
- Decrease in axillary, pubic, and scalp hair. Women may have increased facial hair as estrogen function is lost; men have increased nasal and ear hair growth.
- Nails grow more slowly and become thicker and more brittle.
- Specific skin lesions are more common in elderly persons, including actinic keratoses, basal cell carcinomas, seborrheic keratoses, stasis ulcers, senile pruritus, and keratotic horns.

Age-Related Skin Disorders	
AGE	**DISORDER**
Children	Impetigo
	Atopic dermatitis or eczema
	Pityriasis rosea
	Juvenile plantar dermatosis
	Rashes secondary to bacterial or viral infections
	Pediculosis capitis
	Varicella
Adolescents/ Young Adults	Acne
	Pityriasis rosea
	Tinea versicolor
Adults	Psoriasis
	Seborrheic dermatitis
	Malignant melanoma
	Herpes simplex virus type 2
	Tinea cruris

(continued)

Age-Related Skin Disorders (*Continued*)

AGE	DISORDER
	Seborrheic intertrigo
	Rosacea
Older Adults	Actinic keratosis
	Seborrheic keratosis
	Basal cell carcinoma
	Squamous cell carcinoma
	Xerosis
	Herpes zoster
Children and Adults	Nummular eczema/dermatitis
	Scabies
	Insect bites, poisonous plants
	Contact dermatitis
	Herpes zoster
	Tinea pedis

Cultural Considerations

- The oral mucosa is best for assessing color changes in dark-skinned persons.
- Assessing the sclera for jaundice, rather than the skin, is more accurate in Asians.
- Fair-skinned persons of Irish, German, or Polish descent have an increased risk for skin cancer with prolonged sun exposure.
- African-Americans have a higher incidence of keloids, pseudofolliculitis, and mongolian spots.
- Asians often have black, straight, silky hair, and Chinese men have very little facial hair.
- Hair texture of African-Americans is often thick and kinky.
- Asians produce less sweat and so have less body odor.

Assessment

History

SYMPTOMS ("PQRST" ANY + SYMPTOM)
- Change in mole or lesion
  - When did you first notice a change in the mole or lesion?
  - What changes did you notice?
  - Have you ever had any severe sunburns?
  - Do you use sun block? If yes, what type?
  - Do you have a family history of skin cancer?
- Pruritus
  - Do you have any allergies?
  - Have you noticed any rashes?
  - Do you have any medical problems?
  - Are you on any medications?
  - Do you typically have any sinus congestion, runny nose, or watery eyes?
  - Have you noticed any change in your overall skin coloring?
  - Have you had any loss of appetite or nausea?
  - Have you recently experienced any abdominal pain?
  - Have you had a change in your energy level?
- Nonhealing lesion or ulceration
  - How long have you had the sore/ulcer?
  - Do you remember bumping or hurting the area?
  - What have you used to treat the sore?
  - Does the sore hurt?
  - Is there drainage? If yes, does it have an odor?
  - Do you have any history of vascular disease or diabetes?
- Rashes
  - Do you have any allergies?
  - Do you have any medical problems?
  - Are you taking any medications, prescribed or over the counter?
  - Have you been exposed to anything different or new, such as soaps or detergents?
  - Have you experienced any fevers?

- Have you noticed any swollen lymph nodes?
- Have you had any associated symptoms such as runny nose, sore throat, or headache?
- Have you had any pain in your joints or muscles?
- Changes in hair
  - Can you describe the changes in your hair?
  - Do you have any medical problems?
  - Are you taking any medications, either prescribed or over the counter?
  - What are your usual patterns of hair care—washing, perms, curling, and so forth?
- Changes in nails
  - Have you noticed any changes in color of your nails?
  - Are your nails brittle?
  - What are your usual patterns of nail care?
  - Do you smoke?
  - Do you bite your nails?

Seasonal Skin Disorders

SEASON	SKIN DISORDERS
Spring	Pityriasis rosea Chickenpox Acne flare-ups
Summer	Contact dermatitis Tinea *Candida* Impetigo Insect bites
Fall	Senile pruritus/winter itch Pityriasis rosea Urticaria Acne flare-ups
Winter	Contact dermatitis of hands Senile pruritus/winter itch Psoriasis Eczema

FOCUSED INTEGUMENTARY HISTORY
- Do you have changes in your skin, hair, or nails?
- Do you have any food, drug, or environmental allergies?
- Do you have any medical problems? Endocrine problems, diabetes, peripheral vascular disease, or cardiovascular disease?
- Are you taking any medications, either prescribed or over the counter (Table 2–1)?

Table 2–1. *Drugs That Adversely Affect the Integumentary System*

DRUG CLASS	DRUG	POSSIBLE ADVERSE REACTIONS
Adrenocortico-steroids	methylpred-nisolone, prednisone	Urticaria, skin atrophy and thin-ning, acne, facial erythema, striae, allergic dermatitis, petechiae, ecchymoses
Anticonvulsants	carbamaze-pine	Pruritic rash, toxic epidermal necrolysis, Stevens-Johnson syndrome
	lamotrigine	Same as carbamazepine
	valproate	Alopecia
	phenytoin sodium	Morbilliform (measles-like) rash, excessive hair growth
	ethosuximide	Urticaria, pruritic (itchy) and ery-thematous (reddened) rashes
Antimalarial	chloroquine phosphate	Pruritus; pigmentary skin changes, eruptions resembling lichen planus (with prolonged therapy)
Antineoplastic agents	bleomycin sulfate	Skin toxicity may be accompanied by hypoesthesia that may progress to hyperesthesia, urticaria, ery-thematous swelling, hyperpig-mentation, patchy hyperkeratosis, alopecia
	busulfan	Cheilosis, melanoderma, urticaria, dry skin, alopecia, anhidrosis
	cyclophos-phamide	Skin and fingernail pigmentation, alopecia
Barbiturates	pentobarbi-tal sodium, phenobarbi-tal	Urticaria; maculopapular, morbilli-form, or scarlatiniform rash

(continued)

Table 2–1. *Drugs That Adversely Affect the Integumentary System (Continued)*

DRUG CLASS	DRUG	POSSIBLE ADVERSE REACTIONS
Cephalosporins	cefazolin sodium, cefoxitin sodium, cefuroxime sodium, ceftriaxone sodium, cefotaxime sodium	Rash, pruritus, urticaria, erythema multiforme
Gold salts	auranofin, gold sodium thiomalate	Rash, pruritus, photosensitivity, urticaria
Nonsteroidal anti-inflammatory agents	diflunisal	Rash, pruritus, erythema multiforme, Stevens-Johnson syndrome
	ibuprofen	Rash, erythema multiforme, Stevens-Johnson syndrome
	sulindac	Rash, pruritus, photosensitivity, erythema multiforme, Stevens-Johnson syndrome
Oral anti-diabetic agents	all types	Photosensitivity, various skin eruptions
Penicillins	amoxicillin trihydrate, ampicillin, penicillin G potassium, penicillin V potassium, nafcillin, mezlocillin	Urticaria, erythema, maculopapular rash, pruritus
Phenothiazines	chlorpromazine hydrochloride, thioridazine hydrochloride, trifluoperazine hydrochloride	Dermatoses, pruritus, marked photosensitivity, urticaria, erythema, eczema, exfoliative dermatitis

(continued)

Table 2–1. *Drugs That Adversely Affect the Integumentary System (Continued)*

DRUG CLASS	DRUG	POSSIBLE ADVERSE REACTIONS
Sulfonamides	co-trimoxazole, sulfamethoxazole, sulfasalazine, sulfisoxazole	Rash, pruritus, erythema nodosum, erythema multiforme, Stevens-Johnson syndrome, exfoliative dermatitis, photosensitivity
	griseofulvin	Rash, urticaria, photosensitivity, lupus erythematosus, or lupus-like syndrome
Tetracyclines	demeclocycline hydrochloride, doxycycline hyclate, tetracycline hydrochloride	Photosensitivity
Miscellaneous agents	allopurinol	Pruritic maculopapular rash, exfoliative dermatitis, erythematous dermatitis
	captopril	Maculopapular rash, pruritus, erythema
	corticotropin (ACTH)	Urticaria, pruritus, scarlatiniform exanthema, skin atrophy and thinning, acne, facial erythema, hyperpigmentation
	oral contraceptives (estrogen)	Chloasma or melasma, rash, urticaria, erythema
	thiazide diuretics	Photosensitivity
	lithium	Acne
	warfarin	Skin necrosis

Assessment of Integumentary System's Relationship to Other Systems

Remember, all systems are related! As you assess the integumentary system, look at the relationship between it and all other systems.

SUBJECTIVE DATA	OBJECTIVE DATA
Area/System: General	
Ask about:	*Inspect for:*
Changes in energy level	Signs of distress
Weight changes	*Measure:*
Fevers	Vital signs
	Height and weight
Area/System: HEENT	
Head and Neck	
Ask about:	*Inspect for:*
Lumps or swelling in neck	Facial expression
Difficulty swallowing	Neck vein distention
History of endocrine problems	Enlarged accessory muscles
	Palpate for:
	Lymph node enlargement
	Thyroid gland enlargement
Eyes	
Ask about:	*Inspect for:*
Watery eyes and allergies	Red eyes
Changes in eye color	Icteric eyes
Ears, Nose, and Throat	
Ask about:	*Inspect for:*
Ear, throat, or sinus infections	Red, swollen nasal and oral
Sore throat	mucous membranes
Nasal discharge	
Area/System: Respiratory	
Ask about:	*Inspect for:*
Cough, breathing difficulty	Signs of hypoxia
History of respiratory disease	Asymmetric chest movement
	Auscultate for:
	Abnormal/adventitious breath
	sounds
Area/System: Cardiovascular	
Ask about:	*Inspect for:*
History of cardiovascular	Signs of impaired circulation
disease	Skin changes in extremities
Leg pain	*Palpate for:*
	Pedal pulses
	Edema
	Auscultate for:
	Irregular rhythms, rales, and extra
	sounds
Area/System: Gastrointestinal	
Ask about:	*Inspect for:*
History of liver disease	Ascites
Nausea/vomiting, loss of	*Palpate for:*
appetite	Liver enlargement, tenderness

(continued)

SUBJECTIVE DATA	OBJECTIVE DATA
Change in stool to clay color	*Percuss for:* Liver size
Area/System: Genitourinary/Reproductive	
Ask about:	*Inspect for:*
Changes in urine color	Lesions on external genitalia skin
Urinary tract infections	
Incontinence	
History of sexually transmitted diseases	
Safe-sex practices	
Area/System: Musculoskeletal	
Ask about:	*Inspect for:*
History of joint disease,	Joint deformity
rheumatoid arthritis	Decreased ROM
	Skin changes over joints
Area/System: Neurological	
Ask about:	*Test for:*
Loss of sensation	Sensory perception changes, both
	superficial and deep sensations
	Percuss for:
	Deep tendon reflexes
Area/System: Endocrine	
Ask about:	
History of thyroid disease, diabetes	
Area/System: Immune/Hematologic	
Ask about:	*Inspect for:*
Immune disorders	Ecchymoses or petechiae
Use of immunosuppressive drugs	
Bleeding	
Use of anticoagulants or aspirin	

HEENT = head, eyes, ears, nose, and throat; ROM = range of movement

Physical Assessment

APPROACH: Inspection, palpation
Assessment can be approached in any of three ways:

- Using a head-to-toe approach
- Observing all skin on the anterior, posterior, and lateral surfaces of the body
- Inspecting the skin by regions, as you assess the other body systems

POSITION: Dependent on approach used
TOOLBOX: Gloves; flexible, transparent ruler; marker; penlight; glass slide; and magnifier

AREA/PA SKILL	NORMAL FINDINGS	ABNORMAL FINDINGS
Skin		
Inspection		
Note color, odor, and integrity. Cold or hot weather can affect surface characteristics of skin and nails. Differentiate central (mouth and conjunctiva) vs. peripheral cyanosis (extremities).	Uniform skin color with slightly darker exposed areas. No jaundice, cyanosis, pallor, erythema, or hyper/hypopigmentation. Ethnic/racial differences account for many variations in color. Mucous membranes and conjunctiva pink. No unusual odors	Color changes may be benign or may indicate underlying pathology (see Table 2–2) Unusual body odor: Poor hygiene or underlying disease. If from poor hygiene, may be related to self-care deficit that warrants nursing intervention. Odors from excessive sweating (hyperhidrosis): Possible thyrotoxicosis. Odors from night sweats: Possible tuberculosis. Urine odor: Incontinence problem. Stale urine odor may be associated with uremia. Mousy odor: Liver disease
Identify any lesions: primary, secondary, or vascular. (See Tables 2–3 through 2–5.)	Skin intact, no suspicious lesions	Primary lesions: See Table 2–3. Secondary lesions: See Table 2–4. Vascular lesions: See Table 2–5.
Assess for pressure ulcers (see Table 2–6).		Pressure ulcers: See Table 2–6.

(continued)

AREA/PA SKILL	NORMAL FINDINGS	ABNORMAL FINDINGS

Skin
Inspection

☐ **Pressure ulcers often develop over bony prominences, such as the sacrum and heels, so inspect these areas carefully.**

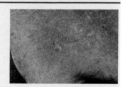

Actinic keratosis

☐ *With pressure ulcers, extensive undermining often occurs, extending through the dermal layer to the bone. The visible pressure ulcer may be only the "tip of the iceberg."*

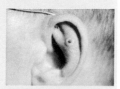

Basal cell carcinoma

Risk factors for pressure ulcers: Impaired mental status, impaired nutritional status, sensory deficits, immobility, mechanical forces, shearing and friction, and excessive exposure to moisture from bodily secretions.

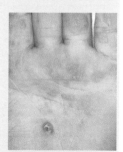

Kaposi's sarcoma

Describe morphology, distribution, pattern, and location of lesions. (See Tables 2–7 through 2–9.)

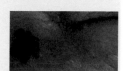

Malignant melanoma

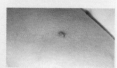

Squamous cell carcinoma

(continued)

AREA/PA SKILL	NORMAL FINDINGS	ABNORMAL FINDINGS
Skin *Inspection*		
Assess for malignant lesions. A = asymmetry B = border irregularity C = color variation D = diameter >0.5 cm		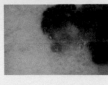
Skin *Palpation*		
Maintain universal precautions. Wear gloves if assessing an open area. Temperature **(use dorsal part of hand)** Palpate for tenderness and surface characteristics of any lesions. Check for pulsations and blanching of vascular lesions.	Skin warm Temperature varies depending on area being assessed; for example, exposed areas may be cooler than unexposed areas	Local area with increased temperature: Inflammatory process, infection, or burn; caused by increased circulation to area Generalized increase in temperature: Fever Local area with decreased temperature: Decreased circulation to area, arterial occlusion Generalized decrease in skin temperature: Exposure or shock

AREA/PA SKILL	NORMAL FINDINGS	ABNORMAL FINDINGS
Skin *Palpation (Continued)*		
Moisture	Skin warm and dry. Moisture dependent upon body area. Exposed areas tend to be drier	Increased moisture: Fever or thyrotoxicosis Decreased moisture: Dehydration, myxedema, chronic nephritis
Texture	Texture varies from soft/fine to coarse/thick depending upon area and age of client. Skin coarser on extensor surfaces	Coarse, thick, dry skin: Hypothyroidism Skin more fine-textured: Hyperthyroidism Smooth, thin, shiny skin: Arterial insufficiency Thick, rough skin: Venous insufficiency
Turgor **(test unexposed area such as below clavicle)**	Good skin turgor, no tenting	Decreased turgor or tenting: Dehydration or normal aging Increased turgor and tension: Scleroderma and edema

(continued)

AREA/PA SKILL	NORMAL FINDINGS	ABNORMAL FINDINGS
Nails *Inspection*		
Note color, condition, angle of attachment, and presence of focal or generalized abnormalities, e.g., ridges, clubbing.	Color varies from pink to light brown in darker-skinned individuals.	Color changes in nails: Local or systemic problem Yellow nails: Cigarette smoking, fungal infections, psoriasis Very distal band of reddish-pink or brown covering <20% of nail (Terry's nails): Cirrhosis, disorders causing hypoalbuminemia Distal band of reddish-pink or brown covering 20%–60% of nails (Lindsay's nails or half-and-half nails): Renal disease, hypoalbuminemia Blue (cyanotic) nails: Peripheral disease or hypoxia Green nails: *Pseudomonas* infections White nails (leukonychia): Trauma, cardiovascular, liver, or renal disease Black nails: Trauma Splinter hemorrhages: Bacterial endocarditis or trauma

ABNORMAL

Fungal infection

Blue nails

Half-and-half nails

Onycholysis

Leukonychia

Psoriasis

Splinter hemorrhages

Paronychia

(continued)

AREA/PA SKILL	NORMAL FINDINGS	ABNORMAL FINDINGS
Nails *Inspection*		
Shape Normal angle 160° **ABNORMAL** Finger clubbing >180° *Nail clubbing*	Angle of attachment 160 degrees. Nails convex	Angle of nail attachment 180 degrees or more: Clubbing: Congenital heart disorders, cystic fibrosis, and chronic pulmonary diseases Spooning or concave nail (koilonychia): Severe iron deficiency anemia, hemochromatosis, thyroid and circulatory diseases, in response to some skin diseases and local trauma
Nail and cuticle	Nails well groomed. Cuticle pink and intact	Onycholysis, separation of the nail from nail bed: Fungal infections, psoriasis, thyrotoxicosis, eczema, systemic diseases, following trauma, or as allergic response to nail products/contactants Pitting: Psoriasis Red and inflamed perionychium (paronychia): Infection or ingrown nail

(continued)

AREA/PA SKILL	NORMAL FINDINGS	ABNORMAL FINDINGS
Nails *Palpation*		
Texture **ABNORMAL** *Pitted nails* *Longitudinal ridges* *Beau's lines*	Nails smooth and firm, no ridges, adhere well to nailbed	Soft, boggy nails: Clubbing due to poor oxygena-tion Brittle nails: Hyper-thyroidism, malnu-trition, calcium and iron deficiency, repeated use of harsh nail contac-tants or products Pitted nails: Psoria-sis, eczema, alope-cia areata Beau's lines (transverse ridges): Serious illness that causes nail growth to slow or halt Thick, brittle nails: Arterial insuffi-ciency
Capillary refill	Brisk capillary refill <3 seconds	Poor capillary refill: Cardiopulmonary problems or anemia

(continued)

AREA/PA SKILL	NORMAL FINDINGS	ABNORMAL FINDINGS
Hair and Scalp *Inspection*		
Note quantity and distribution of hair, condition of scalp, presence of lesions or pediculosis. Gender, genetics, and age affect hair distribution.	Hair evenly distributed over scalp, no alopecia Normal balding patterns common to men and elderly persons No lesions or pediculosis	Generalized hair loss: Nutritional deficiencies, hypothyroidism, lupus erythematosus, thyroid disease, serious illnesses, or side effects of medications
Note actual hair loss, with smooth skin beneath, or whether hair has been broken off near the scalp, with palpable stubble over the skin.		Patchy alopecia: Alopecia areata, trichotillomania, and fungal infections such as tinea capitis Scaling of scalp: Dandruff, seborrhea, psoriasis, certain tineas, and eczema (atopic dermatitis)

ABNORMAL

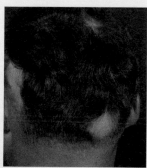
Alopecia areata

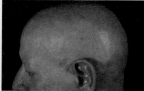
Alopecia

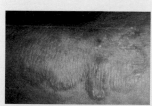
Tinea capitis

(continued)

AREA/PA SKILL	NORMAL FINDINGS	ABNORMAL FINDINGS
Hair and Scalp *Inspection*		
Assess the body for normal distribution of hair.	Fine body hair (vellus) noted over most of body	Hirsutism, hair in male patterns in a woman (e.g., excess facial or trunk hair): Endocrine disorders or medications such as steroids *Hirsutism*
Note color of hair.	Hair color appropriate, thins and grays with age	Localized areas of white or gray hair: Recovering from alopecia areata, or having vitiligo and piebaldism Diffuse white hair: Albinism Green hair: Copper exposure and pernicious anemia
Palpation		
Palpate scalp for tenderness, masses, and mobility. Note texture of hair.	Scalp mobile, nontender Hair texture varies (fine, medium, coarse) depending on genetics and treatments, (e.g., perms)	Dry, coarse hair: Hypothyroidism Fine, silky hair: Hyperthyroidism

PA = physical assessment

Table 2-2. *Skin Color Variations*

COLOR	CAUSE/DESCRIPTION
Bronzing/ tanning 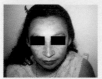 *Addison's disease*	Addison's disease/adrenal insufficiency: Generalized, most evident over exposed areas Hemochromatosis: Generalized, may be gray-brown coloring
Tan 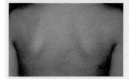 *Chloasma* 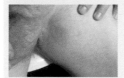 *Tinea versicolor*	Ichthyosis: With coarse scaliness Sprue: Tan/brown patches of any area Scleroderma: Generalized tanning/yellowing of skin, associated with loss of elasticity Chloasma: "Mask of pregnancy" (on face) Lupus: Butterfly rash on face Tinea versicolor: Fawn color or yellow patchy
Yellow 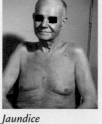 *Jaundice* 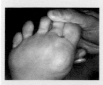 *Carotenemia*	Uremia: Generalized Liver disease, such as hepatitis, cirrhosis, liver cancer, or gallbladder disease with obstructive jaundice: Generalized carotenemia: Not found in conjunctiva or sclera **Jaundice from liver disease is seen in the sclera and conjunctiva. Pseudojaundice—yellow color variations associated with carotenemia—is seen on the skin but not in the eyes.**

(continued)

Table 2–2. *Skin Color Variations (Continued)*

COLOR	CAUSE/DESCRIPTION
Dusky blue 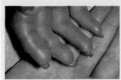 *Cyanosis*	Arsenic poisoning: Paler spots on trunk and extremities Central cyanosis with hypoxia; peripheral cyanosis from vasoconstriction: Caused by cold exposure or vascular disease **To differentiate peripheral cyanosis (caused by vasoconstriction or decreased circulation) from central cyanosis (caused by hypoxia), check the oral mucous membranes and conjunctiva. Cyanotic mucous membranes and conjunctiva indicate a central process.**
Pallor 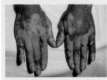 *Vitiligo* 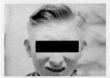 *Albinism*	Anemia: Also on conjunctiva and mucous membranes Vitiligo: Patchy Albinism: Generalized
Red 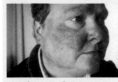 *Erythema of rosacea*	Polycythemia Erythema: Dilated superficial capillaries, such as in rosacea Cherry red: Carbon monoxide poisoning

Table 2–3. *Primary Lesions*

SURFACE CHARACTERISTICS	LESION	EXAMPLES
Flat, nonpalpable	**Macule** <1 cm	Cherry angioma, freckle, flat mole, measles, melanoma
	Patch >1 cm	Vitiligo, tinea versicolor, mongolian spot

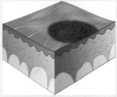
Macule

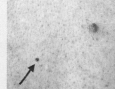
Cherry angioma

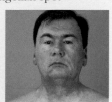
Vitiligo

| Palpable, raised, but superficial | **Papule** <1 cm | Raised mole, wart, lichen planus |
| | **Plaque** >1 cm | Seborrheic keratosis, psoriasis |

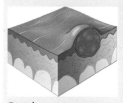
Papule

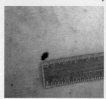
Mole

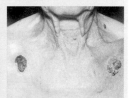
Seborrheic keratosis

| Raised, superficial | **Wheal/hive** Hives (urticaria) are groups of wheals | Transient lesion |

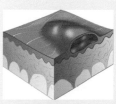
Wheal/Hive

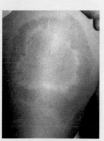
Transient lesion (hive)

(continued)

Table 2–3. *Primary Lesions (Continued)*

SURFACE CHARACTERISTICS	LESION	EXAMPLES
Palpable, solid with depth into dermis	**Nodule** <2 cm If fluid filled and encapsulated, callcd a cyst **Cyst** **Tumor** >2 cm	Erythema nodosum, fibroma, xanthoma, keratogenous cyst

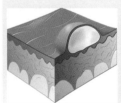

Cyst

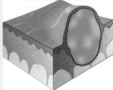

Keratogenous cyst

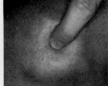

Neoplasm (lipoma)

Palpable, fluid filled	**Vesicle (serous)** <1 cm **Bulla (serous)** >1 cm Pustule (pus filled)	Blister, herpes simplex, contact dermatitis Blister, contact dermatitis, burns Acne, impetigo

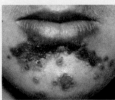

Vesicle (serous)

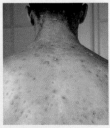

Herpes simplex

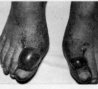

Blister

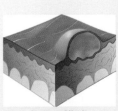

Pustule (pus filled)

Acne vulgaris

Table 2–4. *Secondary Lesions*

SURFACE CHARACTERISTICS	LESION	EXAMPLES
Secondary lesions that add to:		
Thickening and scaling with increased skin markings	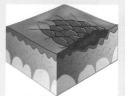 *Lichenification*	Eczema, contact dermatitis 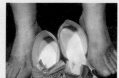 *Contact dermatitis*
Shedding, dead skin cells; scales can be either dry or oily, adherent or loose, variable in color	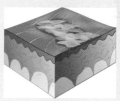 *Scales*	Dandruff, psoriasis 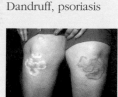 *Psoriasis*
Dried exudates	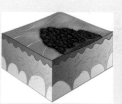 *Crust*	Impetigo, dried herpes simplex 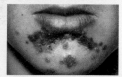 *Dried herpes simplex*
Replacement connective tissue formations	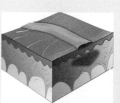 *Scar*	Surgical site, trauma sites 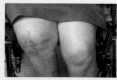 *Surgical site*

(continued)

Table 2–4. *Secondary Lesions (Continued)*

SURFACE CHARACTERISTICS	LESION	EXAMPLES
Hypertrophic scarring caused by excess collagen formation; raised and irregular	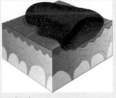\n\n*Keloid*	Surgical site, tattoo, ear-piercing site\n\n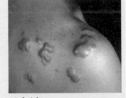\n\n*Keloids*

Secondary lesions that take away from:

Abrasions or other loss that does not extend beyond the superficial epidermis	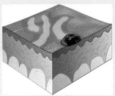\n\n*Excoriation*	Scratch marks, scabies, vascular rupture sites\n\n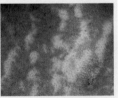\n\n*Excoriation from uremic pruritus*
Loss of superficial epidermis	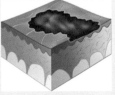\n\n*Erosion*	Abrasion; some fungal infections such as candidiasis can cause erosion\n\n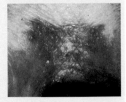\n\n*Candidiasis*

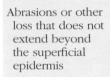
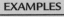

(continued)

Table 2–4. *Secondary Lesions (Continued)*		
SURFACE CHARACTERISTICS	**LESION**	**EXAMPLES**
Linear breaks in the skin with well-defined borders, may extend to the dermis	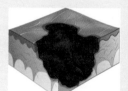 *Fissure*	Athlete's foot, syphilis, cheilitis 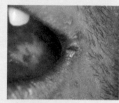 *Cheilitis*
Irregularly shaped loss extending to or through the dermis; may be necrotic	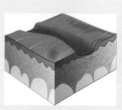 *Ulcer*	Stasis ulcer, pressure ulcer 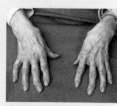 *Stasis ulcer*
Thinning of skin with transparent appearance and loss of markings	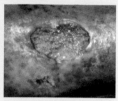 *Atrophy*	Arterial insufficiency, aging 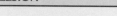 *Aging*

Table 2–5. *Vascular Lesions*

LESION	EXAMPLE	CHARACTERISTICS
Ecchymosis	*Ecchymosis*	Extravasation of blood into skin layer Caused by trauma/injury Does not blanch
Petechiae or purpura	*Petechiae*	Extravasations of blood into skin Caused by steroids, vasculitis, systemic diseases Does not blanch
Venous star	*Venous star*	Blue color Irregularly shaped, linear, spider Does not blanch Caused by increased pressure on superficial veins
Telangiectasia	*Telangiectasia*	Red color Very fine and irregular vessels Blanches Seen with dilation of capillaries
Spider angioma	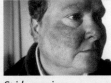 *Spider angioma*	Red color, type of telangiectasia Looks like a spider, with central body and fine radiating legs Blanches Seen in liver disease, vitamin B deficiencies, idiopathic origin

(continued)

Table 2–5. *Vascular Lesions (Continued)*

LESION	EXAMPLE	CHARACTERISTICS
Capillary hemangioma	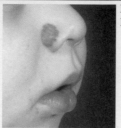 *Capillary hemangioma*	Red color Irregular-shaped macular patch
Port-wine stain	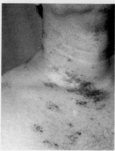 *Port-wine stain*	Red color Does not blanch Seen with dilation of dermal capillaries

Table 2–6. *Staging Criteria for Pressure Ulcers*

STAGE	APPEARANCE	CHARACTERISTICS
Stage I	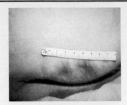	Nonblanchable erythema of intact skin; indicates potential for ulceration
Stage II	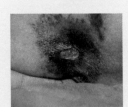	Partial-thickness loss involving both epidermis and dermis. Ulcer is still superficial and appears as a blister, abrasion, or very shallow crater
Stage III	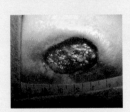	Full thickness loss involving subcutaneous tissue. Ulcer may extend to but not through fascia. A deep crater that may undermine adjacent tissues
Stage IV	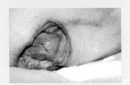	Full thickness loss with extensive involvement of muscle, bone, or supporting structures. This deep ulcer may involve undermining and sinus tracts of adjacent tissues
Stage V	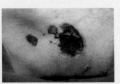	Ulcers that are covered with eschar cannot be staged without debridement

Table 2–7. *Clinical Description of Lesions*

CHARACTERISTICS	SIGNIFICANCE
Size	Major determinant of correct category for primary lesions. Pigmented lesions are typically <0.5 cm. If larger, consider potential for malignancy. Depth of pressure ulcers is major determinant of assigned grade. (See Table 2–6.)
Shape	Macules, wheals, and vesicles are circumscribed. Fissures are linear. Irregular borders associated with melanoma.
Color	Varies widely, and many changes are diagnostic of specific skin diseases. Variegated-colored lesions may signal melanoma. Pustules are usually yellow-white. New scars are red and raised; old scars, white or silver. Petechiae are red. Purpura are red to purplish. Vitiligo is white.
Texture	Macules are smooth. Warts are rough. Psoriasis is scaly.
Surface Relationship	Surface characteristics help differentiate between potential causes of a change and between various primary and secondary lesions. *Flat (nonpalpable):* Macules, patches, purpura, ecchymoses, spider angioma, venous spider *Raised (palpable) solid:* Papules, plaques, nodules, tumors, wheals, scale, crust *Raised (palpable) cystic:* Vesicles, pustules, bullae, cysts *Depressed:* Atrophy, erosion, ulcer, fissures *Pedunculated:* Skin tags, cutaneous horns
Exudate	*Clear or pale, straw-yellow exudate:* Serous oozing/weeping from noninfected lesion *Thicker, purulent discharge:* Infected lesion.

(continued)

Table 2-7. *Clinical Description of Lesions (Continued)*

CHARACTERISTICS	SIGNIFICANCE
	Clear serous exudates: Vesicles, as seen with herpes simplex; or bullae, larger than vesicles, as seen with second-degree burns
	Yellow pus exudates: Pustules, as seen with impetigo or acne
Tenderness/Pain	Tenderness or pain associated with a lesion depends on the underlying cause. May be associated with bullae from a burn or ecchymosis (bruise)

Table 2–8. *Pattern and Configuration of Lesions*

PATTERN		EXAMPLE

Round/Oval

Coin- or oval-shaped, such as in nummular eczema

Discrete

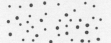

Lesions that remain separate and apart are common to many skin disorders. Moles (nevi) are an example

Grouped

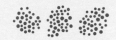

Lesions that are grouped, or clustered, such as herpes simplex

Confluent

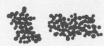

Lesions that run together or are confluent are common in childhood diseases such as rubella

Linear

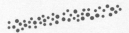

Lesions arranged in lines are common with contact dermatitis due to poison ivy or herpes zoster

Annular/Circular

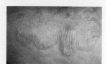

Ring-shaped lesions may be ringworm

Arciform

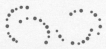

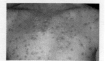

Lesions arranged in partial rings, or arcs, occur in syphilis

Iris

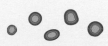

A bull's-eye lesion, or round lesion with central clearing, is typical of erythema multiforme and Lyme disease

(continued)

Table 2–8. *Pattern and Configuration of Lesions (Continued)*

PATTERN	EXAMPLE
Reticular 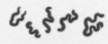	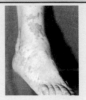

Meshlike pattern as in lichen planus

| **Gyrate** | |

Lesions have serpentine configuration as in gyrate erythema

| **Polycyclic** | 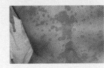 |

Coalesced, concentric circles such as urticaria

Table 2–9. *Distribution of Skin Lesions*

AREA	EXAMPLE

Diffuse/Generalized

Lesions distributed over entire body, such as urticaria from allergic reactions

Scattered

 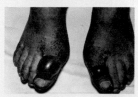

Lesions that are sparsely distributed, as in seborrheic keratosis

Localized

 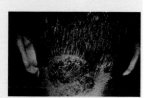

Lesions in a very limited, discrete area. Location may indicate contact with an allergen or a wheal from insect bite

Regional

Head
Confined to a specific body area
Tinea capitis

(continued)

Table 2–9. *Distribution of Skin Lesions (Continued)*

AREA	EXAMPLE
Torso	

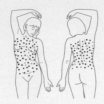 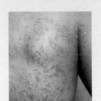

Pityriasis rosea

Extensor surfaces

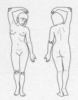 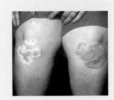

Psoriasis

Flexor surfaces

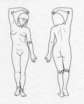 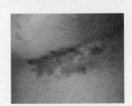

Intertrigo

Dermatome

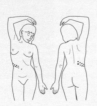 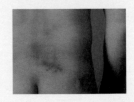

Herpes zoster

(continued)

Table 2–9. *Distribution of Skin Lesions (Continued)*

AREA	EXAMPLE

Hairy areas

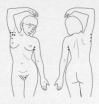 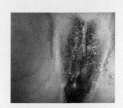

Herpes II, pediculosis pubis

Intertriginous areas (folds of skin)

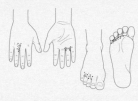 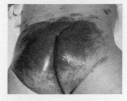

Contact dermatitis, diaper rash, intertrigo (erythema   and scaling of body folds)

Sun-exposed areas

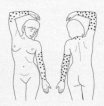 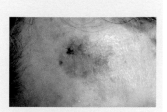

Actinic keratosis

■□■□ CHAPTER 3

ASSESSING THE HEAD, FACE, AND NECK

Primary Functions

The head, face, and neck are not systems but regions of the body in which most of the systems are included.

- Integumentary system: Covers and protects the head, face, and neck.
- Respiratory system: Begins at the nose.
- Cardiovascular (CV) system: Major CV vessels (carotids and jugulars) provide blood supply to the brain.
- Gastrointestinal system: Begins at the mouth.
- Musculoskeletal system: Facial, mouth, and neck muscles allow for movement, eating, and communication; the skull protects the brain.
- Neurological system: Skull houses brain; cranial nerves innervate head, face, and neck.
- Endocrine system: The thyroid, the largest endocrine gland, is located in the neck.
- Lymphatic system: The cervical lymph nodes are located in the neck.

Developmental Considerations

Infants and Children

- Molding of the head occurs during vaginal delivery, yet the head assumes a symmetrical, rounded shape within several days of birth.

- Fontanels ("soft spots") allow for growth.
- Sinuses are not fully developed until age 7.
- Children have 20 deciduous teeth.
- Lymphatic tissue (nodes and tonsils) is larger in children than in adults.

Pregnant Clients
- The thyroid is more active during pregnancy, and is often palpable.
- Chloasma occurs on face.
- Gums may hypertrophy.

Older Adults
- Gum disease and tooth loss are often problems.
- Salivation decreases.
- Senses of taste and smell may diminish.

Cultural Considerations

- African-Americans may develop pseudofolliculitis.
- Chinese-Americans have very little facial hair.
- Irish-Americans are at increased risk for skin cancer on sun-exposed areas.
- Filipino-Americans have almond-shaped eyes, mildly flared nostrils, and a low, flat nose bridge.

Assessment

History
SYMPTOMS ("PQRST" ANY + SYMPTOM)
- Head pain
  - How long have you had this pain?
  - Have you had any recent head trauma or other injury/accident?
  - What have you done to treat the pain?
- Jaw tightness/pain
  - How long have you had this tightness or pain?
  - When does it usually occur?
  - Do you have a personal or family history of heart disease?
  - Please describe the discomfort, using your own words.

- Neck pain/stiffness
  - How would you describe the stiffness or pain?
  - How has the pain or stiffness affected your usual activities?
  - What do you believe may have caused the pain/stiffness?
  - Have you recently had any injury or done any unusual activity?
  - Have you had similar symptoms before?
  - Have you been sick—upper respiratory infection (URI), sore throat?
- Neck mass
  - When did you first notice the mass?
  - Have you had any recent illness, sore throat, rashes, or other symptoms?
  - Do you have a personal or family history of malignancies?
- Nasal congestion
  - Have you ever had similar congestion before?
  - What other symptoms have you recently noticed?
  - When is the congestion at its worst?
- Nosebleeds (epistaxis)
  - When did you first have a nosebleed?
  - Describe the typical episode.
  - Are there any particular settings or situations in which the bleeding is most likely to occur?
  - Do you have a personal or family history of a bleeding disorder or high blood pressure?
  - Have you had any recent trauma, injury, or procedure to your nose or sinuses?
- Mouth lesions
  - When did you first notice the sore?
  - Does the area hurt or have other related symptoms?
  - How has it changed since you first noticed it?
  - What do you think caused the sore?
  - Do you use tobacco or alcohol?
- Mouth/dental pain
  - Describe the pain you are having in your own terms.
  - When did the pain first occur?
  - Does the pain occur in certain situations more frequently than in others?

- Do you have any family or personal history of cancer or heart disease?
- Sore throat
  - Please describe the pain or discomfort in your own words.
  - Where, exactly, is the pain located?
  - How would you describe the onset/frequency of the pain?
  - Are there any other symptoms?
- Hoarseness
  - Tell me about the progression of the hoarseness since the time you first noticed it.
  - Do you use tobacco or alcohol?
  - Is there any family or personal history of cancer or throat disease?
  - Have you had any problems with heartburn, wheezing, or indigestion?
  - What, if any, other symptoms have you recently noticed?
  - Have you recently had an injury to the throat area, surgery, or any other procedure?

FOCUSED HEAD, NECK, AND THROAT HISTORY
- Do you have any problems or complaints related to your head, face, nose, mouth, throat, or neck? Some examples might be head pain, nasal congestion, nosebleeds, nasal discharge, mouth sores or pain, sore throat, postnasal drip, difficulty swallowing, or neck pain.
- Do you have any allergies to any medications, foods, or environmental factors?
- What, if any, health problems do you have?
- What, if any, over-the-counter or prescribed medications do you take (Table 3–1)?
- Is there anything specific that you think I should know in relation to your overall health or this specific complaint?

Table 3-1. *Drugs That Adversely Affect the Head, Face, and Neck*

DRUG CLASS	DRUG	POSSIBLE ADVERSE REACTIONS
Anticholinergics	atropine, scopolamine, glycopyrrolate, propantheline, belladonna alkaloids, dicyclomine, hyoscyamine	Decreased salivation, dry mouth
Anticonvulsants	phenytoin sodium	Gingival hyperplasia
Antidepressants	tricyclics, including amitriptyline and nortriptyline, paroxetine	Dry mouth
Antihistamines	diphenhydramine, brompheniramine, chlorpheniramine	Dry mouth
Antihypertensives	guanabenz, clonidine, methyldopa, nifedipine (all calcium channel blockers)	Dry mouth
Antilipemic	clofibrate	Dry brittle hair, alopecia
Antineoplastics	bleomycin sulfate	Ulcerated tongue and lips, alopecia
-	dactinomycin	Mouth lesions, alopecia
	melphalan	Mouth lesions
	mitomycin	Mouth lesions, alopecia
	methotrexate	Gingivitis, mouth lesions, alopecia
	cyclophosphamide	Mouth lesions, alopecia
	vincristine sulfate	Mouth lesions, alopecia
	chlorambucil	Mouth lesions
	uracil mustard	Mouth lesions
	cisplatin	Gingival platinum line, alopecia
	hydroxyurea	Mouth lesions
	fluorouracil	Alopecia, epistaxis
	doxorubicin	Mouth lesions, alopecia
	cytarabine	Mouth lesions, alopecia
	daunorubicin	Mouth lesions, alopecia
	etoposide	Alopecia
Cardiac agents	disopyramide phosphate	Dry mouth

(continued)

Table 3-1. *Drugs That Adversely Affect the Head, Face, and Neck* *(Continued)*

DRUG CLASS	DRUG	POSSIBLE ADVERSE REACTIONS
Genitourinary smooth-muscle relaxants	flavoxate, oxybutynin, propantheline	Dry mouth
Gold salts	gold sodium thiomalate	Gingivitis, mouth lesions
	auranofin	Mouth lesions
Nonsteroidal anti-inflammatory agents	indomethacin	Gingival lesions
	ibuprofen	Dry mouth, gingival lesions
Miscellaneous agents	lithium salts	Dry mouth, dry hair, alopecia
	metoclopramide	Dry mouth, glossal or periorbital edema
	penicillamine	Mouth lesions
	isotretinoin	Inflamed lips, epistaxis, dry mouth
	allopurinol	Alopecia
	propranolol	Hyperkeratosis and psoriasis of the scalp, alopecia
	guanethidine sulfate	Nasal stuffiness, dry mouth
	edrophonium	Increased salivation
	pyridostigmine	Increased salivation, increased tracheo-bronchial secretions
	fluorides	Staining or mottling of teeth
	warfarin sodium	Epistaxis with excessive dosage
	amphetamines	Dry mouth, continuous chewing or bruxism (tooth grinding) with prolonged use
	tetracycline	Enamel hypoplasia and permanent yellow-gray to brown tooth discoloration in children under age 8 and in offspring of pregnant clients
	cyclosporin	Gingival hyperplasia
	valproic acid	Alopecia

Assessment of Head, Face, and Neck's Relationship to Other Systems

Remember, all systems are related! As you assess the head, face, and neck, look at the relationship between them and all other systems.

SUBJECTIVE DATA	OBJECTIVE DATA
Area/System: General	
Ask about:	*Inspect:*
Changes in energy level	Features for symmetry and propor-
Weight changes	tion
Fevers	*Measure:*
Night sweats	Vital signs
	Height and weight
Area/System: Integumentary	
Ask about:	*Inspect:*
Changes in skin, hair, and	Skin for color changes (e.g.,
nails	cyanosis, pallor), lesions, hair
Rashes, itching	distribution
	Palpate:
	Skin for temperature, turgor,
	texture
	Nails and hair texture
Area/System: HEENT	
Head and Neck	
Ask about:	*Inspect:*
Head or neck pain	Size, shape, symmetry of head and
Masses or swollen nodes	facial features
	Facial expression
	Palpate:
	Thyroid
	Lymph nodes
Eyes	
Ask about:	*Inspect:*
Vision changes	Conjunctiva
Drainage, itching, pain	Palpebral fissures
	For lid lag, exophthalmos
	Test:
	Visual acuity
Ears, Nose, and Throat	
Ask about:	*Inspect:*
Changes in hearing	Gross hearing
Ear drainage, itching, pain	Structures of the mouth and throat

(continued)

SUBJECTIVE DATA	OBJECTIVE DATA
Nasal congestion, drainage, sinus pain Nosebleeds Mouth sores or dental pain Jaw pain	External ear and tympanic membrane

Area/System: Respiratory

Ask about:	*Measure:*
Cough, congestion, wheezing, mucus production	Respiratory rate *Auscultate:* Breath sounds

Area/System: Cardiovascular

Ask about:	*Measure:*
History of cardiovascular disease (e.g., coronary artery disease, hypertension) Chest pain, palpitations	Heart rate Pulse amplitude *Palpate:* Pulse *Auscultate:* Heart sounds, bruits

Area/System: Gastrointestinal

Ask about:	*Inspect:*
Changes in appetite Bowel changes Nausea, vomiting	Abdomen for size, shape, and symmetry *Palpate:* For organomegaly *Auscultate:* Bowel sounds

Area/System: Genitourinary/Reproductive

Ask about:	*Inspect:*
History of sexually transmitted diseases Changes in libido *For women:* Last menstrual period Menstrual changes Vaginal discharge or sores *For men:* Penile discharge or sores	External genitals for lesions or discharge

Area/System: Musculoskeletal

Ask about:	*Inspect:*
Joint pain Muscle weakness Limited movement	Range of motion of head and neck *Palpate:* For muscle strength, joint deformities

(continued)

SUBJECTIVE DATA	OBJECTIVE DATA
Area/System: Neurological	
Ask about:	*Test:*
Nervousness	Level of orientation
Difficulty staying focused	Thought process and memory
Forgetfulness	Cranial nerves
Changes in level of	Sensation
consciousness	*Inspect:*
Numbness and tingling	For abnormal movements
Headaches, head injury	
Area/System: Endocrine	
Ask about:	*Inspect:*
Changes in shoe size or	For masses, goiters
ring size	*Palpate:*
Changes in facial features	For thyroid enlargement and
Changes in energy level	nodules
Weight changes	*Auscultate:*
Sleep problems	Thyroid, if palpable
Area/System: Immune/Hematological	
Ask about:	*Inspect:*
Unusual bleeding, bruising	For ecchymoses, petechiae
Current/recent infection	*Palpate:*
History of cancer	For lymph node enlargement

HEENT = head, eye, ear, nose, and throat

Physical Assessment

ANATOMICAL LANDMARKS: Palpebral fissures and nasolabial folds; anterior and posterior triangles

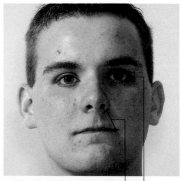

Palpebral fissures and nasolabial folds

Nasolabial fold
Palpebral fissure

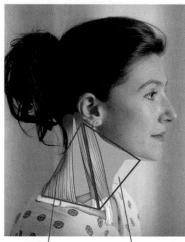

Anterior and posterior triangles

Posterior   Anterior

APPROACH (ANTERIOR AND POSTERIOR): Inspection, palpation, percussion, auscultation
POSITION: Sitting
TOOLBOX: Penlight or otoscope for focused light, tongue blades, gauze, stethoscope, transilluminator, cup of water, gloves, and nasal speculum

AREA/PA SKILL	NORMAL FINDINGS	ABNORMAL FINDINGS
Inspection *Head*		
Note size, shape, symmetry, and position. Assess fontanels and head circumference in infants.	Normocephalic, erect, midline	Increasing head circumference in children: Hydrocephalus Increasing head size in adolescents or adults: Acromegaly

Acromegaly

(continued)

AREA/PA SKILL	NORMAL FINDINGS	ABNORMAL FINDINGS
Inspection *Head (Continued)*		
Face		Asymmetry: Trauma or congenital deformity
Assess facial expression.	Facial expression appropriate	Facial appearance inconsistent with gender, age, or racial/ethnic group: Inherited or chronic disorder with typical facies (e.g., Graves' disease, hypothyroidism with myxedema, Cushing's syndrome, or acromegaly) 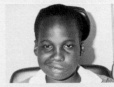 *Cushing's syndrome*
Check for symmetry of facial features. Nasolabial folds and palpebral fissures are good places to check for symmetry.	Nasolabial folds and palpebral fissures symmetrical	Asymmetry of features: Previous trauma, surgical alterations, congenital deformity, paralysis, or edema. Also seen with Bell's palsy and cerebrovascular accident (CVA) *Bell's palsy*

(continued)

AREA/PA SKILL	NORMAL FINDINGS	ABNORMAL FINDINGS
Inspection *Face (Continued)*		
Inspect for abnormal movements, lesions, and hair distribution.	Hair distribution appropriate for client's age, sex, and ethnicity No lesions or abnormal movements	Asymmetry of movement: Neuromuscular disorder or paralysis. Tics usually occur in the head and face Hirsutism in women: Steroid use or Cushing's syndrome
Nose		
Note position, deformities, septal deviation, discharge, flaring.	Nose midline, symmetrical, no deviation, no flaring	Misalignment of nose, or shape inconsistent with client's history: Previous trauma, congenital deformity, surgical alteration, or mass; also associated with typical facies, including acromegaly or Down syndrome **Nasal flaring: Suggests respiratory distress, especially in infants, who are obligatory nose breathers**
Assess for color, intactness, lesions, edema, and discharge (types of discharge: clear, bloody, purulent).	Nasal mucosa pink, moist; no lesions, edema, or discharge	Drainage: Clear, bilateral: Allergic rhinitis **Clear, unilateral: May be spinal fluid as a result of head trauma or fracture** Clear, mucoid· Viral rhinitis

(continued)

AREA/PA SKILL	NORMAL FINDINGS	ABNORMAL FINDINGS
Inspection *Nose (Continued)*		
Inspect for color and edema of turbinates.	Septum intact and midline	Yellow or green: Upper respiratory infection Bloody: Trauma, hypertension, or bleeding disorders Bright red nasal mucosa: Inflammation from rhinitis or sinusitis; also suggests cocaine abuse Pale/gray mucosa: Allergic rhinitis Copious or colored discharge: Allergic or infectious disorder, epistaxis, head or nose trauma Clustered vesicles: Herpes infection Ulcers or perforations: Chronic infection, trauma, or cocaine use Dried crusted blood: Previous nosebleed Polyps (elongated, rounded projections): Allergies 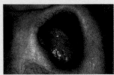 *Polyps* Deviated septum: Normal variant or following trauma Enlarged, boggy turbinates: Allergic disorder

(continued)

AREA/PA SKILL	NORMAL FINDINGS	ABNORMAL FINDINGS
Inspection *Nose (Continued)*		
		Deviated septum
		Pale or gray mucosa overlying turbinates: Allergic disorder
Frontal and Maxillary Sinuses		
Frontal sinuses above eyes; maxillary below eyes		
Assess for periorbital edema, dark circles under eyes.	No periorbital edema	Periorbital edema and dark under-eye circles: Sinusitis
Transilluminate sinuses if indicated.	Sinuses clear, presence of transillumination	Absence of transillumination over one sinus when opposite structure transilluminates: Mucosal thickening or sinus fullness with sinusitis Absence of transillumination must be considered with other findings
Parotid and Submandibular Glands		
Parotid glands in front of ears; submandibular under mandible		
Assess for edema, redness.	No edema or redness over glands	Fullness or inflammatory changes of glands: Blockage of duct by calculi, infection, malignancy

(continued)

AREA/PA SKILL	NORMAL FINDINGS	ABNORMAL FINDINGS
Inspection *Lips*		
Note color, condition, lesions.	Lips pink (or consistent with ethnic group/race), moist, intact, no lesions	Asymmetry of placement: Congenital deformity, trauma, paralysis, or surgical alteration Pallor: Anemia Redness: Inflammatory or infectious disorder Cyanosis: Vasoconstriction or hypoxia Lesions: Infectious or inflammatory disorder Cheilitis, drying, and cracking: Dehydration, allergy, lip licking Cheilosis: Deficiency of B vitamins or maceration related to overclosure 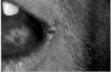 *Cheilitis and cheilosis* Chancre: Single, painless ulcer of primary syphilis 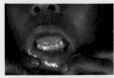 *Chancre*

(continued)

AREA/PA SKILL	NORMAL FINDINGS	ABNORMAL FINDINGS
Inspection *Lips (Continued)*		
		Angioedema: Allergic response Clustered area of fullness/nodularity that forms vesicles, then ulceration: Herpes simplex viral infection *Angioedema: Allergic response* *Herpes viral infection* *Cancer on lip*
Assess for breath odor and pursed-lip breathing.	No unusual odors (halitosis) No pursed-lip breathing	Halitosis: Infections or gastrointestinal (GI) problems
Oral Mucosa		
Note color, condition, lesions.	Oral mucosa pink (or consistent with ethnic group/race), moist, intact, no lesions	Abrasions, erosion of underlying mucosa. In denture wearers, poorly fitted dentures

(continued)

AREA/PA SKILL	NORMAL FINDINGS	ABNORMAL FINDINGS
Inspection *Oral Mucosa (Continued)*		
		Painful, reddened mucosa, often with mildly adherent white patches: *Candida albicans*
		Reddened, inflamed oral mucosa, sometimes with ulcerations: Allergic stomatitis
		Small, painful vesicles, often with reddened periphery and a white or pale yellowish base: Aphthous ulcer caused by viral infection, stress, or trauma
		Nodular, macular, or papular lesions widely involving the integument and oral mucosa: Kaposi's sarcoma

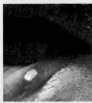

Aphthous ulcer

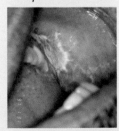

Lichen planus

(continued)

AREA/PA SKILL	NORMAL FINDINGS	ABNORMAL FINDINGS
Inspection *Oral Mucosa (Continued)*		Inflammatory changes of the integument, often found on oral mucosa as chronic gray, lacy patches with or without ulceration: Lichen planus. May progress to neoplasm
		Reddened mucosal change that may progress to form cancer: Erythroplakia
		White, adherent mucosal thickening: Leukoplakia. Precancerous lesion, warrants follow-up

ABNORMAL

Cancer on oral mucosa

Fordyce granules

Torus palatinus

Leukoplakia

Torus mandibularis

Parotitis

(continued)

AREA/PA SKILL	NORMAL FINDINGS	ABNORMAL FINDINGS
Inspection *Oral Mucosa (Continued)*		
		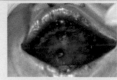 *Cocaine use* 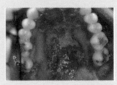 *HIV palatal candidiasis*
Assess for inflammation of Stensen's and Wharton's ducts **(Stensen's ducts opposite second upper molars; Wharton's ducts on floor of mouth under tongue).** *Gingivae*	Stensen's and Wharton's ducts patent, no inflammation	
Assess for color, condition, retraction, hypertrophy, edema, bleeding, and lesions.	Gingivae pink, moist, intact; no bleeding edema, recession, hypertrophy, or lesions	Inflamed, bleeding gingivae: Leukemia and human immunodeficiency virus (HIV). Also, poorly fitted dentures in denture wearers

ABNORMAL

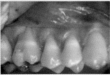 *Gingival recession*

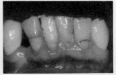 *Chronic gingivitis*

(continued)

AREA/PA SKILL	NORMAL FINDINGS	ABNORMAL FINDINGS
Inspection *Gingivae (Continued)*		

Hyperplasia of gums: Side effect of medications, e.g., dilantin or calcium channel blockers

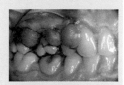

Gum hyperplasia

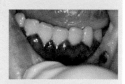

Leukemia

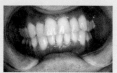

Early HIV periodontitis

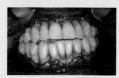

Advanced HIV periodontitis

(continued)

AREA/PA SKILL	NORMAL FINDINGS	ABNORMAL FINDINGS
Inspection *Gingivae (Continued)*		
		Gum recession or inflammatory gum changes: Poor dental hygiene or vitamin deficiency Pale/gray gingivae: Chronic gingivitis
Teeth		
Assess for number, color, condition. Note any missing or loose teeth.	32 teeth in adults (28 without wisdom teeth), 20 in children; white; edges smooth; in good repair; no caries; no missing or loose teeth	Various abnormalities include loose, poorly anchored teeth, malalignment, dental caries **A loose tooth poses a threat of airway obstruction.**

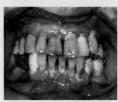

Dental caries

Discoloration of teeth: Chemicals or medications (tetracycline may discolor teeth gray if administered before puberty)

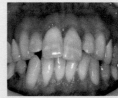

Tetracycline staining

(continued)

AREA/PA SKILL	NORMAL FINDINGS	ABNORMAL FINDINGS
Inspection ***Teeth (Continued)***		
		Mottled enamel: Fluorosis *Fluorosis*
Check occlusion.	Good occlusion	*Malocclusion*
Tongue		
Assess color, texture, position, and mobility (tests cranial nerve [CN] XII). Note any involuntary movements or lesions.	Tongue pink, moist, intact; papillae intact; midline with full mobility (CN XII intact) No lesions or involuntary movements Geographic tongue is normal variation *Geographic tongue*	Absence of papillae, reddened mucosa, ulcerations: Allergic, inflammatory, or infectious cause Color changes may indicate underlying problems (e.g., red "beefy" tongue is seen with pernicious anemia) *Red "beefy" tongue*

(continued)

AREA/PA SKILL	NORMAL FINDINGS	ABNORMAL FINDINGS
Inspection *Tongue (Continued)*		Black hairy tongue: Fungal infections
		Hypertrophy and discoloration of the papilla: Antibiotic use
		Reddened, smooth, painful tongue, with or without ulcerations: Anemia, chemical irritants, medications
		Cancers may form on the tongue and on other oral mucosa

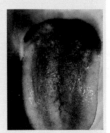

Black, hairy tongue

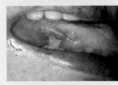

Glossitis

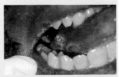

Cancer of the tongue

(continued)

Inspection
Oropharynx, Hard/Soft Palate, Tonsils, and Uvula

AREA/PA SKILL	NORMAL FINDINGS	ABNORMAL FINDINGS
Assess for color, condition, lesions, drainage, exudates, and edema.	Hard and soft palate pink and intact Tonsils pink, symmetrical, + 1, no exudates	Reddened, hypertrophic tonsil, with or without exudates: Acute infection or tonsillitis with lymphoid cobblestoning Enlarged tonsils with exudates Erythema, exudate, lesions: Infectious process Perforation of palate: Congenital defect, cleft palate, trauma, drug use

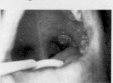
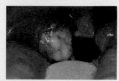

Herpangioma

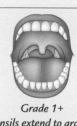
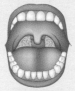
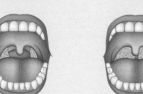
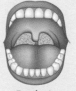

Grade 1+
Tonsils extend to arches.

Grade 3+
Tonsils approximate the uvula.

Grade 2+
Tonsils extend to just beyond arches.

Grade 4+
Tonsils meet midline ("kiss").

Enlarged tonsils with exudates. See box for specific tonsil grades.

AREA/PA SKILL	NORMAL FINDINGS	ABNORMAL FINDINGS
Look for symmetrical rise of the uvula. Test swallow reflex (CN IX, X)	Symmetrical rise of uvula + swallow and gag reflex	Asymmetrical rise of uvula: Problem with CN IX and X

(continued)

AREA/PA SKILL	NORMAL FINDINGS	ABNORMAL FINDINGS
Palpation *Neck, Thyroid, Cervical Lymph Nodes*		
Inspect neck in neutral position, hyperextended, and as client swallows. Assess symmetry, neck ROM, and condition of skin.	Neck symmetrical, active range of motion [AROM], no masses, skin intact Larynx and trachea rise with swallowing	Enlargements: Lymphadenopathy, lymphoma or other malignancy Torticollis: Scars, tonsillitis, adenitis, disease of cervical vertebrae, enlarged cervical glands, cerebellar tumor, rheumatism, retro-pharyngeal abscess
Note any thyroid and lymph node enlargement.		Enlarged, visible thyroid: Goiter or malignant mass

☐ *Palpation (Maintain universal precautions—wear gloves when palpating the mouth or if lesion is suspected.)*

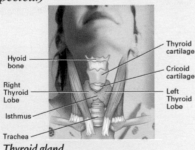

Thyroid cartilage
Hyoid bone
Cricoid cartilage
Right Thyroid Lobe
Left Thyroid Lobe
Isthmus
Trachea

Thyroid gland

Cervical adenitis

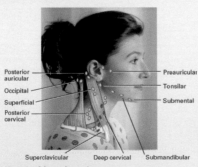

Posterior auricular
Occipital
Superficial
Posterior cervical
Preauricular
Tonsilar
Submental
Superclavicular   Deep cervical   Submandibular

Cervical lymph nodes

(continued)

AREA/PA SKILL	NORMAL FINDINGS	ABNORMAL FINDINGS
Palpation *Head*		
Assess for masses and tenderness. Assess scalp mobility. Palpate fontanels in infants. Anterior fontanel closes between 18 and 24 months; posterior by 2 months.	Head symmetrical, no masses, nontender; scalp freely movable	Bulging fontanels and tight scalp: Hydrocephalus, increased intracranial pressure (ICP) Masses, tenderness: Trauma, cysts
Face		
Note condition, symmetry, tenderness. Assess muscle tone and temporomandibular joint (TMJ) function.	Facial bones smooth, intact, symmetrical, nontender Facial muscles with good tone TMJ with AROM; no crepitus or tenderness	Contour abnormalities, including bulges or projections: Previous trauma or surgery, or congenital deformity Tenderness: Trauma, TMJ syndrome, temporal arteritis, or inflammatory process
Nose		
Assess for patency, tenderness, deformity.	Nares patent; no nasal tenderness or deformity	Deviations or masses: Previous trauma or infection
Frontal and Maxillary Sinuses		
Palpate for tenderness.	Sinuses nontender	Tenderness: May indicate infectious or allergic sinusitis
Parotid and Submandibular Glands		
Palpate for tenderness and enlargement.	Parotid and submandibular glands nontender and not enlarged	Enlarged, tender parotid glands: Parotitis, blocked ducts, infection, or malignancy
Lips and Tongue		
Assess for tenderness, muscle tone, and lesions.	Soft, nontender, with good muscle tone No lesions	Areas of induration, thickening, nodularity, or masses: Neoplasm, potential malignancy

(continued)

AREA/PA SKILL	NORMAL FINDINGS	ABNORMAL FINDINGS
Palpation *Lips and Tongue (Continued)*		
		Tender induration that soon develops vesicles: Herpes simplex Areas of induration, thickening, nodularity: Potential malignancy
Oropharynx		
Test gag reflex.	Presence of gag reflex	**Absent gag reflex: Damage to CN IX, X; CVA poses risk for aspiration**
Thyroid Gland		
Locate thyroid isthmus below cricoid cartilage. Palpate for size, shape, symmetry, consistency, tenderness, and nodules.	Thyroid nonpalpable, nontender, or small; smooth edge of thyroid palpable	Enlarged thyroid: Tumor, goiter Nodular thyroid tissue Tender thyroid: Inflammatory process such as acute thyroiditis
Cervical Lymph Nodes		
Use light palpation with your finger pads in a circular movement. Palpate for size, shape, symmetry, consistency, mobility, tenderness, and temperature.	Cervical nodes nonpalpable, nontender; or superficial or shotty node palpable, <1 cm, mobile, soft to firm, nontender	Palpable nodes (1 cm or greater): Malignancy, inflammatory or infectious process of glands or area they drain Significant lymphadenopathy: Mononucleosis and various forms of lymphoma

(continued)

AREA/PA SKILL	NORMAL FINDINGS	ABNORMAL FINDINGS
Percussion *Frontal and Maxillary Sinuses*		
Percussion (Use direct percussion.)		
Assess for tenderness.	Sinuses nontender, resonant	Tenderness: Sinusitis Dull tone: Thickening or fullness of sinus cavity or cavities, associated with chronic or acute sinusitis
Auscultation (Use the bell of the stethoscope and have client hold breath.) *Thyroid*		
Listen for bruits.	No bruits over thyroid	*Bruit:* Increased vascularity of hyperthyroidism

PA = physical assessment

CHAPTER 4

ASSESSING THE EYES AND EARS

EYES

Primary Function

- Vision

Developmental Considerations

Infants

- Normal spacing measurements are plotted between the 10th and 90th percentile.
- The color of the iris after birth is normally blue/gray in light-skinned infants, brown in darker-skinned infants. Permanent color is usually established by 9 months of age.
- Brushfield spots can be a normal variant or a sign of Down syndrome.
- Edema of the lids and irritation of the conjunctiva may be caused by birth trauma or silver nitrate prophylaxis.
- The sclera is very thin at birth, so it may have a slightly blue undertone.
- The pupils should normally constrict in response to light. After 3 weeks, if no pupillary light reflex is present, blindness is indicated. However, the presence of pupillary reaction alone does not confirm an infant's ability to see. A

blink reflex in response to bright light and observing the infant for ability to follow objects or light with the eyes confirm that some degree of vision is intact.

- By 2 to 4 weeks, an infant should be able to fixate on an object; by 1 month, to fixate on and follow an object.
- An infant's visual acuity is usually about 20/200; 20/20 vision is usually achieved by school age.
- During the first 1 to 2 months, infants' eye movements are often disconjugate, making screening for strabismus difficult. Persistence of disconjugate eye movements after this time may indicate strabismus and warrants referral to a specialist.
- Absence of a red reflex may indicate congenital cataracts or retinal detachment. The general background in infants is typically paler than that in adults. The macula also is not fully developed until about 1 year of age.

Toddlers
- Visual acuity in toddlers is determined by the Allen test.
- Untreated strabismus can lead to permanent visual damage.

Preschoolers
- By age 3 to 5, the Snellen E chart can usually be used to determine visual acuity.
- Normal visual acuity for a 3-year-old is approximately 20/40 or better.
- By the time the child is 4 years old, visual acuity should be about 20/30 or better.

School-Age Children
- By the time the child is about 5 to 6 years old, visual acuity approximates that of the adult—20/20 in both eyes. Use the Snellen E chart until the child has acquired reading skills and can easily verbalize the letters seen on the Snellen chart.
- Screen for color blindness between 4 and 8 years of age.

Older Adults
- Both central and peripheral visual acuity may be diminished with advanced age.

- Changes in near vision occur around the 4th and 5th decade, often resulting in presbyopia.
- Lids lose elasticity and fatty deposits, causing the eyes to appear sunken.
- Ectropion is significant because the punctum is no longer in contact with the globe, resulting in constant tearing.
- Entropion is significant because the punctum may not be able to drain tears and the lashes may rub the conjunctiva and cornea, causing pain and injury to the cornea.
- A decrease in tear production may result in dry eyes.
- Lens becomes more opaque and yellowish, obscuring the transfer of light rays to the retina.
- Arcus senilis may appear.
- Senile cataracts may appear.
- Pupil size at rest is generally smaller than in younger adults.
- Pupillary reaction to light and accommodation slows.
- General fundoscopic background is paler, and the blood vessels of the eye may show signs of the same atherosclerotic processes that are occurring elsewhere throughout the body.
- Visual fields may be less than normal.
- Color vision may be less vivid.
- Night vision may be impaired.
- Macular degeneration and glaucoma are the two leading causes of blindness in older adults.

Cultural Considerations

- Persons of Asian origin typically have an epicanthal fold at the medial canthus.
- In blacks and others with normally dark skin, muddy sclera is common.
- In dark-skinned people, the color of the optic disc is typically darker orange and the retinal background is darker red than in fair-skinned people.
- A black person's sclera also may have a blue/gray appearance or a yellowish cast at the peripheral margins.
- Incidence and severity of glaucoma are greater in blacks than in people of other races.
- Cataracts occur with greater frequency in people living in sunny climates.

Assessment

History

SYMPTOMS ("PQRST" ANY + SYMPTOM)
- Vision loss
  - Have you noticed any changes in your vision?
  - Have you experienced any decrease or loss of vision?
  - Was the loss of vision sudden or gradual?
  - Was the loss of vision painful?
- Eye pain
  - Do you have any pain or discomfort in your eyes?
  - Did the pain occur suddenly or gradually?
  - Do you have any other symptoms associated with the eye pain?
  - Does light bother your eyes?
  - Is the pain associated with movement of the eye? With blinking?
  - What makes your eye pain better? What makes it worse?
- Diplopia
  - Does the double vision get worse when you are tired?
  - Did the double vision occur suddenly or gradually?
  - Did the double vision occur after a head injury?
- Eye tearing
  - Have you noticed any tearing of the eyes?
  - Is the tearing associated with pain? With direct contact with chemicals, irritants, or environmental allergens?
- Dry eye
  - Have you noticed any dryness or discomfort of the eye when blinking?
  - Do you wear contact lenses?
  - Do you have a history of corneal abrasion or burns?
  - Medications?
- Eye drainage
  - What does the drainage look like?
  - Is the drainage associated with redness? Or with itching?
- Eye appearance changes
  - Have you noticed any recent changes in the appearance of your eyes?

- Describe how the appearance of your eyes has changed.
- Blurred vision
  - Do you wear corrective lenses?
  - Is the blurred vision worse for near or for far objects?
  - When was your last eye examination?

Focused Eye History

- Have you noticed any changes in your vision?
- Do you wear glasses or contact lenses?
- Have you ever had an eye injury?
- Have you ever had eye surgery?
- Have you ever had blurred vision?
- Have you ever seen spots or floaters, flashes of light, or halos around lights?
- Do you have a history of frequent or recurring eye infections, styes, tearing, or dryness?
- When was your last eye examination?
- Do you have a history of diabetes or high blood pressure?
- What medications, prescription or over the counter, are you currently taking (Table 4–1)?
- Do you use any prescription or over-the-counter eye drops?

Table 4–1. *Drugs That Adversely Affect the Eyes*

DRUG CLASS	DRUG	POSSIBLE ADVERSE REACTIONS
Aminoglycosides	all aminoglycosides	Optic neuritis with blurred vision, scotomas, enlargement of the blind spot
Antiarrhythmics	quinidine sulfate	Blurred vision, color perception disturbances, night blindness, mydriasis, photophobia, diplopia, reduced visual fields, scotomas, optic neuritis
	flecainide acetate	Blurred vision, difficulty focusing, spots before eyes, diplopia, photophobia, nystagmus
Anticholinergic agents	all types	Blurred vision, cycloplegia, mydriasis, photophobia
Anti-infectives	chloramphenicol	Optic neuritis, decreased visual acuity
	norfloxacin	Visual disturbances
	sulfisoxazole	Periorbital edema, conjunctival and scleral injection
Antineoplastics	cisplatin	Optic neuritis, papilledema, cerebral blindness
	methotrexate	Conjunctivitis
	tamoxifen	Retinopathy, corneal opacities, decreased visual acuity
Antitubercular agents	isoniazid, pyrazinamide, ethambutol	Optic neuritis, decreased visual acuity, loss of red-green color perception, central and peripheral scotomas (ethambutol only)
Cardiotonic glycosides	digitalis leaf, digoxin, digitalis	Altered color vision, photophobia, diplopia, halos or borders on objects
Diuretics	amiloride	Visual disturbances
	hydrochlorothiazide	Altered color vision, transient blurred vision
Genitourinary smooth muscle relaxants	flavoxate	Blurred vision, disturbed accommodation
	oxybutynin	Transient blurred vision, cycloplegia, mydriasis

(continued)

Table 4–1. *Drugs That Adversely Affect the Eyes (Continued)*

DRUG CLASS	DRUG	POSSIBLE ADVERSE REACTIONS
Glucocorticoids	prednisone and others	Exophthalmos, increased intraocular pressure, cataracts, increased susceptibility to secondary fungal and viral eye infections
Antipsychotics	all phenothiazines	Abnormal corneal lens pigmentation
	chlorpromazine	Cataracts, retinopathy, visual impairment
	quetiapine	Lens changes
Miscellaneous agents	carbamazepine	Blurred vision, transient diplopia, visual hallucinations
	oral contraceptives (estrogen with progesterone)	Worsening of myopia or astigmatism, intolerance to contact lenses, neuro-ocular lesions
	isotretinoin	Conjunctivitis, dry eyes, corneal opacities, eye irritation
	loxapine	Blurred vision, pigmentary changes
	metrizamide	Diplopia, amblyopia, photophobia, eye flickering, blurred vision
	Pentazocine hydrochloride	Blurred vision, focusing difficulty, nystagmus, diplopia, miosis, photophobia, calcific conjunctivitis (with vitamin D intoxication)

Assessment of Eyes' Relationship to Other Systems

Remember, all systems are related! As you assess the eyes, look at the relationship between them and all other systems.

SUBJECTIVE DATA	OBJECTIVE DATA
Area/System: General	
Ask about:	*Inspect:*
General state of health	General appearance
Recent infections/illnesses	Level of consciousness
Vision problems	
Area/System: Integumentary	
Ask about:	*Inspect for:*
Allergies	Skin lesions on lids
Rashes	Periorbital edema
Area/System: HEENT	
Ask about:	*Inspect for:*
Headaches/migraines	Masses
Head trauma	Abnormalities in oral, nasal, and
Ear infections	ear structures
Runny nose	*Palpate:*
Thyroid disease	Head
	Thyroid
Area/System: Respiratory	
Ask about:	*Inspect for*
Breathing problems	Cyanotic color changes
Lung disease	*Auscultate:*
	Breath sounds
Area/System: Cardiovascular	
Ask about:	*Measure:*
History of hypertension (HTN)	Blood pressure
Vascular disease	*Palpate:*
	Pulses
	Auscultate:
	Heart sounds
	Bruits
Area/System: Abdomen	
Ask about:	*Palpate:*
History of liver disease	Abdomen
History of renal disease	Liver
Area/System: Musculoskeletal	
Ask about:	*Inspect:*
Muscle weakness	Joints for deformities
Joint swelling, pain, rheumatoid	Range of motion
arthritis	*Palpate:*
	Joints for nodules
	Muscle strength
Area/System: Neurological	
Ask about:	*Test:*
History of multiple sclerosis,	Sensory function
myasthenia gravis, or neuro-	CN II, III, IV, VI
logical problems	

Physical Assessment

ANATOMICAL LANDMARKS: 6 cardinal fields; fundoscopic structures

APPROACH: Inspection, palpation, ophthalmoscopy, visual acuity, extraocular muscles, external structures, fundoscopy

POSITION: Sitting

TOOLBOX: Visual acuity charts (Snellen and Snellen E charts, Allen cards, Jaeger chart), Ishihara cards, ophthalmoscope, penlight, cotton-tipped swab, and cotton ball

AREA/PA SKILL	NORMAL FINDINGS	ABNORMAL FINDINGS
Inspection *Visual Acuity*		
(Measure each eye separately, then together, with and without corrective lenses. Tests CN I.) *Far Vision*		
Depending on client's age and literacy level, use Snellen eye chart, Snellen E chart, or STYCAR chart. **Numerator = 5 distance client stands from chart (20 feet). Denominator = distance in feet at which person with normal vision could read any given line on chart. No more than 2 mistakes permitted per line.**	20/20 right eye (OD), left eye (OS), both eyes (OU)	A smaller fraction (e.g., 20/30, 20/40): Diminished distant visual acuity Myopia: Impaired far vision

(continued)

AREA/PA SKILL	NORMAL FINDINGS	ABNORMAL FINDINGS
Inspection *Near Vision*		
Assess client's ability to read newsprint held 13 to 15 inches from eyes. Use print-size pictures if client is unable to read.	Near vision intact	A smaller fraction (e.g., 14/18): Diminished near vision (hyperopia or, if it occurs with aging, presbyopia)
Color Vision		
Screen for color vision by assessing ability to differenti-ate patterns of colors on Ishihara cards or identify color bars on Snellen eye chart.	Color vision intact	Inability to detect embedded number or letter in Ishihara cards: Color blind-ness. Often inherited in an X-linked recessive pattern predominantly affecting males. Can result from macular degenera-tion or other dis-eases affecting the cones that mediate color vision
Peripheral Vision		
Assess client's ability to detect movement coming in from the periphery (inferior, superior, temporal, and nasal fields).	Peripheral vision intact OU, all fields.	Diminished visual fields seen with glaucoma and cataracts ***Sudden loss of peripheral vision needs immediate ophthalmology referral—may be a sign of acute closed-angle glau-coma, a medical emergency.***

(continued)

AREA/PA SKILL	NORMAL FINDINGS	ABNORMAL FINDINGS

Inspection

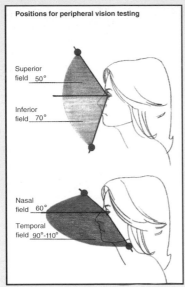

Positions for peripheral vision testing

Superior field _50°_

Inferior field _70°_

Nasal field _60°_

Temporal field _90°-110°_

Positions for peripheral vision testing

Extraocular Muscles

AREA/PA SKILL	NORMAL FINDINGS	ABNORMAL FINDINGS
Inspect eyes for parallel alignment.	Eyes in parallel alignment	Asymmetrical corneal light reflex: Weak extraocular muscles or strabismus
Perform corneal light reflex test. **(Look for the sparkle in your client's eyes!)**	Corneal light reflex symmetrical	
Put eyes through range of motion (ROM), six cardinal fields of vision **(tests CN III, IV, VI).**	Extraocular motion intact OU, no lid lag or nystagmus	

(continued)

AREA/PA SKILL	NORMAL FINDINGS	ABNORMAL FINDINGS
Inspection *Extraocular Muscles (Continued)*		
Perform the cover/ uncover test, check for drifting.	No wandering with cover/uncover test	Shift in gaze: One or more eye muscles are weak. When uncovered eye shifts in response to covering opposite eye, covered eye is dominant. When covered eye shifts after being uncovered, it indicates weakness in that eye
		Limited or disconjugate movement in one or more fields of gaze, nystagmus in fields other than extreme lateral, ptosis, and lid lag: Damage, irritation, or pressure on corresponding extraocular muscle or cranial nerve that innervates the muscle

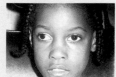

Exotropia (divergent strabismus)

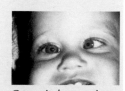

Congenital exotropia

(continued)

AREA/PA SKILL	NORMAL FINDINGS	ABNORMAL FINDINGS
Inspection *External Structures*		
General Appearance		
Appearance and parallel alignment 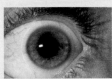 *Soft contact lenses*	Eyes clear and bright, in parallel alignment 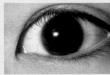 *Hard contact lenses*	Glazed eyes: Febrile state Unequal parallel alignment: Exotropia
Eyelids		
Note color, lesions, edema, symmetry of palpebral fissures **(opening of the eyes between upper and lower lids),** and lid lag.	Color consistent with client's complexion, no lesions or edema, palpebral fissures symmetrical, no lid lag	Visible sclera between iris and upper lid (exophthalmos): Hyperthyroidism or hydrocephalus (setting-sun sign) Asymmetry of lids: CN III damage, CVA Ptosis of both lids: Myasthenia gravis Various lesions may be found on lids 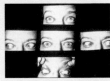 *Exophthalmos* 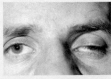 *Ptosis*

(continued)

AREA/PA SKILL	NORMAL FINDINGS	ABNORMAL FINDINGS

Inspection
External Structures

Eyelids (Continued)

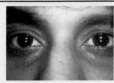

Xanthelasma

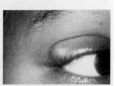

Chalazion

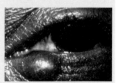

Hordeolum

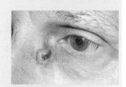

Basal cell carcinoma

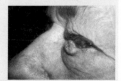

Squamous cell carcinoma

(continued)

AREA/PA SKILL	NORMAL FINDINGS	ABNORMAL FINDINGS
Inspection *External Structures*		
Eyelashes		
Note symmetry and distribution.	Eyelashes evenly distributed, no ectropion or entropion	Absence of lashes: Alopecia universalis
		Lice or ticks at base of lashes: Infestation
		Blepharitis (inflammation of lashes and meibomian glands of eyelids)
		Entropion can scratch the cornea
		Ectropion can lead to excessive drying of the eyes

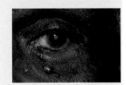

Blepharoconjunctivitis

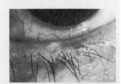

Entropion

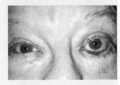

Ectropion

(continued)

AREA/PA SKILL	NORMAL FINDINGS	ABNORMAL FINDINGS
Inspection *External Structures*		
Eyelashes (Continued)		
		Dacryocystitis *Lice*
Eyeball		
Inspect for protrusion of eyeball.	No protrusion beyond frontal bone (mild protrusion seen in some African-Americans)	Protrusion: Hyperthyroidism or inherited disorders of mucopolysaccharide metabolism
Lacrimal ducts, puncta		
Note color, edema, excessive tearing or drainage.	Puncta pale pink and patent, no excessive tearing or dryness, drainage, or edema	Swelling, redness, drainage, or tenderness: Obstruction or inflammation
Conjunctiva		
Assess color, moisture, lesions, and foreign bodies. **Palpebral conjunctiva covers the lids; bulbar conjunctiva, the eyeball.**	Conjunctiva clear, pink, and moist; no lesions	Reddened palpebral and bulbar conjunctiva: Conjunctivitis Pale pink conjunctiva: Anemia *Acute allergic conjunctivitis*

(continued)

AREA/PA SKILL	NORMAL FINDINGS	ABNORMAL FINDINGS

Inspection
External Structures

Conjunctiva (Continued)

| | | Growth and thickening of conjunctiva from inner canthal area toward iris: Pterygium or pinguecula
Subconjunctival hemorrhage: Eye injury
Conjunctival nevus or papilloma |

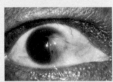

Pterygium

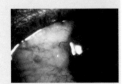

Pinguecula

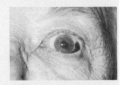

Subconjunctival hemorrhage

(continued)

AREA/PA SKILL	NORMAL FINDINGS	ABNORMAL FINDINGS
Inspection *External Structures*		
Conjunctiva (Continued)		
		 Nevus *Papilloma*
Sclera		
Note color, moisture, and lesions or tears	Sclera white and intact, no lesions or tears	Bluish sclera: Osteogenesis imperfecta Yellow sclera at the limbus: Jaundice Bitot's spots: Vitamin A deficiency Episcleritis: Inflammation of sclera *Diffuse episcleritis*
Cornea		
Note clarity and lesions or abrasions. *Examine cornea from oblique angle.*	Cornea clear without opacities, lesions, or abrasions Arcus senilis: Common finding and normal variant in older adults	Clouding of cornea: Infection (hypopyon: Pus in the anterior chamber) or vitamin A deficiency

(continued)

AREA/PA SKILL	NORMAL FINDINGS	ABNORMAL FINDINGS
Inspection *External Structures*		
Cornea (Continued)		
		Roughness or irregularity of cornea: Corneal abrasions and ulcers

Normal lens

Corneal abrasion

Arcus senilis

Healing corneal ulcer

AREA/PA SKILL	NORMAL FINDINGS	ABNORMAL FINDINGS
Test corneal reflex (CN V and VII) **Instead of touching the cornea with a wisp of cotton, use a needleless syringe and shoot a small amount of air over the cornea, or gently touch lashes and look for blink reflex.**	+ corneal reflex	Kayser-Fleischer ring: Wilson's disease Cataracts may also be seen through transparent cornea

Mature cataract

Anterior Chamber

AREA/PA SKILL	NORMAL FINDINGS	ABNORMAL FINDINGS
Inspect for clarity, bulging of the iris, and blood.	Anterior chamber clear, no blood or bulging of the iris	Hypopyon: Corneal ulceration or other infection

(continued)

AREA/PA SKILL	NORMAL FINDINGS	ABNORMAL FINDINGS

Inspection
External Structures

Anterior Chamber (Continued)

Inspect with client's eyes looking straight ahead, while you look across the eye from the side.	Normal Shallow	Hyphema: Trauma or intraocular hemorrhage Crescent-shaped shadow on nasal side of iris: Protrusion of iris into anterior chamber from increased intraocular pressure; seen in narrow-angle glaucoma

Hypopyon

Hyphema

Acute angle closure

(continued)

AREA/PA SKILL	NORMAL FINDINGS	ABNORMAL FINDINGS
Inspection *External Structures*		
Iris		
Note color, size, shape, and symmetry.	Irides round and symmetrical	Brushfield spots: Common in persons with Down syndrome (but sometimes a normal variant) Red, bloodshot appearance of vessels in iris: Iritis New blood vessel on anterior surface of iris: Diabetes Heterochromia iridis: Previous damage in lighter colored eye or (rarely) Waardenburg syndrome Aniridia: Congenital absence of part or all of iris Keyhole wedges in iris: Previous eye surgery
Pupils		
Note size, shape, reaction to light (direct and consensual); test for accommodation **(tests CN III).** **Consensual reaction: The pupil not receiving light stimulus reacts the same as the pupil receiving stimulus.**	**Pupil size 3 to 5 mm in adults. (Normal size depends on age: Larger in children, smaller in older adults.) No miosis or mydriasis** PERRLA—Pupils equal, round, reactive to light (pupils constrict) and accommodation (pupils converge and constrict) direct and consensual	Miosis: Brain injury to the pons; use of narcotics, atropine, and other drugs Mydriasis: Brain herniation, anoxia, use of marijuana or mydriatic eye drops *Changes in pupils, such as unequal or dilated, may be a sign of increased intracranial pressure (IICP).* Anisocoria: Unilateral brain herniation; IICP

(continued)

AREA/PA SKILL	NORMAL FINDINGS	ABNORMAL FINDINGS
Inspection *External Structures*		
Pupils (Continued)		
	Older client may have decreased accommodation. Anisocoria <0.5 mm can be normal variation	Tonic pupil slow to react to light: Adie's pupil Pupils unequal, affected pupil small but reacts to light: Horner's syndrome

ABNORMAL

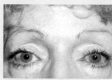

Anisocoria

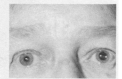

Adie's pupil

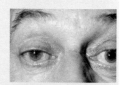

Horner's syndrome

Sluggish or fixed pupil reaction to light: Lack of oxygen to optic nerve or brain, or topical or systemic drug effects

Absence of consensual response: Conditions that compress or deprive optic nerve and brain of oxygen

One or both pupils fail to dilate or constrict to near or distant objects

(continued)

AREA/PA SKILL	NORMAL FINDINGS	ABNORMAL FINDINGS
Inspection *External Structures*		
Pupils (Continued)		
		Sluggish accommodation in the absence of advanced age may be caused by drugs
Palpation *External Structures*		
(Maintain universal precautions. Wear gloves if there is eye drainage.) *Eyeball*		
Gently palpate globe with fingertips or thumb on upper lids over sclera. Note consistency and tenderness. *Do not palpate eyeball in clients with eye trauma or known glaucoma.*	Eyeball firm and nontender	Excessively firm or tender globe: Glaucoma
Lacrimal Apparatus (Tear Gland and Ducts)		
Palpate below eyebrow and inner canthus of eye. Note tenderness or excessive tearing or discharge from punctae. **Ophthalmoscopy (Perform in dark room. Examine same eye to same eye, your right to your client's right. Use small white light aperture for undilated pupil. See Box 4.1.)**	Lacrimal gland nontender, no drainage or excessive tearing	Swelling and tenderness: Inflammation

(continued)

AREA/PA SKILL	NORMAL FINDINGS	ABNORMAL FINDINGS

Inspection
External Structures

Lacrimal Apparatus (Tear Gland and Ducts) (Continued)

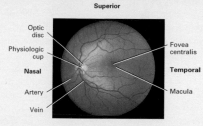

Normal fundoscopic structures of the left eye with fields (Courtesy of Wills Eye Hospital, Philadelphia, PA)

Red Reflex

Note presence, opacities. **Approach from an oblique angle about 14 inches from client.**	+ Red reflex, no opacities	Opaque/blackened area of red reflex: Cataracts Dark spots or shadows that interrupt red reflex: Opacities in lens or vitreous

Optic Disc and Physiological Cup (located nasally)

Note size, shape, borders, color, cup-disc ratio.	Optic disc round, with sharp margins, cup-disc ratio 1:2. Color depends on client's pigmentation: Yellow to orange with white cup	Whitish or gray color of the optic disc: Partial or complete death of optic nerve (optic atrophy) Blurred margins other than nasally: HTN, glaucoma, or papilledema Excessive cup-disc ratio greater than 1:2: Open-angle glaucoma

Retinal Vessels

(Arteries and veins come out of disc in pairs.)		

(continued)

AREA/PA SKILL	NORMAL FINDINGS	ABNORMAL FINDINGS
Inspection *Retinal Vessels (Continued)*		
Assess size ratio of arteries and veins (A/V ratio), color, arteriole light reflex, crossings. **Veins normally darker and larger than arteries.**	Vessels noted. A/V ratio 2:3 or 4:5. + Arteriole light reflex. AV crossings smooth, no nicking or narrowing	Large A/V ratio: HTN Narrowed arteries: Severe hypertension, retinitis pigmentosa, and central retinal artery occlusion AV crossings more than 2 DD from optic disc or nicking or pinching of underlying vessel: HTN
Retina		
Assess color, texture, exudates, lesions, hemorrhages, or aneurysms.	Color varies depending on pigmentation of client, from pale yellow to orange-red The darker the person, the darker the background Texture finely granular No lesions, hemorrhages, exudates, aneurysms	Cotton wool spots: Microinfarctions that occur with diabetes, hypertension, lupus, papilledema Dot hemorrhages: Deep intraretinal hemorrhages seen with diabetes Flame-shaped hemorrhages: Superficial retinal hemorrhages that occur in hypertension
Macula and Fovea Centralis		
(Always examine last!) **Note, color, size, location, lesions. Macula is darker area temporal to disc.**	Macula darker area on retina, 2 DD temporal to OD, 1 DD in size, no lesions + fovea light reflex	Excess or clumped pigment: Trauma or retinal detachment Hemorrhage or exudate in the macula: Macular degeneration

(continued)

AREA/PA SKILL	NORMAL FINDINGS	ABNORMAL FINDINGS

Inspection
Macula and Fovea Centralis (Continued)

Abnormalities of the Optic Disk

Acute papilledema

Chronic papilledema

Glaucomatous optic nerve

Optic neuritis

Optic nerve pallor

Hypertensive changes

Diabetic retinopathy

Malignant hypertension

Age-related macular degeneration ("dry")— vision 20/20

Advanced macular degeneration ("wet")— vision 20/400

PA = physical assessment

BOX 4.1. Ophthalmoscope Apertures

Aperture Type	Purpose
Small white aperture	Best for examining the undilated eye. Start the eye exam with this setting.
Large white aperture	For general examination of the eye and when pupils are dilated.
Red-free filter	A green light for differentiating hemorrhages, which appear black, from melanin, which looks gray. Also differentiates arteries, which appear black, from veins, which appear blue.
Blue light	When fluorescein dye is injected into client intravenously, a blue filter enables examiner to see movement of dye into eye vessels. Useful for detecting hemorrhages, leaking vessels, or vessel abnormalities.
Grid	Used to measure size or location of lesions.
Slit or streak	Used to determine levels or depth of lesions.

EARS

Primary Function

- Hearing
- Balance/equilibrium

Developmental Considerations

Infants and Children

- Abnormalities in the structure and positioning of the ears are more common in infants who have a hearing deficit.
- Low-set ears, ears positioned at greater than a 15-degree angle, or malformed ears are often associated with genetic disorders and developmental delay.
- Infants and children are more prone to inner ear infections than adults because of the shape and position of the external auditory canal and eustachian tube.
- By school age, the external auditory canal has assumed a straighter, adult configuration.

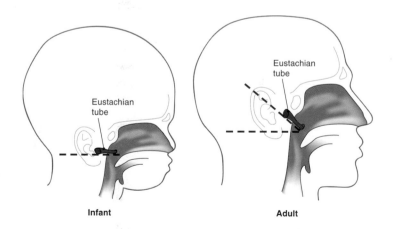

Infant   Adult

Young and Middle-Aged Adults

- Noise-induced hearing loss from exposure to loud music or machinery is the most common cause of hearing loss for adults aged 20 to 40 years old.

Older Adults

- Hearing loss in older adults is extremely common and can be associated with sensorineural loss or conductive loss.
- Presbycusis occurs around the 5th decade and gradually progresses. Typically, presbycusis involves hearing loss for high-pitched sounds such as consonants and affects men more often than women.
- Older adults are prone to stiffening of the cilia in the external canal, which impedes the transmission of sound waves and causes cerumen to accumulate more readily and obstruct the membrane. Excess accumulation of cerumen impairs hearing by air conduction and is one of the most common correctable causes of conductive hearing loss in older adults.

Cultural Considerations

- Incidence and severity of otitis media for Native American, Hispanic, and Alaskan infants are even higher than for the general population.
- Cerumen is dry, white, and flaky in the majority of Asians and Native Americans.
- Cerumen is brown, wet, and sticky in the majority of blacks and whites.
- People living in highly industrialized communities are routinely exposed to sounds above 80 dB, such as traffic and occupational machinery, and are more prone to hearing loss.

Assessment

History

SYMPTOMS ("PQRST" ANY + SYMPTOM)
- Hearing loss
  - Was your hearing loss sudden or gradual?
  - Is your hearing loss in one or both ears?
  - Can you hear better when it is noisy?
  - Have you ever been given an antibiotic called gentamicin or streptomycin?
  - Are you, or have you been, exposed repeatedly to continuous or loud noise?

- Vertigo
  - Do you ever feel as though the room is spinning when you are at rest?
  - If so, was the spinning sensation brought on or worsened by a change in position?
  - Does the spinning sensation change if you change position?
  - Is the sensation associated with blurred vision? Nausea? Vomiting? Weakness? Ringing in the ears?
- Tinnitus
  - Is the ringing or buzzing continuous or intermittent?
  - Does anything in particular seem to bring on the ringing or buzzing sound?
  - Does the ringing or buzzing sound pulsate?
- Drainage from ear (otorrhea)
  - Have you had any drainage from the ear?
  - If so, what does it look like (color, clarity)?
  - Does the drainage have an odor?
  - Have you had a recent ear or throat infection?
  - Do you have any dizziness? Ear pain? Change in your hearing?
  - Have you had a recent head or ear injury?
- Ear pain (otalgia)
  - Is the pain associated with decreased hearing?
  - Have you had any recent trauma to the ear?

FOCUSED EAR HISTORY

- Do you have any problems with your ears? Ringing? Hearing?
- Do you have any balance problems?
- Do you have any drainage from your ears? If yes, amount, color?
- Have you had recent head trauma?
- Do you have any health problems?
- Are you exposed to noise pollution in your job or environment?
- Are you taking any medications, prescribed or over the counter (Table 4–2)?
- Do you have allergies?

Table 4–2. *Drugs That Adversely Affect the Ears*

DRUG CLASS	DRUG	POSSIBLE ADVERSE REACTIONS
Aminoglycosides	all aminoglycosides	Tinnitus, vertigo, hearing loss
Anti-inflammatory agents	all nonsteroidal anti-inflammatory agents (e.g., diflunisal, ibuprofen, and indomethacin)	Tinnitus, vertigo, hearing loss
Antimalarials	quinine	Tinnitus, vertigo, hearing loss
Diuretics	furosemide and bumetanide	Tinnitus, vertigo, hearing loss (with too-rapid I.V. administration)
Non-narcotic analgesics and antipyretics	all salicylates and all combination products containing salicylates	Tinnitus, vertigo, hearing loss (with high dose or long-term therapy)
Miscellaneous agents	capreomycin, cisplatin, erythromycin, ethacrynic acid, quinidine sulfate, and vancomycin	Tinnitus, vertigo, hearing loss

Assessment of Ears' Relationship to Other Systems

Remember, all systems are related! As you assess the ears, look at the relationship between them and all other systems.

SUBJECTIVE DATA	OBJECTIVE DATA
Area/System: General	
Ask about:	*Inspect for:*
General state of health	Ear guarding, inattentiveness,
Recent infections/illnesses	inappropriate responses, bal-
Hearing difficulty	ance problems
	Measure:
	Vital signs
Area/System: Integumentary	
Ask about:	*Inspect:*
Lesions on ears (sun-exposed	Lesion, areas of inflammation
area, common site for skin	*Palpate for:*
cancer)	Tenderness
Area/System: HEENT	
Head and Neck	
Ask about:	*Palpate for:*
Pain	Lymph node enlargement, sinus
Swollen nodes	tenderness
Nose and Throat	
Ask about:	*Inspect:*
Sore throat	Oral and nasal structures
Nasal congestion	
Area/System: Respiratory	
Ask about:	*Measure:*
Cough, congestion	Respiratory rate
Mucus production	*Auscultate:*
	Lung sounds
Area/System: Cardiovascular	
Ask about:	*Measure:*
History of vascular disease	Heart rate
	Palpate:
	Pulses, carotid thrills
	Auscultate:
	Heart sounds, bruits
Area/System: Musculoskeletal	
Ask about:	*Inspect:*
History of gout	Ear lobes for tophi
Hearing problems	
Area/System: Neurological	
Ask about:	*Test:*
History of transient ischemic	Romberg's
attacks	
Balance problems	
Neurological problem	

HEENT = head, eyes, ears, nose, and throat

Physical Assessment

ANATOMICAL LANDMARKS: Position of ears; tympanic membrane

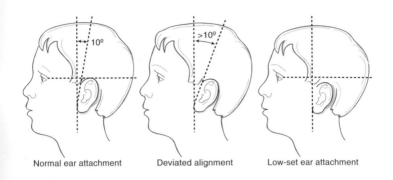

Normal ear attachment   Deviated alignment   Low-set ear attachment

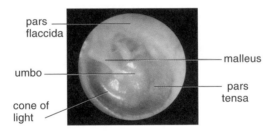

Tympanic membrane, left ear

APPROACH: Inspection and palpation of external structures; otoscopy of external auditory canal and TM; hearing tests

POSITION: Sitting; supine for infants to immobilize head

TOOLBOX: Tuning fork (500 to 1000 cycles per second), otoscope with pneumatic attachment, thermometer, and watch

AREA/PA SKILL	NORMAL FINDINGS	ABNORMAL FINDINGS
Inspection *External Ear*		
Note position, shape, size, symmetry, angle of attachment, color, lesions, and drainage (clear, bloody, or purulent) **To assess angle of attachment, draw imaginary line from top of helix to external canthus of eye and then a perpendicular line in front of ear.**	Vertical ear position with <10-degree lateral posterior slant. Ears aligned with eyes, symmetrical, no redness, lesions, or drainage	Microtia: Small ears <4 cm vertical height in adults. Seen in some genetic disorders Macrotia: Large ears >10 cm vertical height in adults Landmarks missing or malformed: Associated with hearing deficit Creased ear lobe: Associated with heart conditions Ear pits or sinuses usually located anterior to the tragus: Associated with internal ear anomalies Low-set ears or ears rotated posteriorly more than 15 degrees: Associated with mental retardation

Congenital ear anomaly

Darwinian tubercle

Low-set ears

(continued)

AREA/PA SKILL	NORMAL FINDINGS	ABNORMAL FINDINGS
Inspection *External Ear (Continued)*		
		If clear drainage noted from nose or ears, secondary to head trauma, suspect cerebrospinal fluid 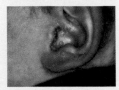 *Impacted cerumen*
Palpation (**Maintain universal precautions. Wear gloves if drainage is present.**) *External Ear*		
Assess consistency, tenderness, lesions. Palpate tragus and mastoid process.	Helix soft and pliable, nontender, no nodules or lesions	Tenderness of mastoid, helix, tragus, or pinna: Ear infections or tophi

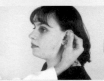

Palpating the ear

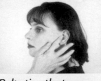

Palpating the tragus

Palpating the mastoid

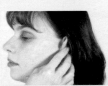

Pulling helix forward

(continued)

AREA/PA SKILL	NORMAL FINDINGS	ABNORMAL FINDINGS
Palpation *External Ear (Continued)*		
Before starting oto-scopic examina-tion, palpate tragus and mastoid, pull helix forward. If tender, proceed carefully with insertion of oto-scope—patient may have ear in-fection.		
Otoscopic Exam **Use the largest and shortest speculum that the ear canal can accommodate (4, 5, or 6 mm, ½″). Have client tilt head to opposite side to that being examined. Pull helix up and back for an adult and down for a child. Always look into canal before insert-ing the otoscope. Insert ½″ for adult, ¼″ for child Avoid the inner ⅔ of the canal—it is over the temporal bone and is very sensitive.** *External Ear Canal*		
Note color, drainage, patency, edema, lesions, or foreign objects.	Ear canal light-colored and patent, small amount of yellow cerumen and hair; no lesions, exudates, or foreign objects	Ear canal may be blocked by a foreign object or cerumen Reddened canal: Otitis externa

(continued)

AREA/PA SKILL	NORMAL FINDINGS	ABNORMAL FINDINGS

Otoscopic Exam
External Ear Canal (Continued)

Cerumen is the only normal drainage in the ear.	*Color and amount of cerumen vary depending on ethnicity*	Excessive impacted cerumen in older adults can contribute to conductive hearing loss
		Exudate and an edematous canal: External otitis
		Drainage: Bloody drainage can result from trauma; purulent from infection; and clear may be spinal fluid from head injury
		Exostosis often results from swimming in cold water.

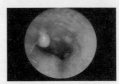

Exostosis

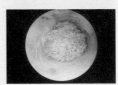

Foreign body

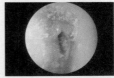

External otitis

(continued)

AREA/PA SKILL	NORMAL FINDINGS	ABNORMAL FINDINGS

Otoscopic Exam
Tympanic Membrane (TM)

Note position of landmarks (cone of light, pars flaccida, pars tensa, malleus, and umbo).	TM shiny, pearly gray, intact, and mobile. No lesions or exudates	Yellowish membrane with fluid and air bubbles visible behind TM: Serous otitis
Ears are mirror images, so cone of light is at 7 o'clock in left ear and 5 o'clock in right ear.	Landmarks appropriately noted. No bulging or retraction of the TM	Reddish TM with absent or distorted light reflex: Otitis media
Note intactness of TM, color, lesions, and exudates.		Round/oval-shaped dark area: Perforated TM
Assess mobility of TM in children using pneumatic attachment.		White irregular-shaped area: Scar tissue
Never irrigate the ear canal unless you are sure the TM is intact.		

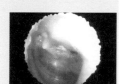

Serous otitis

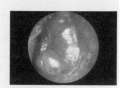

Otitis media

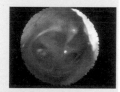

Perforated TM

(continued)

AREA/PA SKILL	NORMAL FINDINGS	ABNORMAL FINDINGS

Otoscopic Exam
Tympanic Membrane (TM) (Continued)

Blue to black TM: Hemotympanum; bleeding usually results from trauma

Golden-brown TM with caramel-color, thick, elastic (like rubber cement) drainage: Secretory, adhesive otitis media; associated with viral infection

Cystic mass of epithelial cells in middle ear: Cholesteatoma, a complication of chronic otitis media

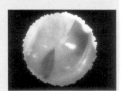

Hemotympanum

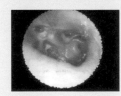

Adhesive otitis media

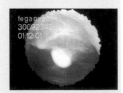

Cholesteatoma

(continued)

AREA/PA SKILL	NORMAL FINDINGS	ABNORMAL FINDINGS

Otoscopic Exam
Tympanic Membrane (TM) (Continued)

		Tubes placed in ear to promote drainage and equalize pressure
		Change in position or shape of cone of light reflex and absence or exaggeration of bony landmarks: Imbalance in middle ear pressure. Bony landmarks are more prominent if negative pressure in inner ear, less prominent in infections or conditions in which fluid or pus collects behind membrane

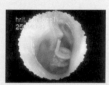

Pressure equalization tube

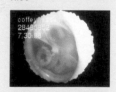

Tympanotomy

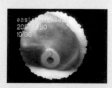

Intact patient pressure equalization tube

(continued)

AREA/PA SKILL	NORMAL FINDINGS	ABNORMAL FINDINGS
Otoscopic Exam *Tympanic Membrane (TM) (Continued)*		
		Limited mobility of drum: Associated with bulging drum
Hearing Exam *Gross Hearing*		
Use whispered voice test to assess for low-pitch deficits **(1 to 2 feet from ear).**	Gross hearing intact bilaterally	Inability to repeat whispered words: Low-tone frequency loss
Use ticking watch to assess for high-pitch deficits **(5 inches from ear).** *Weber Test*		Inability to hear watch ticking: High-tone frequency loss
Place vibrating tuning fork on forehead or top of head to assess bone con-duction. ***Be careful not to touch the prongs of tuning fork—it will dampen vibration.*** *Rinne Test*	Negative lateralization of sound: Heard equally in both ears	Lateralization of sound: Either con-ductive or sensori-neural loss
Compare bone con-duction (BC) to air conduction (AC). Place vibrating tuning fork on mastoid (BC) until no longer heard, then move fork to in front of ear (AC). Time how long the sound is heard.	Sound transmission through air is normally twice as long as sound trans-mission through bone AC>BC	AC-to-BC ratios that differ markedly in each ear: Unilateral hearing deficit AC < twice BC: Hearing loss by AC, possibly caused by ear wax, otitis media, serous otitis, or damage to ossi-cles of middle ear

(continued)

AREA/PA SKILL	NORMAL FINDINGS	ABNORMAL FINDINGS
Hearing Exam *Balance*		
Perform Romberg test with patient's eyes open and then closed.	Negative Romberg	Positive Romberg test, loss of balance: Inner ear problem, cerebellar dysfunction, or ingestion of drugs or alcohol

PA = physical assessment

CHAPTER 5

ASSESSING THE RESPIRATORY SYSTEM

Primary Function

- Exchange of oxygen and carbon dioxide through respirations
- Plays important role in maintaining acid-base balance

Developmental Considerations

Infants

- Obligatory nose breathers
- Irregular respiratory patterns with patterns of apnea
- Abdominal breathers
- AP:lateral ratio 1:1

Pregnant Clients

- Increased tidal volume
- Increased costal angle
- Diaphragm rises
- Increased oxygen demands

Older Adults

- Decreased surface area
- Decreased breathing and lung capacity
- Increased dead space
- Decreased vital capacity

Cultural Considerations

- Chinese-Americans have smaller chests than Caucasians.
- African-Americans in urban areas have higher incidence of respiratory disease.
- Appalachians have higher incidence of black lung, tuberculosis (TB), and emphysema.
- Irish have higher incidence of respiratory problems related to coal mining.
- Navajo Indians have increased risk for respiratory problems related to close living quarters.

Assessment

History

SYMPTOMS ("PQRST" ANY + SYMPTOM)
- Cough
  - How long have you had the cough?
  - When does your cough occur: On awakening, late afternoon, in the evening, after eating, during the night?
  - Do you cough when sitting up, or just when lying down?
  - Do you cough when you exercise?
  - Are you allergic to pollens, animals, or dust?
  - When you cough, what does it sound like? Is it dry or moist sounding? Wheezy?
  - Do you have trouble catching your breath when you start coughing?
  - Do you bring up mucus or sputum when you cough?
  - What color is the sputum? Does it smell or taste bad?
  - Is your sputum thick and hard to get up? Or is it thin? Is it frothy or bubbly?
- Dyspnea
  - Do you ever feel you don't have enough air or you can't catch your breath? If so, please describe what you are doing when this happens, whether it occurs suddenly or over time, and how it affects your activities.
  - How many pillows do you sleep with?
  - Do you experience shortness of breath, or breathless-

ness, with activity or exercise? How much can you do before you become short of breath?

- Can you breathe better after you rest or when you are quiet?
- Do you wake up at night feeling breathless?
- Do you have pain associated with the shortness of breath?
- How long have you noticed this problem of breathlessness?

- Chest pain
  - Do you experience pain in your chest, especially when you take a deep breath?
  - If you have shortness of breath, is it accompanied by pain?
  - Do you have pain when you cough?
  - Where in your chest do you feel the pain?
  - Please describe your pain: Is it aching, sharp, stabbing, gripping? How severe is it on a scale of 1 to 10?
  - Is your chest wall tender or sore when touched?
- Other related symptoms
  - Do you have swelling of your abdomen, legs, ankles, or feet?
  - Do you have enough energy to do your usual daily activities?
  - Do you need to sleep or rest more than usual?

FOCUSED RESPIRATORY HISTORY

- Do you have a history of respiratory disease? If yes, are you taking any medications for it? If yes, what are you taking and why?
- Do you have any other medical problems? (Especially note cardiac problems.)
- Do you have allergies? If yes, describe reaction.
- Do you have a cough, shortness of breath, or chest pain?
- Do you smoke? If yes, what do you smoke, how much, and for how long?
- What is your occupation?
- Where do you live?
- When was your last purified protein derivative test, and what were the results?
- Have you ever had a chest x ray? If yes, what were the results?

- Have you been immunized for influenza or pneumonia?
- Are you taking any medications, prescribed or over the counter (OTC) (Table 5–1)?

Table 5–1. *Drugs That Adversely Affect the Respiratory System*

DRUG CLASS	DRUG	POSSIBLE ADVERSE REACTIONS
Adrenergic agents (sympatho-mimetics)	epinephrine hydrochloride	Dyspnea, paradoxical bronchospasms
Adrenergic blockers (sympatholytics)	methysergide maleate	Nasal congestion; pulmonary fibrosis, resulting in dyspnea, tightness, chest pain, pleural friction rubs, effusion
Alkylating agents	busulfan	Irreversible pulmonary fibrosis (busulfan lung)
	carmustine	Pulmonary infiltrates, fibrosis
	cyclophosphamide	Pulmonary fibrosis (with high doses)
	melphalan	Pneumonitis
Antiarrhythmics	amiodarone hydrochloride	Interstitial pneumonitis, pulmonary fibrosis
Antibiotic anti-neoplastic agents	bleomycin sulfate	Fine crackles, dyspnea (early signs of pulmonary toxicity); interstitial pneumonitis
	mitomycin	Dyspnea, cough, hemoptysis, pulmonary infiltrates
Antihypertensives	enalapril maleate	Cough
	guanethidine sulfate	Nasal congestion
	guanabenz acetate	Nasal congestion
	reserpine	Nasal congestion
Anti-infectives	polymyxin B sulfate	Respiratory paralysis
Antimetabolites	methotrexate sodium	Pneumonitis
Beta blockers	all beta blockers	Bronchospasm, particularly in clients with a history of asthma; dyspnea, wheezing
Cholinergic agents	bethanechol chloride, donepezil	Dyspnea, sore throat, bronchoconstriction (with subcutaneous administration)

(continued)

Table 5–1. *Drugs That Adversely Affect the Respiratory System (Continued)*

DRUG CLASS	DRUG	POSSIBLE ADVERSE REACTIONS
	neostigmine bromide	Increased bronchial secretions, bronchospasm
Gold salts	aurothioglucose, gold sodium thiomalate	Pulmonary infiltrates, interstitial pneumonitis, interstitial fibrosis, "gold" bronchitis
Narcotic analgesics	all types	Respiratory depression
Nonsteroidal anti-inflammatory agents	aspirin	Bronchospasm
	ibuprofen	Bronchospasm, dyspnea
	indomethacin	Bronchospasm, dyspnea
Penicillins	all types	Anaphylaxis
Sedatives and hypnotics	all types	Respiratory depression, apnea
Urinary tract antiseptics	nitrofurantoin, nitrofurantoin macrocrystals	Pulmonary sensitivity reactions, such as cough, chest pain, dyspnea, pulmonary infiltrates; interstitial pneumonitis (with prolonged use)
Miscellaneous agents	cromolyn sodium	Cough, wheezing
	levodopa	Excessive nasal discharge, hoarseness, episodic hyperventilation, bizarre breathing patterns
	thiamine hydrochloride	Tightness of throat, respiratory distress, cyanosis, pulmonary edema (with I.V. administration)

Assessment of Respiratory System's Relationship to Other Systems

Remember, all systems are related! As you assess the respiratory system, look at the relationship between it and all other systems.

SUBJECTIVE DATA	OBJECTIVE DATA
Area/System: General *Ask about:* Changes in energy level Activity intolerance Fatigue Weight changes	*Inspect for:* Signs of acute distress, such as shortness of breath, dyspnea on exertion Posture: Tripod; Position: Orthopnea *Measure:* Height, weight (check for changes) Temperature, pulse, respirations, blood pressure (check for increases)
Area/System: Integumentary *Ask about:* Skin color changes Fevers, night sweats	*Inspect for:* Skin color changes (e.g., cyanosis, pallor, ruddiness) Central (mucous membranes) vs. peripheral cyanosis Nail clubbing *Palpate:* Skin temperature, turgor, edema Capillary refill
Area/System: HEENT *Ask about:* Lumps or swelling in neck Excessive eye tearing Ear infections, sore throats, upper respiratory infections (URIs), sinus problems Difficulty swallowing or breathing	*Inspect for:* Facial expression (e.g., anxious) Neck vein distention, hypertrophy, and use of accessory neck muscles Color of conjunctiva Ear or nose drainage, nasal flaring Color of mucous membranes, color of tonsils and enlargement *Palpate:* Sinus tenderness, lymph nodes, tracheal position, thyroid gland, patent nares, tonsillar glands *Examine:* Fundus, optic disk External ear and tympanic membrane (otoscopic exam) Internal nasal mucosa and structures

(continued)

SUBJECTIVE DATA	OBJECTIVE DATA
Area/System: Cardiovascular	
Ask about:	*Inspect for:*
Chest pain	**Edema**
Palpitations	*Palpate for:*
Swelling, tight shoes	**Edema, Homans' sign**
	Auscultate:
	Right side S4 and S3
Area/System: Gastrointestinal	
Ask about:	*Palpate for:*
Changes in appetite	**Enlarged liver, ascites**
Gastrointestinal (GI) complaints	
Right upper quadrant (RUQ) pain	
Area/System: Genitourinary/Reproductive	
Ask about:	
Nocturia	
Changes in sexual activity	
Safe-sex practices	
Pregnancy	
Area/System: Musculoskeletal	
Ask about:	*Inspect for:*
Weakness	**Hypertrophy and use of accessory muscles, muscle atrophy, spinal deformities**
	Measure:
	Muscle strength, checking for weakness
Area/System: Neurological	
Ask about:	*Inspect for:*
Memory changes	**Impaired mental status, AAO × 3**
Morning headaches	**Asterixis (flapping tremors)**
Tremors	
Area/System: Endocrine	
Ask about:	
Thyroid disease	
Area/System: Lymphatic/Hematological	
Ask about:	
Bleeding, anemia	
Allergies	

HEENT = head, eyes, ears, nose, and throat

Physical Assessment

ANATOMICAL LANDMARKS

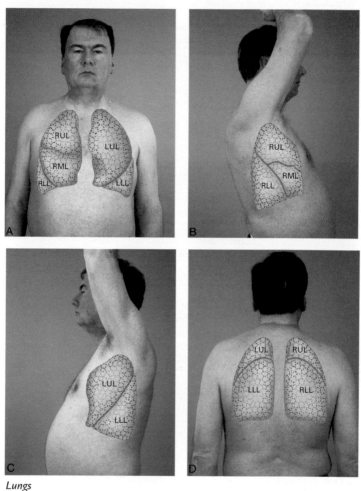

Lungs

APPROACH: Inspection, palpation, percussion, auscultation from anterior, posterior, and lateral approaches. Compare side to side, work apex to base.

POSITION: Sitting.

TOOLBOX: Stethoscope, felt-tipped marker, and metric ruler.

AREA/PA SKILL	NORMAL FINDINGS	ABNORMAL FINDINGS
Inspection *Chest*		
Assess respiratory rate, rhythm, depth. Respiratory rate varies with age.	Look for symmetry of chest movement Respirations quiet, symmetrical, with regular rhythm and depth	Altered respiratory rate and pattern
Check anteroposterior (AP):lateral ratio, costal angle.	AP:lateral 1:2; costal angle 90 degrees	
Inspect for spinal deformities.	No barrel chest or spinal deformities No retraction or use of accessory muscles	Altered shape— Barrel chest 1:1 with costal angle >90 degrees: Chronic obstructive pulmonary disease (COPD) Altered chest symmetry: Spinal deformities, kyphosis, scoliosis
Note muscles used for breathing.	Women are more thoracic breathers, men and infants more abdominal breathers	Altered breathing symmetry: Fractured ribs, flail chest, pneumothorax, atelectasis Sternal and intercostal retraction: Hypoxia and severe respiratory distress, especially with airway obstruction Intercostal bulging: COPD
Note condition of skin.	Skin intact	Blue skin color (cyanosis): Hypoxia or extreme cold temperature Scars: Previous trauma or surgery

(continued)

AREA/PA SKILL	NORMAL FINDINGS	ABNORMAL FINDINGS

Inspection
Chest (Continued)

When assessing a client's respirations, the nurse should determine their rate, rhythm, and depth. These schematic diagrams show different respiratory patterns.

Eupnea
Normal respiratory rate and rhythm

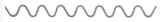

Tachypnea
Increased respiratory rate

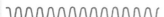

Bradypnea
Slow but regular respirations

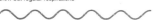

Apnea
Absence of breathing (may be periodic)

Hyperventilation
Deeper respirations; normal rate

Cheyne-Stokes
Respirations that gradually become faster and deeper than normal, then slower; alternates with periods of apnea

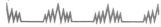

Biot's
Faster and deeper respirations than normal, with abrupt irregular pauses between them

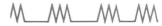

Kussmaul's
Faster and deeper respirations without pauses

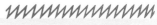

Apneustic
Prolonged, gasping inspiration followed by extremely short, inefficient expiration

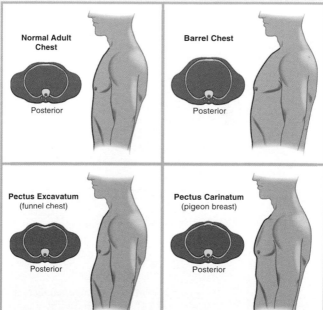

Normal Adult Chest

Posterior

Barrel Chest

Posterior

Pectus Excavatum
(funnel chest)

Posterior

Pectus Carinatum
(pigeon breast)

Posterior

Chest shapes

(continued)

AREA/PA SKILL	NORMAL FINDINGS	ABNORMAL FINDINGS
Palpation		
Trachea		
Note position.	Midline, no deviation	Tracheal deviation: Tumor or thyroid enlargement; tension pneumothorax deviates trachea to unaffected side, severe atelectasis to affected side
Chest		
Palpate for tenderness, masses, crepitus.	Chest nontender, no masses or crepitus	**Crepitus: Subcutaneous emphysema**
Note excursion.	Symmetrical excursion at bases anterior and posterior, no lags	Asymmetrical excursion: Thoracotomy, complete or partial obstruction, effusion, or pneumothorax
Assess for tactile fremitus. **Use balls or ulnar surface of your hand as client says "99."**	Equal tactile fremitus anterior and posterior	Increased fremitus: Consolidating pneumonia, atelectasis, fibrosis, pulmonary edema, or infarction Decreased fremitus: Emphysema, asthma, effusion, pneumothorax, or airway obstruction
Percussion Use indirect (mediate) percussion.		
Chest		
Assess density of underlying lung tissue. Identify extent of lung fields.	Anterior chest: Resonance to 2nd intercostal space (ICS) on left, to 4th ICS on right Lateral: Resonance to 8th ICS Posterior: Resonance to T10 and T12 on deep inspiration	**Dullness: Tumors, fluid, pleural effusion, pneumonia, pulmonary edema** Hyperresonance: Air trapping of emphysema

(continued)

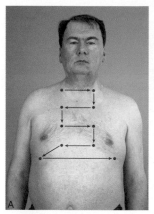

Palpation sequences

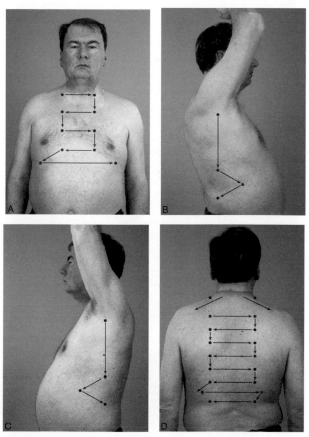

Percussion sequences

AREA/PA SKILL	NORMAL FINDINGS	ABNORMAL FINDINGS
Percussion *Chest (Continued)*		
Assess diaphragmatic excursion.	Diaphragmatic excursion 3 to 6 cm	Decreased excursion: Paralyzed diaphragm, atelectasis, COPD
Auscultation (Use the diaphragm of the stethoscope. Have client take slow deep breaths through mouth.) *Chest*		
(Listen through one full respiratory cycle.) Note relationship of inspiration to expiration, pitch, intensity, and location of sound.		
Assess breath sounds. Note abnormal and adventitious breath sounds.	**Lungs clear to auscultation (CTA)** Bronchial sounds over trachea; bronchovesicular over manubrium; vesicular over most of lung fields No adventitious sounds	Decreased breath sounds: Poor inspiratory effort, emphysema, pleural effusion Absent breath sounds: Airway obstruction, pneumothorax Displaced bronchial breath sounds: Pneumonia Crackles/rales: Pulmonary edema, pneumonia, atelectasis, fibrosis Wheezes: Asthma, COPD Rhonchi: Pneumonia, bronchitis

(continued)

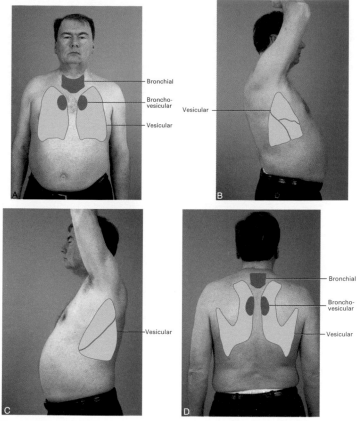

Bronchial
Broncho-vesicular
Vesicular

Vesicular

Vesicular

Bronchial
Broncho-vesicular
Vesicular

Normal breath sounds

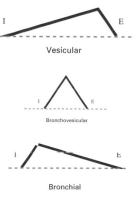

I   E
Vesicular

I   E
Bronchovesicular

I   E
Bronchial

AREA/PA SKILL	NORMAL FINDINGS	ABNORMAL FINDINGS
Auscultation *Chest (Continued)*		
		Stridor: Laryngeal or tracheal obstruction, epiglottitis, viral croup
		Pleural friction rub: Inflamed pleura, pleuritis
Note abnormal voice sounds.	**No abnormal voice sounds**	Abnormal voice sounds (egophony, bronchophony, whispered pectorilo- quy): Consolidated lung tissue, pul- monary edema, pul- monary hemorrhage

I   E

Crackles

I   E

Rhonchi

I   E

Mild Wheeze

I   E

Moderate Wheeze

I   E

Severe Wheeze

I   E

Friction Rub

PA = Physical assessment

CHAPTER 6

ASSESSING THE CARDIOVASCULAR SYSTEM

Primary Function

- Delivery of oxygenated blood throughout body
- Removal of metabolic wastes

Developmental Considerations

Infants and Children

- Change from fetal circulation with closure of foramen ovale and ductus arteriosus shortly after birth
- Innocent systolic murmur commonly heard
- Sinus arrhythmia with respirations common
- Point of maximal impulse (PMI) at 4th intercostal space (ICS) to age 7, to left midclavicular line (MCL) till age 4, at MCL at age 6, to right MCL at age 7

Pregnant Clients

- Mammary souffle
- Systolic murmur common
- Displace PMI up and lateral
- Blood pressure lower during first and second trimester with slight increase in rate

Older Adults

- Postural hypotension
- Auscultatory gaps
- Incidence of coronary vascular disease (CVD) increases with age

Cultural Considerations

- Japanese and Puerto Ricans have a lower incidence of hypertension (HTN) and high cholesterol.
- Hispanics have a lower mortality rate from heart disease than non-Hispanics.
- Middle-aged Caucasians have the highest incidence of coronary artery disease (CAD).
- Blacks have an earlier onset and greater severity of CAD than other groups.
- Black women have a greater incidence of CAD than white women.
- Native Americans under age 35 have twice the mortality rate from heart disease as other groups.

Assessment

History

SYMPTOMS ("PQRST" ANY + SYMPTOM)
- Chest pain
  - When did the pain begin?
  - What were you doing before the pain began?
  - Did anything you do make it better or worse?
  - Can you tell me what it feels like?
  - Point to where it hurts!
  - Are you having any breathing difficulties?
- Palpitations
  - Do you ever feel that your heart is racing or skipping beats?
  - Does your heart feel as if there is a butterfly in your chest?
- Syncope
  - Have you ever had a fainting or "blackout" spell?
  - Do you ever feel light-headed or dizzy?
- Edema

- Have you noticed any swelling in your ankles or feet?
  - Are your shoes tight?
  - Have you noticed any recent changes in your weight?
- Fatigue
  - Have you noticed any changes in your energy level?
  - Do you find you don't have enough energy to get through the day?
  - Do you need to take naps throughout the day?
- Extremity changes
  - Do you ever experience numbness or tingling of your arms or legs?
  - Do your hands or feet feel cold?
  - Do you get pain or cramps in your legs while walking?
- Related symptoms
  - Do you have any breathing difficulties?
  - Do you wake up during the night short of breath?
  - How many pillows do you sleep on?
  - Do you get short of breath with activity?
  - Do you have a cough?
  - Is the cough productive? If yes, what color is the mucus?

FOCUSED CARDIAC HISTORY
- Are you having any chest discomfort? If yes, when did it start?
- What were you doing before the pain?
- Did anything make it better or worse?
- Have you ever had this pain before?
- What does it feel like?
- Show me where it hurts.
- On a scale from 1 to 10, how bad is the pain?
- Do you have a history of cardiovascular disease? If yes, are you taking any medications for it? If yes, what are you taking and why?
- Do you have any other medical problems?
- Are you taking any other medications, prescribed or over the counter (Table 6–1)?
- Are you having any breathing difficulties?
- Do you have any allergies? If, yes, describe reaction.

Table 6-1. *Drugs That Adversely Affect the Cardiovascular System*

DRUG CLASS	DRUG	POSSIBLE ADVERSE REACTIONS
Antidepressants	trazodone hydro-chloride	Hypotension, HTN, syncope, chest pain, tachycardia, palpitations, EKG changes
	tricyclic antidepressants	Postural hypotension, HTN, EKG changes, dysrhythmias, syncope, thrombosis, thrombophlebitis, CHF
Antineoplastics	daunorubicin hydrochloride, doxorubicin hydrochloride	Dose-dependent cardiomyopathy manifested by CHF, EKG changes, dysrhythmias
Antipsychotics	phenothiazines, thioridazine, mesoridiazine, ziprasidone	Hypotension, postural hypotension, tachycardia, syncope, EKG changes, dysrhythmias
Anxiolytics	diazepam	Hypotension, bradycardia, cardiac arrest, dysrhythmias (with I.V. route)
	midazolam hydro-chloride	Hypotension, cardiorespiratory arrest
Bronchodilators, antiasthmatic agents	aminophylline, theophylline	Palpitations, sinus tachycardia, extrasystoles, ventricular dysrhythmias, hypotension
Cerebral stimulants	amphetamine sulfate	Tachycardia, palpitations, dysrhythmias, HTN, hypotension
	caffeine	Tachycardia
Hormones	oral contraceptives	HTN, fluid retention, increased risk of CVA, MI, thromboembolism
	conjugated estrogens, estradiol, oral contraceptives	HTN, thromboembolism, thrombophlebitis
	vasopressin	Angina in clients with vascular disease; in large doses, HTN, bradycardia, minor dysrhythmias, MI
Narcotic agents	morphine	Hypotension
Miscellaneous agents	bethanechol chloride	Hypotension, reflex tachycardia

(continued)

DRUG CLASS	DRUG	POSSIBLE ADVERSE REACTIONS
	hydralazine hydro-chloride	Tachycardia, angina pectoris, EKG changes
	levodopa-carbidopa	Orthostatic hypotension
	levothyroxine	With excessive doses, angina pectoris, dysrhythmias, tachycardia, HTN
	phenytoin sodium	Hypotension, ventricular fibrillation (with I.V. route)

Table 6–1. *Drugs That Adversely Affect the Cardiovascular System (Continued)*

Assessment of Cardiovascular System's Relationship to Other Systems

Remember, all systems are related! As you assess the cardiovascular system, look at the relationship between it and all other systems.

SUBJECTIVE DATA	OBJECTIVE DATA
Area/System: General	
Ask about:	*Inspect for:*
Fatigue	Signs of chest pain
Dyspnea on exertion (DOE)	Shortness of breath (SOB)
Activity intolerance	Posture
Recent illness or flu	Orthopnea
Weight changes	Changes in VS
	Measure:
	Height and weight
Area/System: Integumentary	
Ask about:	*Inspect for:*
Skin changes	Color changes (e.g., cyanosis or pallor)
Poor wound healing	Color changes in legs (e.g., red or brown)
Skin temperature changes	Lesions (e.g., petechiae or leg wounds)
Nail color changes	Taut, shiny, hairless skin

(continued)

SUBJECTIVE DATA	OBJECTIVE DATA
Ankle swelling	Nails for clubbing
Tight shoes	*Palpate:*
	Skin temperature, turgor, edema
	Capillary refill
Area/System: HEENT	
Head and Neck	
Ask about:	*Inspect:*
Headaches	Facial expression
Dizzy spells	*Palpate:*
	Thyroid
	Neck vein distention
Eyes	
Ask about:	*Test:*
Blurred or double vision	Visual acuity
Yellow spots	*Inspect for:*
	Periorbital edema
	Xanthelasma
	Arcus senilis
	Sclera icterus
	Exophthalmos
	Examine:
	Fundus for atrioventricular nicking, exudates, cotton wool spots, hemorrhages
Ears, Nose, and Throat	
Ask about:	*Note:*
Ringing in ears	Gross hearing
Frequent "strep" throat	*Inspect:*
Nosebleeds	Oropharynx
	Pink tonsils
Area/System: Respiratory	
Ask about:	*Inspect for:*
Breathing difficulties (e.g., SOB, DOE, paroxysmal nocturnal dyspnea)	Chest deformities
	Respiratory rate
Dry cough	Retraction or use of accessory muscles
History of COPD	
	Auscultate:
	Adventitious sounds such as crackles
Area/System: Gastrointestinal	
Ask about:	*Inspect for:*
Right upper quadrant pain	Ascites
Nausea	*Palpate for:*
Gastrointestinal upset	Hepatomegaly

(continued)

SUBJECTIVE DATA	OBJECTIVE DATA
Area/System: Genitourinary/Reproductive	
Ask about:	
Awakening to urinate (nocturia)	
For men:	
Sexual performance problems	
For women:	
Pre- or postmenopausal	
Birth control pills	
Hormone replacement therapy	
Area/System: Musculoskeletal	
Ask about:	*Test:*
Weakness	Muscle strength
Muscle cramps	*Inspect for:*
	Atrophy
	Wasting
Area/System: Neurological	
Ask about:	*Check:*
Fainting episodes	Mental status (AAO × 3)
Behavioral changes	Immediate, recent, and remote
Confusion	memory
Memory loss	Judgment
	Decreased or diminished sensa-
	tions
Area/System: Endocrine	
Ask about:	*Palpate:*
History of diabetes or thyroid	Thyroid
disease	*Auscultate:*
	Bruits over thyroid
Area/System: Lymphatic/Hematological	
Ask about:	*Inspect:*
Bleeding	Skin for ecchymosis, petechiae
Recent infections	*Palpate for:*
	Enlarged lymph nodes

HEENT = head, eyes, ears, nose, and throat

Physical Assessment

ANATOMICAL LANDMARKS

APPROACH: Inspection, palpation, percussion, auscultation

POSITION: Supine, left lateral recumbent, sitting

TOOLBOX: Stethoscope, sphygmomanometer, thermometer, ruler, marker, scale, and penlight

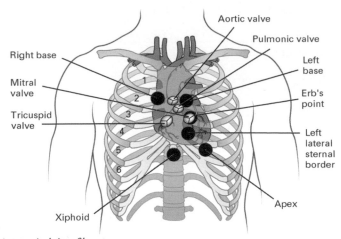

Anatomical site of heart

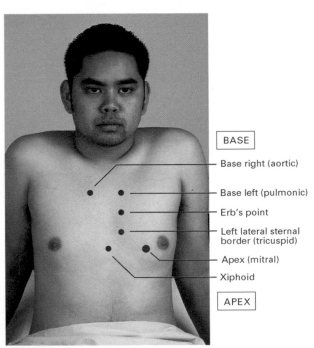

Sites for cardiac assessment

Cardiac Auscultation Sites	
Traditional Sites	**Alternative Sites**
Apex/mitral area	Apex
Left lateral sternal border (LLSB)/tricuspid area	Lower left sternal border
Erb's point	Left base
Base left/pulmonic area	Right base
Base right/aortic area	Xiphoid

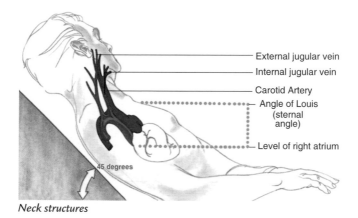

Neck structures

AREA/PA SKILL	NORMAL FINDINGS	ABNORMAL FINDINGS
Inspection *Neck Vessels: Carotid Arteries and Jugular Veins*		
Differentiate carotid and jugular pulsations.	Visible carotid pulsation No neck vein distention	Large, bounding, visible pulsations in neck or at suprasternal notch: Hypertension (HTN), aortic stenosis, or aneurysm
Measure jugular venous pressure (JVP). **Jugular pulsations are easily obliterated, affected by position and respirations, and have undulating waves.**	JVP at 45-degree angle <3 cm Carotid pulsation with one positive wave; jugular pulsation undulated	Elevated JVP: Right-sided congestive heart failure (CHF), constrictive pericarditis, tricuspid stenosis, or superior vena cava obstruction

(continued)

AREA/PA SKILL	NORMAL FINDINGS	ABNORMAL FINDINGS

Inspection
Neck Vessels: Carotid Arteries and Jugular Veins (Continued)

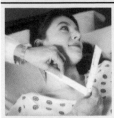

Inspecting the neck

		Low JVP: Hypo-volemia Abnormal venous wave forms Giant A waves: Tricuspid stenosis, right ventricular hypertrophy, or cor pulmonale Absent A wave: Atrial fibrillation

Precordium

Note pulsations in apex, left lateral sternal border, bases, and xiphoid or epigastric areas.	Positive pulsation noted at apex Slight pulsation noted at the bases in thin adults and children Slight epigastric pulsations may be noted	Pulsations to right of sternum or at epigastric area or sternoclavicular areas: Aortic aneurysm Apical pulsation displaced toward axillary line: Left ventricular hypertrophy

Palpation
Neck Vessels: Carotid Arteries and Jugular Veins *(Palpate each carotid separately.)*

Note rate, rhythm, amplitude, contour, symmetry, and elasticity.	Carotids: Rate is age dependent Regular rhythm + 2 amplitude (+ 3 in high output states) Pulses equal Contour has smooth upstroke with less acute descent. (Large pulse wave may be seen in older adults and during exercise) Carotids soft and pliable (May be stiff and cordlike in older adults)	Cardiac rates >100 BPM: Sinus tachycardia, supraventricular tachycardia, paroxysmal atrial tachycardia, uncontrolled atrial fibrillation, ventricular tachycardia. Causes: CHF, drugs (e.g., atropine, nitrates, epinephrine, isoproterenol, nicotine, caffeine), hypercalcemia

(continued)

AREA/PA SKILL	NORMAL FINDINGS	ABNORMAL FINDINGS
Palpation *Neck Vessels: Carotid Arteries and Jugular Veins (Continued)*		
Note any thrills. **If you feel a carotid thrill, listen for a bruit.**	No thrills	Cardiac rates <60 BPM: Sinus brady-cardia, heart block. Causes: myocardial infarction (MI), drugs (e.g., digoxin, quinidine, procaina-mide, beta-adrener-gic inhibitors), hy-perkalemia
		Irregular rhythm: Arrhythmia
		Abnormal pulses
		Bounding, + 3: HTN, aortic regurgitation
		Absent or weak, + 1: Arterial insufficiency or occlusion or de-creased cardiac out-put, as in shock
		Pulsus paradoxus: Chronic obstructive pulmonary disease, cardiac tamponade, CHF
		Pulsus alternans: CHF, digoxin toxicity
		Pulsus bisferiens: Aortic regurgitation
		Pulsus bigeminus: Heart failure, hypoxia
		Small pulse wave: CHF, hypovolemia, aortic stenosis
		Large pulse wave: HTN, exercise, aging
		Corrigan pulse: Aortic regurgitation
		Unequal pulses: Obstruction or occlusion

(continued)

AREA/PA SKILL	NORMAL FINDINGS	ABNORMAL FINDINGS
Palpation *Neck Vessels: Carotid Arteries and Jugular Veins (Continued)*		
Palpate jugular veins and check direction of fill. Check for abdominojugular (hepatojugular) reflux (HJR).	Jugulars are easily obliterated and fill appropriately Negative HJR	Stiff, cordlike arteries: Atherosclerosis Positive abdominojugular reflux: Right-sided CHF, tricuspid regurgitation, tricuspid stenosis, constrictive pericarditis, cardiac tamponade, inferior vena cava obstruction, hypervolemia
Precordium		
Palpate apex, left lateral sternal border, bases, and xiphoid or epigastric areas. Note size, duration, and diffusion of impulses.	PMI at apex 1 to 2 cm, nonsustained, or may normally be nonpalpable Slight epigastric pulsation, no diffusion No pulsations noted at base and lower left sternal border (LLSB) Small nonsustained impulses may be palpable at base and LLSB of thin clients and children. PMI may be displaced laterally and to left during last trimester of pregnancy Increased amplitude in high-output states	Enlargement and displacement of PMI to midaxillary line: Left ventricular hypertrophy with dilation Apical impulse on right side of precordium: Dextrocardia, often associated with congenital heart disease Enlarged apical pulsation without displacement >2–2.5 cm with client supine or >3 cm with the client in the left lateral recumbent position: Ventricular enlargement, HTN, aortic stenosis Sustained pulsation: Hypertrophy, HTN, overload, cardiomyopathy Presystolic impulse: S4, may be seen with aortic stenosis

(continued)

AREA/PA SKILL	NORMAL FINDINGS	ABNORMAL FINDINGS
Palpation *Precordium (Continued)*		
Note thrills, lifts, or heaves. **If you palpate a thrill, listen for a murmur.**	No thrills, lifts, or heaves	Early diastolic impulse: S3, may be seen with CHF Diffuse, sustained impulse displaced downward and laterally: Congestive cardiomyopathy Thrills: Murmur Right ventricular impulse with increased amplitude and duration: Pulmonary stenosis or pulmonary HTN Palpable lifts or heaves: Right ventricular hypertrophy Pulsations felt on fingertips: Right ventricular hypertrophy Large diffuse epigastric pulsation: Abdominal aortic aneurysm Accentuated pulsation in pulmonic area: Pulmonary HTN Accentuated pulsation in the aortic area: HTN or aneurysm
Percussion *Precordium*		
Percuss from anterior axillary line to sternum at 5th ICS.	Dullness noted at 3rd, 4th, and 5th ICS to left of sternum at MCL	Left sternal border extends to midaxillary lines: Enlarged, dilated heart

(continued)

AREA/PA SKILL	NORMAL FINDINGS	ABNORMAL FINDINGS
Auscultation Listen with both bell (light pressure) and diaphragm (heavy pressure) at all sites.		
Neck Vessels: Carotid Arteries and Jugular Veins		
Listen for carotid bruits with the bell.	Negative carotid bruits	Bruit: Carotid stenosis
Have client hold breath when auscultating for carotid bruits.	Carotid bruit may be normal in children and with high-output states	Murmurs can also radiate up to neck from heart, as with aortic stenosis
Listen for jugular venous hums with the bell.	Negative venous hum Venous hum may be normal in children	
Have client hold breath when auscultating for venous hums.		
To differentiate venous hum from a transmitted murmur, venous hum disappears when pressure is applied to jugular vein.		
Precordium		
Auscultate the following sites: Apex: 5th ICS, Left MCL LLSB: 4th to 5th ICS, left sternal border (LSB) Erb's Point: 3rd ICS, LSB Base Left: 2nd ICS, LSB Base Right: 2nd ICS, RSB Xiphoid area **Auscultate with client in sitting, supine, and left lateral recumbent positions.**	Apex: Rate is age dependent, rhythm regular, high-pitched systolic, short duration, 3/6 intensity, S1>S2, accentuated S1 in high-output states	Bradycardia or tachycardia: (See above—abnormal pulses under Palpation of Neck Vessels) Irregular rhythm: Arrhythmia Accentuated S1: High-output states, mitral or tricuspid stenosis Diminished S1: First-degree heart block, CHF, CAD Variable S1: Atrial fibrillation

(continued)

AREA/PA SKILL	NORMAL FINDINGS	ABNORMAL FINDINGS
Auscultation *Precordium (Continued)*		
Listen to S1, S2, splits.	LLSB: S1> or = S2, split S1 possible Base left: S1 <S2, split S2 during inspiration Base Right: S1 <S2	S3, low-pitched early diastolic sound: CHF S4, low-pitched late diastolic sound: CAD, HTN, MI
Note extra sounds: S3, S4, opening snap, ejection clicks. Note murmurs and pericardial rubs. Note rate, rhythm, pitch, intensity, duration, timing in the cardiac cycle, quality, location, and radiation. (See Tables 6–2 and 6–3.) **Erb's Point: Abnormal aortic murmurs heard best.** Grade murmurs on 1–6 scale. *A diastolic murmur or murmur .Grade 3/6 is never innocent.*	No extra sounds	Quadruple rhythm, S3 + S4, with fast rate is called a summation gallop Wide split: Right bundle branch block (RBBB) Midsystolic ejection click (high-pitched systolic sound): MVP Opening snap (high-pitched diastolic sound): Mitral or tricuspid stenosis, ventricular septal defect (VSD), PDA Early systolic murmur: VSD Late systolic murmur or pansystolic (or holosystolic) murmur: Mitral or tricuspid regurgitation Pansystolic murmur: VSD Mid- and late diastolic murmurs: Mitral and tricuspid stenosis Pericardial friction rub (high-pitched systolic and diastolic sound): Pericarditis or post-op cardiac surgery

(continued)

AREA/PA SKILL	NORMAL FINDINGS	ABNORMAL FINDINGS
Auscultation *Precordium (Continued)*		
		Diminished S2: Incompetent aortic or pulmonic valves and low-output states
		Ejection click (high-pitched systolic sound): Aortic or pulmonic stenosis
		Accentuated S2 : HTN or pulmonary HTN
		Wide split S2 : Right bundle branch block, pulmonic stenosis, atrial septal defect (ASD), VSD
		Fixed split S2 (split with no respiratory variation): ASD, VSD, CHF
		Paradoxical split S2 (split occurs during expirations): Left bundle branch block or aortic stenosis
		Midsystolic murmur: Aortic or pulmonic stenosis
		Early diastolic murmur, heard best at Erb's point: Aortic regurgitation
		Early diastolic murmur, heard best at base left: Pulmonic regurgitation
		Pandiastolic murmur: PDA

PA = physical assessment

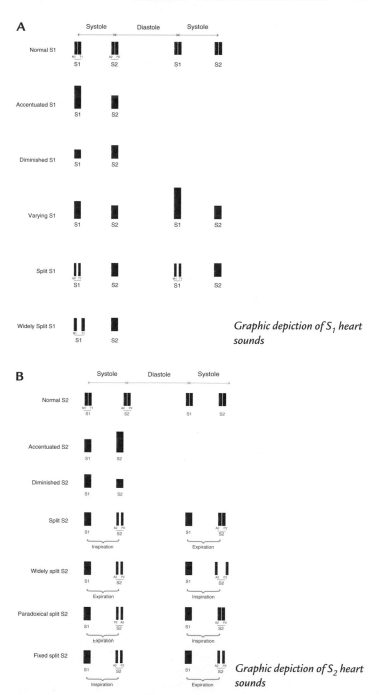

Graphic depiction of S_1 heart sounds

Graphic depiction of S_2 heart sounds

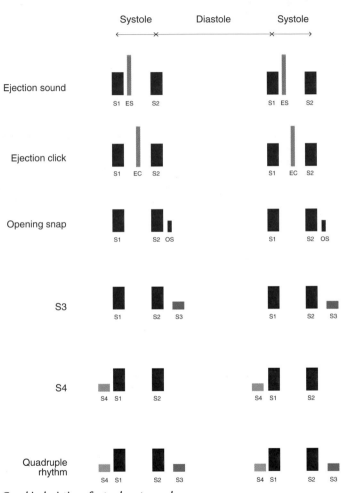

Graphic depiction of extra heart sounds

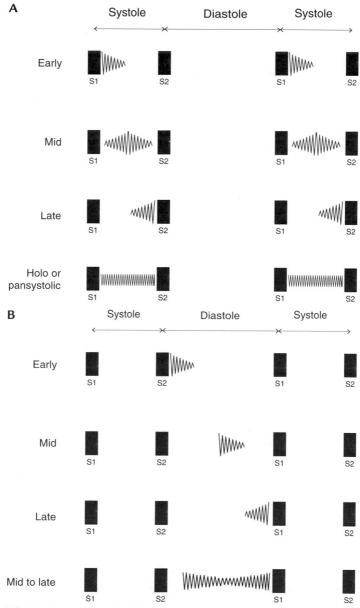

(A) Graphic depiction of systolic murmurs, (B) Graphic depiction of diastolic murmurs

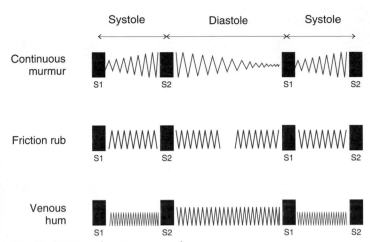

Graphic depiction of continuous sounds

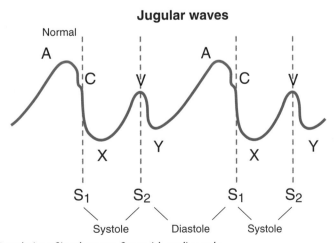

Correlation of jugular wave form with cardiac cycle

Constrictive Pericarditis

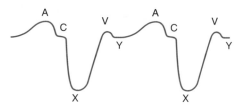

Exaggerated "x" wave

Right Ventricular Hypertrophy

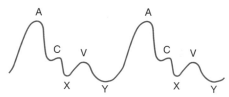

Exaggerated "a" waves

Atrial Fibrillation

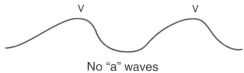

No "a" waves

Tricuspid Regurgitation

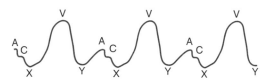

Exaggerated V waves

Abnormal jugular venous waves

Description	Possible Cause

Normal

Small, Weak Pulse

Decreased pulse pressure with a slow upstroke and prolonged peak

Increased peripheral vascular resistance such as occurs in cold weather or severe congestive heart failure; decreased stroke volume such as occurs in hypovolemia or aortic stenosis

Large, Bounding Pulse

Bounding pulse in which a great surge precedes a sudden absence of force or fullness

Increased stroke volume, as in aortic regurgitation; increased stiffness of arterial walls, as in atherosclerosis or normal aging; exercise; anxiety; fever; hypertension

Corrigan's (Water-Hammer) Pulse

Increased pulse pressure with a rapid upstroke and downstroke and a shortened peak

Aortic regurgitation, patent ductus arteriosus, systemic arteriosclerosis

Pulsus Alternans

Regular pulse rhythm with alternation of weak and strong beats (amplitude or volume)

Left ventricular failure

Pulsus Bigeminus

Irregular pulse rhythm in which premature beats alternate with sinus beats

Premature ventricular beats caused by heart failure, hypoxia, or other condition

Pulsus Bisferiens

A strong upstroke, downstroke, and second upstroke during systole

Aortic insufficiency, aortic regurgitation, aortic stenosis

Pulsus Paradoxus

Pulse with a markedly decreased amplitude during Inspiration

Constrictive pericarditis, pericardial tamponade, advanced heart failure, severe lung disease

Abnormal pulses

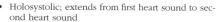

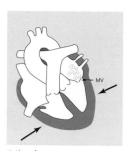

- Holosystolic; extends from first heart sound to second heart sound
- Loudness constant throughout systole
- Heard best at apical area
- May radiate to left lateral chest or, less commonly, to base
- Blowing, rough (harsh), or musical
- If very loud, it may mask first heart sound.

Mitral regurgitation

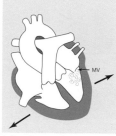

- Occurs in diastolic phase of cardiac cycle.
- With normal sinus rhythm, characteristically a low-pitched rough or harsh murmur beginning immediately after opening snap.
- Extends to sharp first heart sound.
- Demonstrates presystolic (late diastolic) accentuation with normal sinus rhythm and just before termination.
- Presystolic accentuation of mid-late diastolic murmur disappears with atrial fibrillation.
- Best heard in apical area with patient in left lateral position and with bell portion of stethoscope.
- Localized to a very small (quarter-sized) area, so may be hard to find.

Mitral stenosis

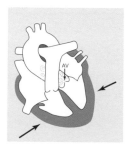

- Midsystolic; characterized by crescendo/decrescendo pattern.
- Begins shortly after first heart sound and ends before second sound.
- Rough (low-pitched).
- Second heart sound at base markedly diminished or absent as a result of poor movement of severely calcified valve leaflets.
- When transmitted to apex, may have musical overtone in addition to rough quality (Gallavardin effect).
- If congenital (represented by two valve leaflets instead of three), early ejection click is often heard shortly after first heart sound.
- Both acquired and congenital murmurs heard best at base in second right interspace. May also be transmitted to apex and neck.

Aortic stenosis

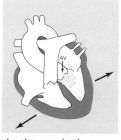

- Onset early in diastole.
- Decrescendo, ending before first heart sound.
- Usually blowing.
- Heard best at base of heart in third left interspace in parasternal line.
- Often transmitted toward apex, if loud enough.
- Loudness varies from Grade 1 to Grade 3 or 4.
- Often is only Grade 1 intensity. If so, to facilitate identification of murmur, have patient sit forward, exhale, and hold his or her breath while you listen in third left interspace in parasternal line.

Aortic regurgitation

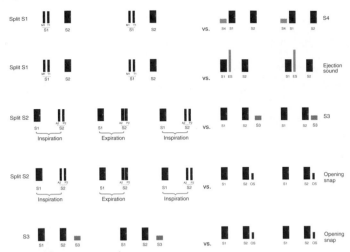

How to differentiate sounds

Table 6–2. *Heart Sounds*

HEART SOUND	LOCATION	PITCH	TIMING IN CARDIAC CYCLE	INTERPRE-TATION
S1	Apex/mitral area	High	Systolic	Normal
S1 split	LLSB/tricus-pid area	High	Systolic	Normal RBBB
S2	Base right/aortic area	High	Systolic	Normal
S2 split	Base left/pulmonic area	High	Systolic	Normal BBB, ASD, VSD, PE, pulmonic stenosis
S3 (Left ventricu-lar origin)	Apex	Low	Diastolic	May be normal under age 30 Left-sided CHF
S3 (Right ventricu-lar origin)	LLSB	Low	Diastolic	Right-sided CHF
S4 (Left ventricu-lar origin)	Apex, LLSB	Low	Diastolic	May be normal in children and young adults MI, HTN, CAD

(continued)

Table 6–2. *Heart Sounds (Continued)*

HEART SOUND	LOCATION	PITCH	TIMING IN CARDIAC CYCLE	INTERPRE-TATION
S4 (Right ventricular origin)	Apex, LLSB	Low	Diastolic	Pulmonary HTN
Opening snap	Apex	High	Diastolic	Mitral stenosis
Ejection click	Base	High	Early systolic	Aortic stenosis, pulmonic stenosis
	Apex	High	Midsystolic	Mitral valve prolapse
Friction rub	LLSB	High	Systolic, diastolic, or both	Pericarditis, pericardial effusion

Table 6–3. *Murmurs*

TYPE	LOCATION	PITCH	QUALITY	INTERPRETATION
Early systolic	LLSB	High/low	Rough	VSD (muscular site)
Midsystolic	Base right Base left	High	Harsh	Aortic stenosis Pulmonic stenosis
Late systolic	Apex LLSB	High	Blowing	MVP Tricuspid regurgitation
Holosystolic	Apex	High		Mitral regurgitation, VSD
	LLSB			Tricuspid regurgitation
Early diastolic	Erb's point Base left	High	Blowing	Aortic regurgitation Pulmonic regurgitation
Mid-diastolic	Apex LLSB	Low	Rumbling	Mitral stenosis Tricuspid stenosis
Late diastolic	Apex LLSB	Low	Rumbling	Mitral stenosis Tricuspid stenosis
Pandiastolic	Base left	Low	Continuous	PDA

CHAPTER 7

ASSESSING THE PERIPHERAL-VASCULAR AND LYMPHATIC SYSTEMS

Primary Function

Primary function of the peripheral-vascular system:

- Transport of oxygenated blood to all organs and tissue and return of unoxygenated blood to the heart

Primary functions of the lymphatic system:

- Movement of lymph fluid in a closed circuit with the cardiovascular system
- Development and maintenance of the immune system
- Reabsorption of fat and fat-soluble substances from the small intestine

Developmental Considerations

Infants and Children

- Infants have immature immune systems, increasing risk for infection; they rely on mother's immunity.
- Amount of lymphatic tissue greatest between ages of 6 and 10 years.
- Thymus largest at birth.
- Tonsils larger during childhood than after puberty.
- Blood pressure (BP) at birth 70/50; slowly increases to adult level, 120/80, during adolescence.

Pregnant Clients

- Increase in leukocytes and decrease in immunoglobulin G (IgG) occur during pregnancy.
- Altered host defense results from decrease in chemotaxis that delays response to infection.
- Decreased systemic vascular resistance results in vasodilation, which may lead to palmar erythema and spider telangiectasis.
- BP decreases during second trimester then increases to prepregnant level.
- 30-mm systolic or 15-mm diastolic increase in BP may indicate preeclampsia.

Older Adults

- Number and size of lymph nodes decrease with age.
- Ability to resist infection decreases.
- Increased fibrosis and decreased elasticity of vessels result in increased peripheral-vascular resistance.

Cultural Considerations

- Hypertension (HTN) is the most serious health problem for African-Americans.
- High incidence of HTN in Puerto Ricans, Cubans, and Mexican-Americans.
- One-sixth of Iranians have HTN, with stress as a major contributing factor.
- Navajo Native Americans have a high incidence of severe combined immunodeficiency syndrome (SCIDS), failure of antibody response, and cell-mediated immunity, unrelated to AIDS.
- African-Americans account for 30 percent of AIDS cases in the United States.

Assessment

History

SYMPTOMS ("PQRST" ANY + SYMPTOM)
- Swelling
  - Where is the swelling located? Does it affect both arms or legs? Does it involve the entire extremity or just a

certain area? How far up the extremity does the swelling go?

- Is the swelling marked or slight? Has the swelling occurred before? If so, is it more or less severe?
- When does the swelling occur? On awakening or at the end of the day? Is it constant or intermittent? How long does it last?
- Do you have an imprint of a sock line or shoe when you take your shoes and socks off?
- Is the swelling associated with pain, warmth, or redness?
- Does anything make the swelling worse, such as sitting for long periods of time or eating salty foods?
- Does anything reduce the swelling, such as elevating your feet or using support hose?

- Limb pain
    - Where is the pain? Is it localized or generalized? Point to where you feel the pain. Is it deep or superficial? Does it radiate to another location?
    - How bad is the pain? On a scale of 0 to 10, with 0 being no pain and 10 being the worst pain, how would you rate your pain? Does the pain interfere with your lifestyle? Can you walk without pain?
    - In what setting does the pain occur? Does it occur only after walking long distances? Does it occur when going up and down stairs? Does it occur after repetitive movements? Does it occur only at night?
    - When did the pain first begin? Did it begin suddenly or gradually? Is it intermittent or continuous? How long does the pain last?
    - Can you describe the pain in your own words? (throbbing, burning?)
    - Is the pain associated with any other problems, such as swelling, tingling, or redness?
    - Does anything make the pain worse? Does anything make it better?

- Change in sensation
    - Where is the sensation? Is it in just one part of the extremity? Does it involve the entire extremity? Does it involve one or both extremities?
    - How intense is the sensation?
    - When or where does it occur? Does it occur when your legs are elevated? When you are bending over?

- When did this problem begin? Was it sudden or gradual? Is this a new or chronic problem?
- Can you describe the type of sensation? Is it associated with weakness or pain?
- What makes the sensory change worse? Cold temperatures? Sitting for long periods?
- What makes the sensation better, rest or leg elevation?
- Fatigue
  - How long have you noticed that you are fatigued?
  - Do you wake up tired or do you become tired during the day?
  - Is your fatigue related to exertion?
  - Have you been overworked at your job or with family commitments?
  - Have you been sleeping well? How many hours do you sleep per night?
  - Do you have trouble getting to sleep or staying asleep?
  - Have you noticed any other associated symptoms along with your fatigue?
  - Does your fatigue interfere with your lifestyle? Does it affect your ability to work or take care of your family?

FOCUSED PERIPHERAL-VASCULAR HISTORY
Arterial occlusion of an extremity can become a situation requiring rapid assessment! Be sure to ask the following questions:

- Have you noticed pain, pallor, pulselessness, polar sensation (cold), paresthesias, or paralysis (the 6 ps of acute occlusion) in an extremity?
- Have you noticed aching, heaviness, throbbing or burning pain, itching, or cramping in your legs?
- Have you noticed ankle swelling? Is it difficult to fit into your shoes or wear your wedding band lately?
- Do you have leg pain when walking? Do you have leg pain at rest? What makes the leg pain better?
- Have you noticed any sores or ulcers on your feet or legs? How long have they been there? What have you used to treat them?
- Do you have a history of high blood pressure?
- Do you have a history of a high cholesterol level?
- Do you have diabetes mellitus?

- Do you have a history of cardiovascular or peripheral-vascular disease?
- Do you smoke? If so, how long and how much?

FOCUSED LYMPHATIC SYSTEM HISTORY
Generally, there is no need to assess this system rapidly. However, these questions will help you narrow your assessment focus.

- Have you noticed any swelling in your neck, armpits, or groin? If so, are the swollen areas sore, hard, or red? Do they appear on both sides of your body?
- Are you unusually tired? If so, are you tired all the time or only after exertion? Do you need frequent naps, or do you sleep an unusually long time at night?
- Have you had a fever recently? If so, how high was it? Was it constant or intermittent? Did it follow a pattern?
- Do you ever have joint pain? If so, which joints are affected? Does swelling, redness, or warmth accompany the pain? Do your bones ache?
- Have you noticed any sores that heal slowly?
- Do you have a history of blood transfusions?
- Have you ever been diagnosed with a chronic infection?
- Are you taking any medications, prescribed or over the counter (Table 7–1)?

Table 7–1. *Drugs That Adversely Affect the Lymphatic System*

DRUG CLASS	DRUG	POSSIBLE ADVERSE REACTIONS
Anticonvulsants	carbamazepine	Aplastic anemia, leukopenia, agranulocytosis, eosinophilia, leukocytosis, thrombocytopenia
	phenytoin	Thrombocytopenia, leukopenia, granulocytopenia, pancytopenia, macrocytosis, megaloblastic anemia
Antidiabetics	acetohexamide, chlorpropamide, glipizide, glyburide, tolbutamide	Leukopenia, thrombocytopenia, pancytopenia, agranulocytosis, aplastic anemia, hemolytic anemia

(continued)

Table 7–1. *Drugs That Adversely Affect the Lymphatic System (Continued)*

DRUG CLASS	DRUG	POSSIBLE ADVERSE REACTIONS
Antihypertensives	captopril	Neutropenia, agranulo-cytosis
	hydralazine	Positive antinuclear anti-body (ANA) titer, sys-temic lupus erythemato-sus-like syndrome
	methyldopa	Positive Coombs' test
Anti-infectives	cephalosporins	Positive Coombs' test; hypothrombinemia, with or without bleeding
	chloramphenicol	Bone marrow depression, pancytopenia, aplastic anemia
	penicillins	Eosinophilia, hemolytic anemia, leukopenia, neu-tropenia, thrombocyto-penia, positive Coombs' test
	pentamidine isethionate	Leukopenia, thrombocy-topenia
	sulfonamides	Granulocytopenia, leuko-penia, eosinophilia, hemolytic anemia, aplastic anemia, thrombocytope-nia, methemoglobinemia, hypoprothrombinemia
Antineoplastics	busulfan	Severe leukopenia, anemia, severe thrombocytopenia
	chlorambucil	Leukopenia, thrombocy-topenia, anemia
	cisplatin, cyclo-phosphamide, doxorubicin hydrochloride	Leukopenia, granulocyto-penia, thrombocytopenia, anemia
	methotrexate	Leukopenia, thrombocyto-penia, anemia, hemor-rhage
	mitomycin	Thrombocytopenia, leukopenia
Antipsychotic agents	chlorpromazine hydrochloride, thioridazine hydrochloride	Agranulocytosis, mild leukopenia

(continued)

Table 7–1. *Drugs That Adversely Affect the Lymphatic System (Continued)*

DRUG CLASS	DRUG	POSSIBLE ADVERSE REACTIONS
Cardiac agents	procainamide hydrochloride	Positive ANA titer; systemic lupus erythematosus-like syndrome
	quinidine	Thrombocytopenia, hypoprothrombinemia, acute hemolytic anemia, agranulocytosis, aplastic anemia, and leukocytopenia can occur as hypersensitivity reactions
Gold compounds	auranofin, gold sodium thiomalate	Leukopenia, thrombocytopenia, anemia, eosinophilia
Nonsteroidal anti-inflammatory agents	ibuprofen	Neutropenia, agranulocytosis, aplastic anemia, hemolytic anemia, thrombocytopenia, decreased hemoglobin and hematocrit
Miscellaneous agents	furosemide	Anemia, leukopenia, neutropenia, thrombocytopenia
	lithium	Leukocytosis

Assessment of Peripheral-Vascular and Lymphatic Systems' Relationship to Other Systems

Remember, all systems are related! As you assess the peripheral-vascular and lymphatic systems, look at the relationship between them and all other systems.

SUBJECTIVE DATA	OBJECTIVE DATA
Area/System: General	
Ask about:	*Inspect for:*
Fatigue	Signs of distress
Fevers	*Measure:*
Weight changes	Vital signs
	Weight
Area/System: Integumentary	
Ask about:	*Inspect for:*
Skin lesions, rashes	Skin lesions
	Hair distribution
	Edema
Area/System: HEENT	
Ask about:	*Inspect:*
Mouth lesions	Oral mucosa, gums, tonsils
Bleeding gums	Nasal mucosa
Sore throat	
Area/System: Respiratory	
Ask about:	*Auscultate:*
History of asthma, allergies	Adventitious breath sounds
Area/System: Cardiovascular	
Ask about:	*Auscultate:*
Chest pain	Heart sounds
History of murmurs	Murmurs, rubs
Area/System: Gastrointestinal	
Ask about:	*Palpate:*
Gastrointestinal (GI) complaints	Organs for enlargement
History of abdominal trauma	
Area/System: Genitourinary/Reproductive	
Ask about:	*Inspect for:*
Urinary tract infections (UTIs)	Discharge
Safe sex practices	STDs, lesions
Sexually transmitted diseases (STDs)	
Area/System: Musculoskeletal	
Ask about:	*Palpate:*
Weakness	Muscle strength
Joint pain	Joints
Area/System: Neurological	
Ask about:	*Test:*
Changes in mental status	Mental status
Loss of sensation	Sensation

HEENT = head, eyes, ears, nose, and throat

Physical Assessment

ANATOMICAL LANDMARKS

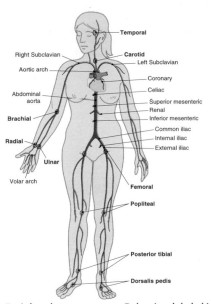

Peripheral venous system. Pulse sites labeled in red

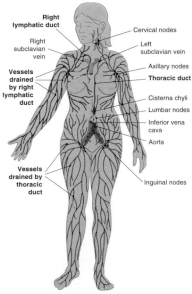

Lymphatic system

APPROACH: *PV system:* Inspection, palpation, auscultation
Lymphatic system: Inspection, palpation

POSITION: Supine and sitting

TOOLBOX: Stethoscope, sphygmomanometer, flashlight, ruler, and tape measure

AREA/PA SKILL	NORMAL FINDINGS	ABNORMAL FINDINGS
Inspection *Upper extremities*		
Inspect for color, edema, erythema, red streaks, lesions. **Look for edema on most dependent parts of body. If edema is present, grade it and weigh patient daily.**	Skin color uniform, no erythema, red streaks, edema, or lesions	Edema: Cellulitis, lymphedema, venous obstruction (thrombophlebitis) Intermittent pallor and cyanosis of hands and fingers: Episodic constriction of peripheral small arteries or arterioles caused by Raynaud's phenomenon or Raynaud's disease. Constriction causes hyperemia and rubor (redness) Ischemic changes and gangrene of hands and fingers: Buerger's disease (thromboangiitis obliterans)
Abdomen		
Note shape, arterial pulsation, increased venous pattern, ascites. **If ascites is present, do fluid wave test or test for shifting dullness.**	Abdomen flat or slightly rounded No increased venous pattern or ascites	Tense, shiny abdominal skin: Ascites or edema Upward or centrifugal venous flow: Inferior vena cava obstruction or portal hypertension

(continued)

AREA/PA SKILL	NORMAL FINDINGS	ABNORMAL FINDINGS
Inspection *Abdomen (Continued)*		
If large, diffuse arterial pulsation is present, do not palpate the abdomen. *Lower Extremities*	Slight arterial pulsation noted in epigastric area at midline	Visible, large, diffuse pulsations: Aneurysm
Note color, condition of skin, hair distribution, edema, erythema, red streaks, lesions. **If edema is present, measure calf circumference.** **If varicosities are present, check venous valve competence with Trendelenburg test or manual compression test.**	Skin color uniform; no erythema, red streaks, edema, or lesions Skin intact, even hair distribution	Streaky redness, tenderness, warmth along course of a vein: Thrombophlebitis Hair loss: Arterial insufficiency Eczema, stasis dermatitis: Chronic venous insufficiency Prominent leg veins, possibly with rope-like, dilated appearance or purplish spiderlike appearance: Chronic venous insufficiency

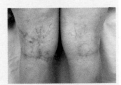

Superficial varicosities

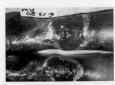

Venous stasis ulcer

(continued)

AREA/PA SKILL	NORMAL FINDINGS	ABNORMAL FINDINGS
Inspection *Lower Extremities (Continued)*		
		Edema: Injury, cellulitis, venous/lymph obstruction, thrombophlebitis, varicosities Skin ulcers: Trauma or venous/arterial insufficiency Venous insufficiency stasis ulcers on ankle Arterial insufficiency ulcers on toes Difference in leg circumference over 1 cm above ankle or 2 cm at calf: Edema

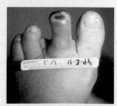

Arterial insufficiency

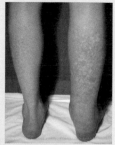

Lymphedema

(continued)

AREA/PA SKILL	NORMAL FINDINGS	ABNORMAL FINDINGS

Inspection
Lower Extremities (Continued)

ASSESSING EDEMA

To assess edema, press your index finger over the bony prominence of the tibia or medial malleolus. Orthostatic (pitting) edema results in a depression that does not rapidly refill and resume its original contour. It is not usually accompanied by thickening or pigmentation of the overlying skin. The severity of edema can be graded on a scale of +1 to +4.

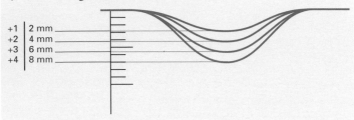

+1	2 mm
+2	4 mm
+3	6 mm
+4	8 mm

- *+1: Slight pitting with about 2-mm depression that disappears rapidly. No visible distortion of extremity.*
- *+2: Deeper pitting with about 4-mm depression that disappears in 10 to 15 seconds. No visible distortion of extremity.*
- *+3: Depression of about 6 mm that lasts more than a minute. Dependent extremity looks swollen.*
- *+4: Very deep pitting with about 8-mm depression that lasts 2 to 3 minutes. Dependent extremity is grossly distorted.*

Palpation
Upper and Lower Extremities

| Palpate for capillary refill, temperature. | + capillary refill <3 seconds
Extremities warm bilaterally | Delayed capillary refill time: Arterial occlusion, hypovolemic shock, hypothermia; also, environmental influences (e.g., decreased ambient temperature), suggesting a problem that may not exist
Cold feet: Arterial insufficiency, especially if unilateral |

(continued)

AREA/PA SKILL	NORMAL FINDINGS	ABNORMAL FINDINGS
Palpation *Upper and Lower Extremities (Continued)*		
	Absence of Homans' sign	Cool extremities: Decreased circulation, vasoconstriction, Raynaud's disease, Buerger's disease, response to cold external temperature Presence of Homans' sign: Deep vein thrombosis (DVT) in 50% of clients. Negative sign does not rule out DVT
Pulse Sites: Carotid, Temporal, Brachial, Radial, Ulnar, Femoral, Popliteal, Dorsalis Pedis, Posterior Tibialis		
Note rate, rhythm, equality, thrills, amplitude. **Pulse amplitude scale:** **0 = absent** **1 = weak** **2 = normal** **3 = full** **4 = bounding** If thrill is present, listen for bruit. If indicated, do Allen's test to assess arterial flow to hands. If indicated, do color change test or measure ankle-brachial index to assess arterial flow to legs. If thrombus or thrombophlebitis is suspected, test Homans' sign.	Pulse rate is age dependent Pulse regular, equal, +2 Arteries soft and pliable No thrills	Alterations in pulse rate/rhythm: Cardiac arrhythmia Unequal pulses: Arterial narrowing or obstruction on one side Diminished or absent pulse: Arterial spasm, partial or complete arterial occlusion of proximal vessel, often caused by arteriosclerosis obliterans ***Sudden absent pulse with cold, mottled extremity: Arterial occlusion, a medical emergency***

(continued)

AREA/PA SKILL	NORMAL FINDINGS	ABNORMAL FINDINGS
Palpation (Continued) *Lymph Node Sites: Cervical, Axillary, Epitrochlear, Inguinal (horizontal and vertical), Popliteal*		
Note size, shape, symmetry, tenderness, mobility, consistency, delineation, location, erythema, warmth, increased vascularity.	**Lymph nodes not palpable, or if palpable, <1 cm, firm, nontender, round, well-defined borders; no erythema, warmth, or increased vascularity**	Tender, palpable lymph nodes: Recent infection Large, well-defined nodes: Acute infection Less-defined node borders: Chronic infection Firm, enlarged, nontender, immobile nodes: Malignancy Involvement of three or more node groups (generalized lymphadenopathy): Autoimmune disease or neoplasm
Auscultation (Use the bell of the stethoscope.) *Arteries and Veins*		
Listen for bruits and venous hums. **Have client hold breath when auscultating for bruits or hums over the neck.** Blood Pressure Measure BP in both arms, with patient supine, sitting, and standing.	No bruits or venous hums	Soft, low-pitched, rushing sound during cardiac cycle: Bruit in temporal or carotid artery. Signifies narrowing of artery
Check BP. **Avoid auscultatory gap by palpating brachial pulse and inflating cuff until obliterated, then reinflating cuff 30 mm Hg above**	Normal BP is age dependent; for adults Systolic <140 mm Hg Diastolic <90 mm Hg	Hypotension: Heart failure, dehydration, endocrine disorders (hypothyroidism), neurogenic vena cava obstruction, cardiac tamponade

(continued)

AREA/PA SKILL	NORMAL FINDINGS	ABNORMAL FINDINGS
Auscultation *Arteries and Veins (Continued)*		
point where pulse was obliterated. Bell of stethoscope is best for detecting Korotkoff sounds. **If BP heard down to "0," retake BP and listen for Korotkoff sounds 1, 4 (first diastolic), and 5; then record all 3.**		
Check pulse pressure **(difference between the systolic and diastolic pressure).**	Pulse pressure is one-third of systolic pressure	
Note orthostatic drops.	No orthostatic drop	Decrease in systolic BP of 10 to 15 mm Hg and drop in diastolic BP on standing, with rise in pulse rate: Orthostatic hypotension caused by antihypertensive medications, volume depletion, peripheral neurovascular disease, or bed rest 3 consecutive BP readings above 140/90: Hypertension Auscultatory gap: Normal variation or sign of systolic hypertension Korotkoff sounds down to zero: Cardiac valve replacement, hyperkinetic states, severe anemia, thyrotoxicosis, or following strenuous exercise

(continued)

AREA/PA SKILL	NORMAL FINDINGS	ABNORMAL FINDINGS
Auscultation *Arteries and Veins (Continued)*		
		Difference of >10 mm Hg between arms: Arterial compression on side of lower reading, aortic dissection, arm pressure > leg pressure, coarctation of aorta
		Widened pulse pressure with increased systolic BP: Exercise, arteriosclerosis, severe anemia, thyrotoxicosis, increased intracranial pressure
		Narrowed pulse pressure with decreased systolic BP: Shock, cardiac failure, pulmonary embolus

PA = physical assessment

CHAPTER 8

ASSESSING THE BREASTS

Primary Function

- Lactation
- Female sexuality

Developmental Considerations

Infants

- At birth, there is an elevation of the nipple.
- Slight secretion of milky material (witch's milk) may occur for 5 to 7 days.
- Palpable breast tissue during infancy is normal; however, not beyond this period.

Children

- A child's breast is underdeveloped compared to the mature breast. Growth of breast tissue generally begins in the prepubertal period.

TANNER STAGES OF BREAST DEVELOPMENT
- Stage 1. Prepuberty, elevation of papilla

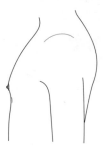

- Stage 2. "Breast bud" stage. There is elevation of breast and nipple and increased diameter of areola.

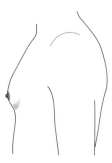

- Stage 3. Areola deepens in color and enlarges further. Glandular tissue begins to develop beneath areola.

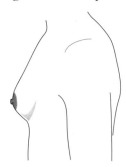

- Stage 4. Areola appears as a mound; breast appears as a mound.

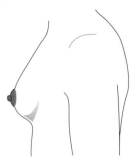

- Stage 5. Mature stage. Areola recesses to general contour of breast; nipple projects forward.

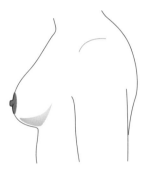

- Adolescent girls may have asymmetrical breasts as they go through puberty.
- Adolescent boys may have gynecomastia.

Pregnant Clients
- Breasts become fuller, firmer; areola and nipples darken and enlarge and venous pattern increases.
- In the third trimester, colostrum occurs. It continues to be secreted after the birth of a baby until milk is produced.

Older Adults
- Ducts become more fibrous.
- Breasts lose elasticity and are less firm and more pendulous.

Cultural Considerations

- Ashkenazi Jews have a greater incidence of breast cancer than other groups.
- African-American women in the South have been known to treat breast lesions with home remedies, which have delayed diagnosis until a more advanced stage.
- African-American men appear to be at greater risk than white men for breast cancer.
- African-American women have lower breast cancer survival rates than white women.
- White women have a higher incidence of breast cancer than nonwhite women.

Assessment

History

SYMPTOMS ("PQRST" ANY + SYMPTOM)
- Lump or mass
  - Where is the lump or mass located?
  - Is there a "mirror" lesion in the opposite breast?
  - Is there pain or tenderness associated with the lump or mass?
  - When did you notice the lump?
  - Have you ever had a similar lump or mass before? When?
  - Does the lump or mass change in size during your menstrual cycle?
  - Have you had a recent injury to the breast?

Breast self-examination needs to be done when the breasts are not under hormonal influence—5 to 7 days after menstruation begins or 3 to 5 days after menstruation ceases.

- Pain
  - Is there pain on palpation?
  - Is there pain in one or both breasts?
  - Can you point to the area of pain?
  - Is the pain associated with a lump or mass?
  - Is pain related to the menstrual cycle? When did you first experience this pain?
  - Do you have any other symptoms? What started first? Second?
  - When was your last menstrual period?

1 First, teach the client how to look at herself in a mirror and, with her arms at her sides, check for any visible abnormalities. She should observe for dimpling, retraction, or breast flattening as she first elevates her arms slowly, then presses her hands against her hips, and finally, bends forward.

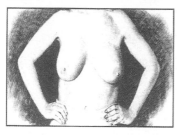

3 Next, show her how to compress the nipple gently between the thumb and index finger as she observes for any discharge.

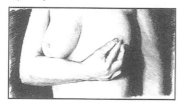

2 Next, by placing your hand over the client's, show her how to use the pads of the middle three fingers of the opposite hand to palpate the breast systematically by compressing the breast tissue against the chest wall. She should palpate all portions of the breast, areola, nipple, tail of Spence, and axilla when she is in the shower or standing before a mirror. She should repeat the procedure lying down with a pillow or folded towel under the shoulder of the side she is examining.

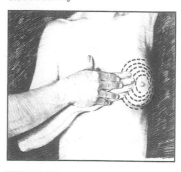

4 Finally, explain that she should report any redness or inflammation, swelling, masses, flattening, puckering, dimpling, retraction, sunken areas, asymmetrical nipple direction, discharge, bleeding, lesions, or eczematous nipple changes to her physician.

- Are you nursing?
- Did you recently complete a pregnancy?
- How would you describe the pain (sharp or dull)?
- Does the pain change, getting better or worse?
- Is it constant or intermittent? (If intermittent, how long does the pain last? How frequent are the episodes of pain?)
- Are there changes in the character of pain with your menstrual cycle?
- How would you rate the pain on a 0 to 10 scale, with 10 being the worst pain?
- What makes the pain worse? What makes it better?
- What have you tried to get rid of the pain? How well did that work?
- Has there been a change in your bra size?
- Have you had nipple piercing?
- Have you lost or gained weight? If yes, how much weight have you lost or gained and over what period of time?

- Are you having any problems with nipple discharge (color, amount, odor) or nipple retraction?

Breast pain (or tenderness) is often a result of the normal physiological cycle. A lump associated with breast cancer is generally painless. Rapidly enlarging cysts may be painful.

- Nipple discharge
  - When did the discharge start?
  - How frequent is the discharge? (continuous, or number of times per day or week)
  - When was the last discharge?
  - Discharge from one or both breasts?
  - What color is the discharge? (clear, bloody, white, yellow)
  - Any changes in the appearance of the discharge? (color, consistency)
  - How much discharge each time?
  - Do you have any other symptoms? (pain in your breast or nipple, change in the direction in which the nipple points, nipples becoming everted or inverted)
  - If you are premenopausal, any change in menstrual cycle?
  - What have you tried to relieve this problem? How well has that worked?
  - Has anything made it worse?
  - Is the discharge spontaneous or when expressed?
  - What medical illnesses do you have?
  - Have you ever had this problem before? When? How was it treated?

FOCUSED BREAST HISTORY
- Address the warning signs and symptoms of breast cancer:
  - Lump or thickening in or near the breast or in the underarm that persists through the menstrual cycle
  - Redness of the skin on the breast or nipple
  - Change in the direction in which one nipple points; inversion, eversion, or discharge from the nipple
  - Change in the size, shape, or contour of the breast
  - Skin changes on the breast or nipple (dimpled, puckered, scaly, or inflamed)
- Ask whether the client is taking any medications, prescribed or over the counter (Table 8–1).

Table 8–1. *Drugs That Adversely Affect the Breasts*

DRUG CLASS	DRUG	POSSIBLE ADVERSE REACTIONS
Androgens	danazol, fluoxy-mesterone, methyl-testosterone, testosterone	*Women:* Decreased breast size *Men:* Gynecomastia
Antidepressants	tricyclic antide-pressants	*Women:* Breast engorge-ment and galactorrhea *Men:* Gynecomastia
Antipsychotics	chlorpromazine hydrochloride, fluphenazine, haloperidol, perphenazine, prochlorperazine maleate, thiorida-zine, thiothixene	*Women:* Galactorrhea, moderate engorgement of breast with lactation, mastalgia *Men:* Gynecomastia, mastalgia
Cardiac glyco-sides	digitoxin, digoxin	*Men:* Gynecomastia
Estrogens	chlorotrianisene, conjugated estro-gens, esterified estrogens, estradiol, estrone, ethinyl estradiol	*Women:* Breast changes, tenderness, enlargement, secretions *Men:* Breast changes, tenderness, gynecomastia
	dienestrol	*Women:* Breast tenderness
	diethylstilbestrol	*Women:* Breast tenderness, enlargement *Men:* Breast tenderness, gynecomastia
Oral contracep-tives	estrogen-progesterone combinations	*Women:* Breast changes, tenderness, enlargement, secretions
Progestins	hydroxyprogeste-rone caproate, medroxyprogeste-rone acetate, norethindrone, norethindrone acetate, norgestrel, progesterone	*Women:* Breast tenderness or galactorrhea
Miscellaneous agents	isoniazid	*Men:* Gynecomastia
	reserpine	*Women:* Breast engorge-ment *Men:* Gynecomastia

(continued)

Table 8–1. *Drugs That Adversely Affect the Breasts (Continued)*		
DRUG CLASS	**DRUG**	**POSSIBLE ADVERSE REACTIONS**
	spironolactone	*Women:* Breast tenderness *Men:* Painful gynecomastia
	cimetidine	*Women:* Galactorrhea *Men:* Gynecomastia

Assessment of Breasts' Relationship to Other Systems

Remember, all systems are related! As you assess the breasts, look at the relationship between them and all other systems.

SUBJECTIVE DATA	OBJECTIVE DATA
Area/System: General	
Ask about:	*Observe:*
General health	Level of consciousness (LOC)
Fever	Affect
Weight changes	*Measure:*
	Vital signs
	Weight
Area/System: Integumentary	
Ask about:	*Inspect for:*
Rashes	Rashes
Lesions	Lesions
Allergies	Color changes
Area/System: HEENT	
If client has breast cancer, *ask about:*	*If client has breast cancer:*
Headaches	Test vision
Changes in mentation	
Area/System: Respiratory	
If client has breast cancer, ask *about:*	*If client has breast cancer:*
Shortness of breath	Auscultate and percuss lungs
Cough	
Breathing difficulty	
Area/System: Cardiovascular	
Ask about:	*Inspect for:*
Cardiovascular medications	Increased vascularity of breasts
	(continued)

SUBJECTIVE DATA	OBJECTIVE DATA
Area/System: Gastrointestinal	
If client has breast cancer, ask about:	*If client has breast cancer:*
Increase in size of abdominal girth	Palpate abdomen
Area/System: Genitourinary/Reproductive	
Ask about:	*Inspect:*
Last menstrual period, whether client is pregnant, number of pregnancies, year of first pregnancy, whether client is pre- or postmenopausal	Perform pelvic exam
Medications (birth control pill, hormone replacement therapy)	
Area/System: Musculoskeletal	
If client has breast cancer, ask about:	*If client has breast cancer:*
Weakness	Test muscle strength
Bone pain	
Fractures	
Area/System: Neurological	
	If client has breast cancer:
	Test LOC, sensory and motor function
Area/System: Endocrine	
Ask about:	*Palpate:*
History of thyroid disease	Thyroid
Area/System: Lymphatic/Hematological	
Ask about:	*Palpate:*
Infection or malignancy	Lymph nodes

HEENT = head, eyes, ears, nose, and throat

Physical Assessment

ANATOMICAL LANDMARKS

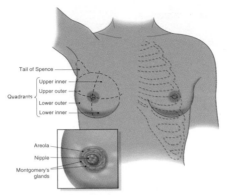

External breast structures and quadrants

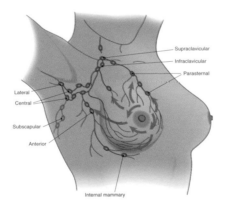

Lymph nodes

APPROACH: **Inspection, palpation; vertical strip, pie wedge, or concentric circles**

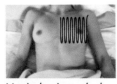

Vertical strip method

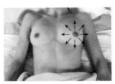

Pie wedge method

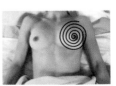

Concentric circles method

POSITION: Supine with pillow under shoulder of breast being examined, sitting with arms at side, sitting with arms over head, sitting with hands on hip or pushed together, sitting leaning forward

TOOLBOX: Small pillow or towel, mirror, centimeter ruler, nonsterile gloves, specimen slide, and specimen culture slide

AREA/PA SKILL	NORMAL FINDINGS	ABNORMAL FINDINGS
Inspection *Breast*		
Assess size, shape, symmetry, color. Note visible masses, lesions, edema, and venous pattern. **Have client press hands together or press hands on hips to check for dimpling or retraction.** Note dominant side.	Breasts lobular, symmetrical, color consistent with body color No masses, lesions, edema, dimpling, retraction, or orange-peel skin Breasts may normally be slightly asymmetrical	Change in breast symmetry: Warrants further investigation Edema and orange-peel skin appearance: Lymphatic obstruction Erythema: Infection, abscess, or inflammatory carcinoma of the breast Dimpling or puckering: Sign of retraction phenomena or abnormal traction on Cooper's ligaments—or attachment to fascia and pectoralis muscle—caused by neoplasm Lesions and asymmetrical increased venous pattern: Signs of breast cancer
Nipple and Areola		
Note color, shape, symmetry, inversions or eversions, discharge, masses, lesions.	Nipples and areola symmetrical, round, and darker than breast tissue Color lighter in fair-skinned and darker in dark-skinned women. No masses, lesions, or discharge	Inverted nipples may make breast-feeding difficult Change in nipple from everted to inverted, or in the direction in which it is pointing: Underlying mass

(continued)

AREA/PA SKILL	NORMAL FINDINGS	ABNORMAL FINDINGS
Inspection *Nipple and Areola (Continued)*		
Note direction of nipples.	Spontaneous discharge normal during pregnancy and lactation Symmetrical nipple direction, usually lateral and upward. Nipples may be everted, flat, or inverted, but should be symmetrical	Flattened or inverted nipples: Shortening of mammary ducts ***Spontaneous discharge not associated with pregnancy or breastfeeding warrants follow-up. Obtain a specimen for evaluation.*** Lesions or erosion and ulceration of areola and nipple: Paget's disease
Inspect for supernumerary nipples.	No supernumerary nipples	Discoloration of areola and nipple that is not associated with pregnancy warrants follow-up Cracks and redness of nipple can occur with breast-feeding.
Axilla		
Note color, lesions, masses, and hair distribution.	Skin intact, no lesions or rashes. Hair growth appropriate for client's age and sex	Rashes, redness, unusual pigmentation: Infection, allergy Malignant acanthosis nigricans, a rare cancer, causes dark pigmentation and velvety skin texture of axilla
Palpation **(Use finger pads of three middle fingers, make small circles with light, medium, and deep pressure.)**		

(continued)

AREA/PA SKILL	NORMAL FINDINGS	ABNORMAL FINDINGS
Palpation *Breasts*		
Palpate from the clavicle to the 6th and 7th intercostal spaces and the sternum to the midaxillary line. Use vertical strip, pie wedge, or circular method.	Breast consistency depends on developmental stage of woman. Premenopausal breast more firm and elastic, pregnancy and lactation firm and tender, postmenopausal less firm and elastic with stringy ducts	Fibroadenoma: Benign breast lumps; usually smooth, firm, round, movable, nontender, 1 to 5 cm in size
Note texture, consistency, tenderness, masses.	Nontender, but premenstrual breast may be tender and nodular	Fibrocystic breast: Benign breast lumps; nodular, tender, movable, soft to firm, change in size with menstrual cycle, increasing before menstruation, and multiple in number
Do not remove finger pads from the skin surface or jump from area to area.	No masses or lesions	
Most breast lesions in women are found in the upper outer quadrant. (This area includes the tail of the breast and contains a greater amount of breast tissue than the other quadrants.)		Breast cancer: Irregular shape, borders irregular and not well defined, nontender, immovable, increases in size as disease progresses
Although the incidence of breast cancer in men is about 1%, you still need to assess the breast. Breast cancer in men most frequently occurs in the areola.		Breast warm and indurated (hard): Mastitis

(continued)

AREA/PA SKILL	NORMAL FINDINGS	ABNORMAL FINDINGS
Palpation *Breasts*		
Nipple and Areola		
Note elasticity, discharge, tenderness.	Nipple elastic, nontender, no discharge or white sebaceous secretion with nipple compression Pregnant or lactating women may have milky discharge	Bloody, purulent discharge: Infection Serous, serosanguineous, or bloody drainage: Intraductal papilloma Thick, gray drainage and fixation of nipple: Ductal ectasia Loss of elasticity: Underlying malignancy
Axilla and Clavicular Nodes: Central, Anterior, Posterior, Lateral, Epitrochlear, Supra- and Infraclavicular		
Note palpable nodes, location, tenderness, size, shape, consistency, mobility, borders, temperature.	Lymph nodes nonpalpable, nontender	Palpable nodes: Infection or metastatic disease Lymph node enlargement caused by infection usually tender; by malignancy, nontender

PA = physical assessment

CHAPTER 9

ASSESSING THE ABDOMEN

Primary Functions

- Every system, except the respiratory system, is found within the abdomen: the gastrointestinal, cardiovascular, reproductive, neuromuscular, and genitourinary systems.
- The primary system is the digestive system, which is responsible for the ingestion and digestion of food, absorption of nutrients, and elimination of waste products.

Developmental Considerations

Infants

- The newborn's bladder is located above the symphysis pubis.
- The liver proportionally takes up more space in the abdomen and may extend 2 cm (¾ inch) below the rib cage.
- The infant's abdominal muscles are weak, so the abdomen normally protrudes.

Children

- A child's abdomen is proportionally larger than an adult's and has a slightly protuberant appearance because of the curvature of the back.

- Abdominal respiration is common in most children.
- Children's abdominal muscles are underdeveloped, so the organs are more easily palpated.
- Children may have diastasis recti.

Pregnant Clients

- For women having multiple pregnancies or a multiple birth, the rectus abdominal muscles may become separated (diastasis recti abdominis).
- As the fetus grows, the stomach rises up and impinges on the diaphragm.
- Bowel sounds are diminished in the pregnant client because the bowels are compressed by the fetus.
- Decreased activity in the lower gastrointestinal (GI) tract, along with ingestion of prenatal vitamins containing large amounts of iron, contributes to constipation.
- Increased venous pressure in the lower abdomen may cause hemorrhoids to develop and create further problems with elimination.
- During pregnancy, the appendix is displaced upward and laterally to the right.
- Linea nigra is a characteristic skin change in most pregnant clients.
- Near the end of pregnancy, the umbilicus may become everted and striae may develop.

Older Adults

- Changes in dentition may affect chewing ability and digestion.
- Poorly fitted dentures may result in painful mastication.
- Reduced saliva, stomach acid, gastric motility, and peristalsis cause problems with swallowing, absorption, and digestion. These changes, along with a general reduction of muscle mass and tone, also contribute to constipation.
- Fat accumulates in the lower abdomen in women and around the waist in men, making physical assessment of the organs a little more challenging.
- The liver becomes smaller and liver function declines, making it harder to process medications.

- Older adults have a diminished response to painful stimuli that may mask abdominal health problems.

Cultural Considerations

- African-Americans have a high incidence of sickle cell anemia, lactose intolerance, and obesity.
- Asian-Americans have a high incidence of GI cancer and lactose intolerance.
- Jewish-Americans have a high incidence of Crohn's disease, ulcerative colitis, and colon cancer.
- Mediterranean-Americans have a high incidence of lactose intolerance and thalassemia anemia.
- Native Americans have a high incidence of alcoholism, liver disease, pancreatitis, diabetes, and gallbladder disease.

Assessment

History

SYMPTOMS ("PQRST" ANY + SYMPTOM)
- Abdominal pain
  - Where is the pain? Would you point to where you feel the pain? (Table 9–1)
  - Does the pain stay in one place or does it move (radiate)? Where does the pain go?
  - When did it start (date)? What were you doing when it started? Gradually or suddenly?
  - Do you have any other symptoms? What started first? Second?
  - Have you ever had this pain before?
  - When was your last menstrual period?
  - How would you describe the pain (sharp or dull)? (Table 9–2)
  - Is the pain getting better or worse?
  - Is it constant or intermittent? (If intermittent, how long does the pain last and how frequent are the episodes of pain?)
  - What makes it worse? What makes it better?
  - What have you tried to get rid of the pain? How well did that work?

Table 9-1. *Significance of Pain by Abdominal Quadrant*	
LEFT UPPER QUADRANT	**RIGHT UPPER QUADRANT**
Heart: Myocardial infarction (MI)/ Ischemia	*Heart:* MI/Ischemia
Lungs: Pulmonary embolism, pneumonia	*Lungs:* Pneumonia
Pancreas: Pancreatitis	*Gallbladder:* Cholelithiasis, cholecystitis
Spleen: Ruptured spleen	*Liver:* Hepatitis, cancer
Stomach: Gastric ulcer, esophagitis, gastroesophageal reflux disease (GERD), hiatal hernia, varices	*Intestines:* Duodenal ulcer
LEFT LOWER QUADRANT	**RIGHT LOWER QUADRANT**
Ovary/Uterus: Ectopic pregnancy, ovarian cyst, pelvic inflammatory disease (PID)	*Ovary/Uterus:* Ectopic pregnancy, ovarian cyst, PID
Intestines: Perforation, constipation, diverticulitis, hernia, ulcerative colitis	*Intestines:* Perforation, obstruction, constipation, Crohn's disease, diverticulitis, hernia, ulcerative colitis, appendicitis
Kidney: Nephrolithiasis (kidney stones), infection	*Kidney:* Nephrolithiasis, infection

- Do you have a fever? Has your appetite changed?
- Have you lost weight? If so, how much weight have you lost and over what period of time?
- Are you having any problems with your bowels? Are there any changes in urination (frequency, burning, color, amount)?
- Have you noticed any bloating in your stomach?
- Are you having any discharge from your private parts? (color, amount, odor?)
- Weight changes
  - How is your appetite? Have you had any changes in your appetite recently?
  - What have you had to eat in the last 24 hours (note 24-hour intake)?

Table 9-2. *Pain Intensity Rating Scales*

SCALE	APPROPRIATE CLIENTS
0–10 Numeric Pain Intensity Scale	Client must be able to:
Horizontal line with 11 marks associated with numbers 0–10	• Process verbal information
0 = no pain; 5 = moderate pain; 10 = worst possible pain	• Communicate verbally or by body movements
Nurse asks client to rate pain on 0–10 scale, either using written instructions on a card or verbally explaining scale.	• Understand numbers 0–10
18 foreign language versions available at: <http://www.partnersagainstpain.com/html/assess/as_scale.htm>	Used with children age 8 and up, teens, and adults.
Wong-Baker FACES Pain Rating Scale (1999)	
Card with six faces with expressions ranging from happy to very sad and crying. Happy face indicates no pain (0); very sad face (5) indicates most severe pain.	Client must be able to see and process information.
Nurse explains process first, then shows client card and asks client to pick face that best reflects pain.	Originally designed for use with children age 3 and over, but is used with adults as well.
Specific tool and instructions available at: <http:www.genx.com/Mosby/Wong/hcom_wong_perm.html>	
Simple Descriptive Verbal Pain Intensity Scale	
Horizontal line with 6 demarcations from left to right with words that describe pain: No Pain—Mild Pain—Moderate Pain—Severe Pain—Very Severe Pain—Worst Possible Pain.	Client must be able to:
	• Speak or understand English
Nurse asks client to select word best describing pain.	• Process information
	• Communicate

- What is your present weight? What is your usual weight?
- Has your weight changed recently?
- How much weight have you lost or gained? Over what period of time?
- Were you trying to lose or gain weight? How did you lose or gain the weight?
- Are you satisfied with your present weight?

- Do you ever eat large amounts of food at one time (like a half gallon of ice cream)?
- Bowel pattern changes
  - When did the changes start?
  - How frequent are your bowel movements usually (per day or week)? Presently?
  - When was your last bowel movement?
  - Do you wake up in the night to have a bowel movement?
  - What color is your stool (black, dark brown, light brown, tan, gray, yellow)? Have there been any changes?
  - Is it soft, hard, formed, loose, liquid? Have there been any changes in consistency?
  - Any mucus or blood?
  - How much are you eliminating at one time? (especially important in diarrhea)
  - Do you have any other symptoms (fullness or pain in your abdomen, bloating, gas, indigestion, nausea, vomiting, fever, weight loss)?
  - What have you tried to relieve this problem? How well has that worked?
  - Has anything made it worse?
  - Is there anything you eat that upsets your stomach or causes changes in your bowel movements? Has your diet changed recently?
  - What medications do you take (medicines, antacids, laxatives, enemas, stool softeners; frequency of medications)?
  - What medical illnesses do you have?
  - Have you ever had this problem before? When? How was it treated?
  - Does anyone you know have similar symptoms? (diarrhea)
  - Have you traveled out of the country recently? (diarrhea)
- Indigestion
  - Where do you feel the indigestion? (point with one finger)
  - Do you have pain anywhere else?
  - Does the pain stay in one place or does it radiate?
  - When did it start?

- What were you doing at that time?
- Have you ever had this before? How long does it last?
- Would you describe the feeling to me (sharp, dull, burning, crushing)?
- Is it constant or intermittent?
- How would you rate the discomfort on a scale of 1 to 10?
- What have you tried to make it better? How did that work?
- What makes it worse?
- Do you have any other symptoms?
- Do you have any difficulty swallowing?

- Nausea
  - When did the nausea start?
  - What were you doing at the time?
  - Does it come on at any particular time of the day?
  - What have you eaten in the last 24 hours? Does anyone in your family have similar symptoms?
  - How would you describe it?
  - Does it come over you in a wave and then dissipate? Or is it constant?
  - Does the nausea interfere with your daily activities?
  - Have you been so nauseated that you have vomited?
  - Have you lost weight?
  - Is there any chance that you are pregnant?
  - Do you have any other symptoms or health problems?
  - What medicines do you take?
  - What have you tried to relieve the nausea? How has that worked?
  - Do you have any other symptoms with the nausea such as fever, chills, headache?

- Vomiting
  - When did the vomiting start?
  - What were you doing at the time?
  - In the last few days, have you been hit on the head?
  - Does anyone else in your house have similar symptoms?
  - What color is the vomit?
  - What is its consistency?
  - How much have you been vomiting at one time?
  - How many times a day are you vomiting?
  - Have you been able to keep any food or fluids down?

- What have you tried to stop the vomiting?
- Did it work? Does anything make it better (lying still, eating crackers, ginger ale)?
- What makes it worse (for example, eating)?
- What other symptoms do you have (retching, nausea, pain, fever, distention, diarrhea, weakness, stiff neck, headache)?

FOCUSED ABDOMINAL HISTORY
- Do you have any abdominal pain?
- Have you ever had the following: stomach ulcer, hemorrhoids, hernia, bowel disease, cancer, hepatitis, cirrhosis, or appendicitis?
- Have you had abdominal surgery? If so, when, what type, and were there any subsequent problems?
- Do you have a family history of ulcer, gallbladder disease, bowel disease, or cancer?
- Do you have any problems with swallowing, heartburn, nausea, yellowing of your skin, gas, bloating, or vomiting (note onset, quality, and quantity)?
- Do you have any food allergies or lactose intolerance?
- Have you noticed any recent weight changes? What is your usual weight and height?
- How is your appetite? What did you eat in the last 24 hours?
- How is your health usually?
- Are you currently being treated for a health problem? If so, what?
- How often do you usually have a bowel movement? Have you noticed any changes in your bowel movements?
- Are you having problems with diarrhea, constipation, hemorrhoids, or fecal incontinence? Have you ever noticed blood in your stool or had black, tarry stools?
- How often do you urinate? Do you have incontinence or burning when you urinate?
- When was your last menstrual period?
- Do you smoke? How many packs a day? (Calculate pack-years.)
- Do you drink alcohol? If so, how often? Do you use street drugs?
- How many cups of coffee, tea, or caffeinated soda do you drink every day?

- Have you been exposed to an infectious disease recently?
- What is your occupation?
- Have you been immunized against hepatitis B?
- Have you ever had a blood transfusion? If so, when?
- Are you taking any medications, prescribed or over the counter (Table 9–3)?
- Do you have any allergies to medications?
- What herbal preparations do you use?
- Do you use antacids, laxatives, enemas, nonsteroidal anti-inflammatory agents (NSAIDs), or aspirin?
- What home remedies do you use?

Table 9–3. *Drugs That Adversely Affect the Gastrointestinal System*

DRUG CLASS	DRUG	POSSIBLE ADVERSE REACTIONS
Analgesics	acetaminophen	Hepatic necrosis with high (toxic) doses
	aspirin	GI disturbances, GI bleeding, ulceration
Antacids	aluminum hydroxide	Constipation
	calcium carbonate	Constipation, gastric hypersecretion, acid rebound
	magnesium hydroxide	Diarrhea
Anticholinergic agents	all anticholinergics	Nausea, vomiting, constipation, xerostomia, bloated feeling, paralytic ileus
Antidepressants	amitriptyline hydrochloride, nortriptyline hydrochloride	Constipation, adynamic ileus, elevated liver enzyme concentrations, jaundice, hepatitis
	selective serotonin reuptake inhibitors	Nausea, vomiting, diarrhea, constipation
Antidiabetic agents	acetohexamide	Nausea, vomiting, diarrhea, heartburn, cholestatic jaundice
	chlorpropamide	Nausea, vomiting, diarrhea, heartburn (pyrosis), jaundice

(continued)

Table 9–3. *Drugs That Adversely Affect the Gastrointestinal System*
(Continued)

DRUG CLASS	DRUG	POSSIBLE ADVERSE REACTIONS
Anti-infectives	ampicillin	Diarrhea, nausea, vomiting, pseudomembranous colitis
	ciprofloxacin	Heartburn
	clindamycin hydrochloride	Nausea, vomiting, diarrhea, tenesmus, pseudomembranous and nonspecific colitis
	erythromycin	Abdominal pain and cramping, nausea, vomiting, diarrhea, hepatic dysfunction, jaundice
	metronidazole	Taste disturbances, abdominal discomfort, diarrhea, nausea, vomiting
	sulfonamides	Nausea, vomiting, hepatic changes
	tetracycline hydrochloride	Nausea, vomiting, diarrhea, stomatitis
Antihypertensives	clonidine hydrochloride	Nausea, vomiting, constipation
	guanethidine sulfate	Increased frequency of bowel movements, explosive diarrhea
	methyldopa	Elevated liver function tests
Antineoplastic agents	all antineoplastics	Nausea, vomiting, stomatitis
Antituberculosis agents	isoniazid	Increased liver enzyme concentrations
	rifampin	Heartburn, nausea, vomiting, diarrhea, increased liver enzyme concentrations
Bisphosphonates	alendronate	Esophagitis, heartburn
Cardiac agents	digoxin	Nausea, vomiting, diarrhea, anorexia with high (toxic) doses
	quinidine sulfate	Nausea, vomiting, diarrhea, abdominal cramps, colic

(continued)

Table 9–3. *Drugs That Adversely Affect the Gastrointestinal System (Continued)*

DRUG CLASS	DRUG	POSSIBLE ADVERSE REACTIONS
Narcotic analgesics	codeine, meperidine hydrochloride, methadone hydrochloride, morphine sulfate, oxycodone	Nausea, vomiting, constipation, biliary spasm or colic
Nonsteroidal anti-inflammatory agents	ibuprofen, indomethacin, salicylates	Nausea, vomiting, dyspepsia, GI bleeding, peptic ulcer
Phenothiazines	prochlorperazine maleate, thioridazine hydrochloride	Constipation, dyspepsia, paralytic ileus, cholestatic jaundice (hypersensitivity reaction)
	acarbose	Diarrhea, flatulence, abdominal pain
Miscellaneous agents	allopurinol	Altered liver function, nausea, vomiting, diarrhea
	aminophylline, theophylline	GI irritation, epigastric pain, nausea, vomiting, anorexia
	barium sulfate	Cramping, diarrhea
	colchicine	Diarrhea, nausea, vomiting, abdominal pain
	estrogen-progestin combinations	Nausea, vomiting, diarrhea, abdominal cramps, altered liver function tests, cholestatic jaundice
	iron preparations	Constipation, nausea, vomiting, black stools
	gold sodium thiomalate, auranofin	Changes in bowel habits, diarrhea, abdominal cramping, nausea, vomiting
	griseofulvin	Nausea, vomiting, diarrhea, flatulence
	levodopa	Nausea, vomiting, anorexia
	lithium	Nausea, vomiting, diarrhea
	phenytoin sodium	Nausea, vomiting, constipation, dysphagia

(continued)

Table 9–3. *Drugs That Adversely Affect the Gastrointestinal System (Continued)*

DRUG CLASS	DRUG	POSSIBLE ADVERSE REACTIONS
	potassium supplements	Nausea, vomiting, diarrhea, abdominal discomfort, small bowel ulceration (with enteric-coated tablets)
	prednisone	Epigastric pain, gastric irritation, pancreatitis
	zidovudine	Nausea, vomiting, anorexia

Assessment of Abdomen's Relationship to Other Systems

Remember, all systems are related! As you assess the abdomen, look at the relationship between it and all other systems.

SUBJECTIVE DATA	OBJECTIVE DATA
Area/System: General	
Ask about:	*Inspect for:*
Weight changes	Orientation
Diet	Facial expression
Fever	Posture
Dizziness	Nutritional status
	Measure:
	Weight
	Vital signs
Area/System: Integumentary	
Ask about:	*Inspect:*
Changes in skin, hair, and nails	Skin, hair, and nails for changes
Rashes, itching, lesion	in color and texture, lesions,
	and edema or ascites
	Skin turgor
Area/System: HEENT	
Head and Neck	
Ask about:	*Inspect for:*
Thyroid disease	Neck masses
Neck masses	*Palpate:*
Recent infections	Thyroid
	Lymph nodes

(continued)

SUBJECTIVE DATA	OBJECTIVE DATA
Eyes	
Ask about:	*Inspect for:*
History of diabetes, renal disease, liver disease	Edema
	Color of sclera
	Retinal changes
Ears, Nose, and Throat	
Ask about:	*Inspect:*
Problems swallowing	Mouth
Sore throat	Throat
Dizziness	Condition of teeth
Last dental examination	*Test:*
	Cranial nerves I, VII, VIII, IX, X, XII
	Balance using Romberg's test
Area/System: Respiratory	
Ask about:	*Measure:*
Breathing problems, shortness of breath (SOB)	Respiratory rate and depth
	Auscultate:
History of chronic obstructive pulmonary disease (COPD)	Breath sounds
Area/System: Cardiovascular	
Ask about:	*Measure:*
History of cerebrovascular disease (CVD), hypertension (HTN), congestive heart failure (CHF)	Vital signs
	Palpate:
	Pulses for thrills
	Auscultate:
	Heart for extra sounds (S3) and bruits
Area/System: Genitourinary/Reproductive	
Ask about:	*Inspect:*
Color of urine	Color of urine
Urinary burning, frequency, hesitancy	External genitalia for lesions or discharge
History of sexually transmitted diseases (STDs)	*Palpate:*
	Bladder for distention
Women:	Kidneys
Last menstrual period (LMP)	Prostate
Vaginal discharge	*Percuss:*
Men:	Costovertebral angle for tenderness
Prostate problems	*Women:*
Penile discharge	Perform pelvic examination
	Men:
	Perform rectal examination

(continued)

SUBJECTIVE DATA	OBJECTIVE DATA
Area/System: Musculoskeletal	
Ask about:	*Measure:*
History of fractures	Height for loss
Joint pain	*Inspect:*
Weakness	Spinal curves
	Joints
	Range of motion (ROM)
	Palpate:
	Muscle strength
Area/System: Neurological	
Ask about:	*Test:*
Alcohol use	Sensation
Numbness	Deep tendon reflex (DTR)
Back problems	
Loss of bowel/bladder control	
Area/System: Endocrine	
Ask about:	
History of diabetes	
Thyroid problems	
Area/System:Immune/Hematological	
Ask about:	*Inspect:*
Food allergies	Lymph nodes for enlargement
Infection	*Palpate:*
Sickle cell anemia	Lymph nodes
	Spleen

HEENT = head, eyes, ears, nose, and throat

Physical Assessment

ANATOMICAL LANDMARKS
Four quadrants; nine regions (Box 9.1 and Table 9–4)

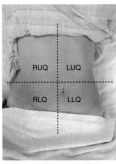

Four-quadrant method

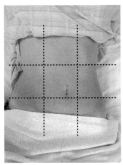

Nine regions of the abdomen

BOX 9.1. Four-Quadrant Method

Right Upper Quadrant	Left Upper Quadrant
Liver	Left lobe of liver
Gallbladder	Spleen
Pylorus	Stomach
Duodenum	Body of pancreas
Head of pancreas	Left adrenal gland
Right adrenal gland	Portion of left kidney
Portion of right kidney	Splenic flexure of colon
Hepatic flexure of colon	Portions of transverse
Portions of ascending	and descending colon
and transverse colon	

Right Lower Quadrant	Left Lower Quadrant
Lower portion of right kidney	Lower section of left kidney
Cecum and appendix	Sigmoid colon
Portion of ascending colon	Descending colon
Bladder (if distended)	Bladder (if distended)
Ovary and salpinx	Ovary and salpinx
Uterus (if enlarged)	Uterus (if enlarged)
Right spermatic cord	Left spermatic cord
Right ureter	Left ureter

Midline

Aorta
Uterus (if enlarged)
Bladder (if enlarged)
Spine

APPROACH: Inspection, auscultation, percussion, palpation

POSITION: Supine, or with knees slightly flexed with a pillow under knees to relax abdominal muscles

TOOLBOX: Stethoscope (bell and diaphragm), pen, metric ruler, and reflex hammer or tongue blade to assess abdominal reflexes. *Remember: Always listen before palpating!*

Table 9-4. *Nine Regions of the Abdomen*

RIGHT HYPOCHONDRIAC	EPIGASTRIC	LEFT HYPOCHONDRIAC
Right lobe of liver	Pylorus	Stomach
Gallbladder	Duodenum	Spleen
Duodenum	Head of pancreas	Pancreas tail
Hepatic flexure	Portion of liver	Splenic flexure
Portion of right kidney		Upper portion of left kidney
Suprarenal gland		Suprarenal gland

RIGHT LUMBAR	UMBILICAL	LEFT LUMBAR
Portion of right kidney	Lower duodenum	Descending colon
Hepatic flexure of colon	Jejunum and ileum	Lower half of left kidney
Ascending colon		Jejunum and ileum
Duodenum		
Jejunum		

RIGHT INGUINAL	HYPOGASTRIC	LEFT INGUINAL
Cecum	Ileum	Sigmoid colon
Appendix	Bladder	Left ureter
Ileum	Uterus (if enlarged)	Left spermatic cord
Right ureter		Left ovary
Right spermatic cord		
Right ovary		

AREA/PA SKILL	NORMAL FINDINGS	ABNORMAL FINDINGS
Inspection (Inspect from side and foot of bed. Have client void before examination.)		

(continued)

AREA/PA SKILL	NORMAL FINDINGS	ABNORMAL FINDINGS
Inspection *Abdomen*		
Note size, shape, and symmetry of abdomen. Note condition of skin, color, lesions, scars, striae, superficial veins, and hair distribution.	Skin color consistent or slightly lighter than exposed areas. No lesions, striae, superficial veins, scars, rashes, or discoloration Hair distribution appropriate for age and gender of client	Jaundice: Liver disease Redness: Inflammation Cyanosis: Hypoxia Cullen's sign: Hemorrhagic pancreatitis or intraperitoneal bleeding Grey-Turner's sign: Pancreatitis or extraperitoneal bleeding Bruises: Recent trauma Pink-purple striae: Cushing's syndrome Spider angioma: Liver failure Caput medusa: Liver failure Dermatomally distributed vesicular rash on lower rib cage in upper quadrants: Herpes zoster

Symphysis pubis   Costal margin

Flat

Scaphoid

Rounded

Protuberant

Shapes of abdomen

AREA/PA SKILL	NORMAL FINDINGS	ABNORMAL FINDINGS
Note abdominal movements: respiratory, peristalsis. Note position, contour, color, and herniation of the umbilicus. Have client raise head off bed and look for bulges (hernias).	Abdomen flat or slightly rounded and symmetrical, no bulges or hernias + respiratory movements, slight pulsation noted in epigastric region, no peristaltic waves Umbilicus midline, inverted, no discoloration or discharge	Hernias are caused by weakness of abdominal muscles. Seen as bulges that occur when client bears down. Occur on old surgical incisions, around umbilicus, or in inguinal area Epigastric or linea alba hernias occur when intestine protrudes through opening in midline of abdomen above umbilicus

(continued)

AREA/PA SKILL	NORMAL FINDINGS	ABNORMAL FINDINGS
Inspection *Abdomen (Continued)*		
		Diastasis recti occurs in pregnant women and newborns Protrusion of umbilicus: Umbilical hernia. Underlying mass causes umbilicus to deviate from midline Asymmetry: Tumors, cysts, bowel obstruction, organomegaly, or scoliosis Abdominal distention is caused by "Nine Fs": fat, fluid, feces, fetus, flatus, fibroid, full bladder, false pregnancy, or fatal tumor Area of abdomen that is distended can pinpoint cause: • Right lower quadrant and left lower quadrant: Pregnancy, ovarian or uterine tumor, bladder enlargement • Left and right upper quadrants: Pancreatic cyst or tumor or gastric distention • Asymmetrical: Tumor, hernia, cyst, bowel obstruction Concave abdomen: Malnutrition Increased peristaltic waves: Intestinal obstruction *(continued)*

AREA/PA SKILL	NORMAL FINDINGS	ABNORMAL FINDINGS
Inspection *Abdomen (Continued)*		
		Reverse peristaltic waves: Pyloric stenosis Shallow respirations in male clients: Abdominal pain Increased/diffuse pulsations: Aortic aneurysm
Auscultation (Use the diaphragm of the stethoscope for bowel sounds and friction rubs. Use the bell for vascular sounds.)		
Abdomen, Liver, and Arteries		
Listen for bowel sounds in each quadrant. Listen for at least 5 minutes before saying that bowel sounds are absent. If you are having difficulty hearing bowel sounds, listen over ileocecal valve to the right of the umbilicus in the right lower quadrant.	Soft, medium-pitched bowel sounds every 5–15 seconds in all four quadrants No borborygmi, bruits, hums, or rubs	Bowel sounds more than 30 clicks/minute: Hyperactive bowel sounds or hyperperistalsis; caused by irritable bowel disease, bowel infection, early bowel obstruction, diarrhea, resolving paralytic ileus, or laxative use Types of hyperperistalsis include borborygmi and succussion splash Bowel sounds <5 clicks/minute but present: Hypoactive bowel sounds or hypoperistalsis; caused by peritonitis, medications such as opioids, bowel obstruction, or postoperative occurrence

(continued)

AREA/PA SKILL	NORMAL FINDINGS	ABNORMAL FINDINGS

Auscultation
Abdomen, Liver, and Arteries (Continued)

Use scratch test to locate the inferior edge of the liver. Auscultate for bruits over the aorta and renal, iliac, and femoral arteries. If indicated, auscultate for venous hum over liver. If indicated, auscultate for friction rubs over organs.	Lower edge of liver located at costal margin by scratch test.	Absent bowel sounds: Late bowel obstruction, peritonitis, paralytic ileus following manipulation of the bowel during surgery A bruit with a systolic and diastolic component is abnormal. Cause depends on area where it is heard: • Aortic: Aortic aneurysm • Epigastric: Renal artery stenosis • Aortic, iliac, or femoral: Arterial insufficiency Venous hums: Venous portal hypertension and liver disease Cruveilhier-Baumgarten murmur: Portal hypertension Friction rub: Inflammation of peritoneal surface of an organ from tumor, infection, or infarct • Splenic friction rubs: Infection, abscess, infarction, or tumor; are best heard at lower rib cage in left anterior axillary line • Liver friction rubs: Liver cancer or abscess; can be auscultated over lower right sternal border

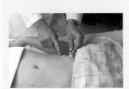

Scratch test

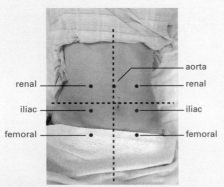

Auscultating sites for vascular sounds

(renal, aorta, renal, iliac, iliac, femoral, femoral)

(continued)

AREA/PA SKILL	NORMAL FINDINGS	ABNORMAL FINDINGS
Percussion Use indirect (mediate) percussion in all four quadrants.		

Abdomen, Organs (liver, gallbladder, spleen, kidneys)

AREA/PA SKILL	NORMAL FINDINGS	ABNORMAL FINDINGS
Note areas of tympany, dullness, tenderness. Percuss tender areas last!	Tympany in all four quadrants, dullness over organs	Extremely high-pitched tympanic sounds: Distention Extensive dullness: Organ enlargement or underlying mass
Measure liver size at the right midclavicular line (RMCL). If enlarged, do measurement at midsternal line. Locate gastric bubble over stomach.	Liver 6–12 cm at RMCL.	Liver span >12 cm: Hepatomegaly
Locate splenic dullness at left midaxillary line (LMAL). If ascites is present, percuss for shifting dullness.	Splenic dullness at 9th, 10th, 11th ribs at LMAL, <7 cm	Splenic upper border percussed beyond 8 cm above costal margin: Enlarged spleen caused by portal hypertension, thrombosis, stenosis, atresia, deformities of splenic vein, cysts, cancer, mononucleosis, trauma, and infection (as long as client does not have a full stomach or intestines) Dullness in suprapubic area: Full bladder (for other causes, see section on Inspection of Abdomen, above)

(continued)

AREA/PA SKILL	NORMAL FINDINGS	ABNORMAL FINDINGS

Percussion
Abdomen, Organs (liver, gallbladder, spleen, kidneys) (Continued)

If indicated, use fist (blunt) percussion to assess for organ (liver or gallbladder) tenderness. Check for kidney tenderness at posterior CVA.	Organs nontender	Severe pain or CVA tenderness: Kidney infection or musculoskeletal problem

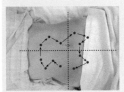

Percussion sites

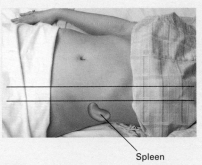

Anterior axillary line
Midaxillary line

Spleen

Percussing at lowest intercostal space at left anterior axillary line

(continued)

AREA/PA SKILL	NORMAL FINDINGS	ABNORMAL FINDINGS
Palpation **Begin with light palpation, then deep, bimanual in all four quadrants.** If client is tense (voluntary guarding), have client slightly flex knees or let client hold your hand as you palpate.		
Abdomen, Organs, and Aorta		
Use light palpation to identify surface characteristics, tenderness, muscular resistance, and turgor, and to put client at ease. Assess the umbilicus for bulges or nodules. **Do not palpate abdomen if large, diffuse pulsations are present or if client has history of organ transplant or known or suspected Wilms' tumor.**	Abdomen soft and nontender, no masses, + skin turgor, no umbilical bulges	Involuntary guarding and rigidity: Peritonitis Areas of tenderness: Underlying problem Masses: Underlying tumor, enlarged uterus, feces-filled colon
Use deep palpation with bimanual technique to palpate organs (liver, spleen, kidneys) and masses. Note tenderness, consistency, pulsations, enlarged organs. Palpate aorta; note pulsation, size, and diffusion.	Liver nonpalpable or liver's edge may be palpable at costal margin, firm, smooth, and nontender Spleen nontender, nonpalpable	Enlarged liver: Cirrhosis, tumor, hepatitis Enlarged spleen: Malignancy, infection, trauma to spleen Lateral diffuse pulsation: Abdominal aortic aneurysm Aortic width >3 cm: Abdominal aortic aneurysm

(continued)

AREA/PA SKILL	NORMAL FINDINGS	ABNORMAL FINDINGS

Palpation
Abdomen, Organs, and Aorta (Continued)

AREA/PA SKILL	NORMAL FINDINGS	ABNORMAL FINDINGS
		Liver palpable below costal margin: CHF, hepatitis, encephalopathy, cirrhosis, cysts, cancer. If liver is enlarged, tender, firm, and nodular or has an irregular border, suspect liver cancer
		Splenic enlargement and tenderness: Infection, CHF, cancer, cirrhosis, trauma
		Enlarged kidneys: Hydronephrosis, neoplasm, polycystic disease
		Kidney tenderness: Trauma or infection
		Nodular or asymmetrical bladder: Possible malignancy
If indicated, assess for rebound tenderness at McBurney's point and perform the iliopsoas test and the obturator test. To test for fluid, perform the fluid wave test. Use ballottement to assess fetal position or masses.	Negative rebound Kidneys nonpalpable. Right kidney may be palpable in thin women + Slight aortic pulsation, no diffusion, aorta 2.5 cm	+ rebound tenderness, iliopsoas, and obturator signs: Peritoneal inflammation, peritonitis, appendicitis + fluid wave, shifting dullness, puddle sign: Ascites Free-floating mass in abdomen: Malignant or benign tumor + Kehr's sign: Splenic injury, renal calculi, ectopic pregnancy

(continued)

AREA/PA SKILL	NORMAL FINDINGS	ABNORMAL FINDINGS
Palpation *Abdomen, Organs, and Aorta (Continued)*		
		+ Ballance's sign: Peritoneal irritation, splenic injury + Murphy's sign: Cholecystitis
Test abdominal reflexes by lightly stroking each quadrant toward the umbilicus. **If client is ticklish, have him or her place a hand over the abdomen, and then place yours over it and do light palpation. When the client starts to feel more relaxed, slip your hand underneath. If you detect a mass, have client tighten his or her abdominal muscles. This helps you feel the mass better. But if the mass is deep in the abdomen below the muscles, it will be difficult to palpate.**	+ abdominal reflexes	Absent abdominal reflexes: Pyramidal tract lesion Absent upper abdominal reflexes: Problems at spinal levels T8 through T10 Absent lower abdominal reflexes: Problems at spinal levels T10 through T12

Palpating the liver

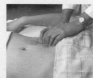

Hooking technique

(continued)

AREA/PA SKILL	NORMAL FINDINGS	ABNORMAL FINDINGS

Palpation
Abdomen, Organs, and Aorta (Continued)

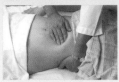

Palpating the spleen

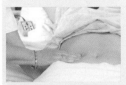

Palpating the kidneys

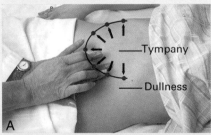

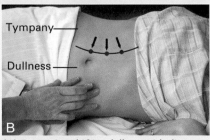

(A) Percussing shifting dullness with client supine, (B) Percussing shifting dullness with client on side

(continued)

AREA/PA SKILL	NORMAL FINDINGS	ABNORMAL FINDINGS

Palpation
Abdomen, Organs, and Aorta (Continued)

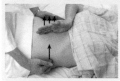
Fluid wave test

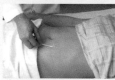
Assessing abdominal reflexes

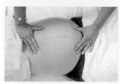
Ballottement

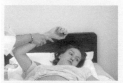
Palpating shoulder to elicit Kehr's sign

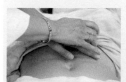
Percussing LUQ to elicit Ballance's sign

(continued)

AREA/PA SKILL	NORMAL FINDINGS	ABNORMAL FINDINGS

Palpation
Abdomen, Organs, and Aorta (Continued)

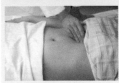

Palpating at right midclavicular line to elicit Murphy's sign

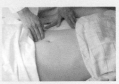

McBurney's point

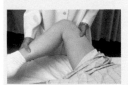

Obdurator muscle test

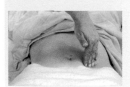

Rovsing's sign

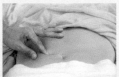

Cutaneous hypersensitivity

(continued)

AREA/PA SKILL	NORMAL FINDINGS	ABNORMAL FINDINGS
Palpation *Abdomen, Organs, and Aorta (Continued)*		

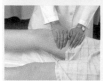

Iliopsoas muscle test

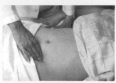

Rebound tenderness test

Inguinal Lymph Nodes

Use light palpation to palpate horizontal and vertical inguinal nodes. Note size, shape, consistency, tenderness, mobility.	Inguinal nodes nonpalpable, nontender	Tender, unmovable nodes >1 cm: Infection, cancer, lymphoma

PA = physical assessment

CHAPTER 10

ASSESSING THE FEMALE GENITOURINARY SYSTEM

Primary Functions

- Manufacturing and protecting ova for fertilization
- Transporting the fertilized ovum for implantation and embryonic/fetal development
- Housing and nourishing the developing fetus
- Regulating hormonal production and secretion of several sex hormones
- Providing sexual stimulation and pleasure
- Providing a drainage site for the excretion of urine (urinary structures)

Developmental Considerations

Infants

- Female infant's genitals are enlarged at birth in response to maternal estrogen.
- Hormonal effect may also cause pseudomenstruation.

Children and Adolescents

- The female child begins puberty changes any time from 8 to 13 years of age.

MATURATION STATES IN GIRLS

Stage 1

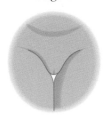

Hair distribution in the preadolescent:
There is no pubic hair except for fine body hair
similar to hair on the abdomen.

Stage 2

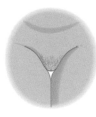

Sparse growth of long, slightly pigmented,
downy hair, straight or only slightly curled,
mostly along the labia.

Stage 3

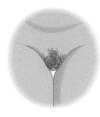

Hair is darker, coarser, and curly and spreads
sparsely over the pubic symphysis.

Stage 4

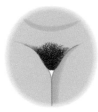

Pubic hair is coarser and curlier, as in adults. It
covers more area than in Stage 3, but not as
great as in the adult.

Stage 5

The quality and quantity are consistent with
adult pubic hair distribution and spread over
medial surfaces of thighs but not over the abdomen.

Pregnant Clients

- The uterus becomes hypertrophied and its capacity increases to 500 to 1000 times its nonpregnant state.
- The vascularity of the cervix increases and contributes to softening of the cervix.
- The vascular congestion creates a blue-purple blemish or change in the cervical color (Chadwick sign).
- Estrogen causes the glandular cervical tissue to produce a thick mucus, which builds up and forms a mucus plug at the endocervical canal.
- The vaginal wall softens and relaxes to accommodate the movement of the infant during birth.

Older Adults

- Around the age of 46 to 55 years, menstrual periods become shorter and less frequent until they stop entirely.
- Menopause is said to have occurred when the woman has not experienced a menstrual period in more than a year.
- Sexual organs atrophy; the clitoris becomes smaller; and vaginal secretions are not as plentiful. Painful intercourse may result.
- Vaginal changes increase the risk for vaginal infections.

Cultural Considerations

Cultural/Ethnic Views of Women

CULTURE	VIEW OF WOMEN
Amish	High status associated with role of wife and mother. Responsibilities include feeding, clothing, and caring for family.
Appalachian	High status associated with motherhood. Having children associated with fulfillment. Responsible for child rearing. Older women preserve culture. Responsible for preparing herbal medicines and folk medicine.
Arab	Women gain status with age. Responsible for caring and educating children and tending to husband's needs.

(continued)

CULTURE	VIEW OF WOMEN
Chinese	Woman's role is to perpetuate male dominance.
Cuban	Women expected to stay at home and care for children.
Egyptian	Status and power increase with pregnancy and birthing, especially of a son. This is expected within 1 year of marriage.
Filipino	Women have equal role with men in health, welfare, and family finance.
Greek	Pregnancy seen as a time of great respect.
Iranian	Prestige associated with having children.
Jewish	Woman runs home and is responsible for children.
Mexican	Woman maintains home and health of family.
Native American (Indian)	Mother is the center of Indian society.
Vietnamese	Women expected to be dutiful and respectful of husband and to make healthcare decisions.

Assessment

History

SYMPTOMS ("PQRST" ANY + SYMPTOM)
- Vaginal discharge
    - When did you first notice the vaginal discharge?
    - Do you have any itching in the genital area?
    - What color is the discharge? Is there an odor to the discharge?
    - Is the amount of discharge small, moderate, or large?
- Lesions
    - When did you first notice the rash, blisters, ulcers, sores, or warts on your genital area or surrounding area?
    - Does your sex partner have any of the same symptoms?
    - Is the lesion painful?
    - Have you ever had a sexually transmitted disease (STD)? If so, what was it? What treatment did you have for it?

- Vaginal bleeding
  - How often do you have any vaginal bleeding outside the time of your normal menstrual period?
  - When did/does it occur?
  - How would you describe the bleeding? Spotty, small, moderate, large amount?
  - Is it more than your normal period?
  - How much bleeding occurs? (Clarify by asking numbers of pads or tampons used in 24 hours.)
  - What method of birth control do you use?
  - When was your last menstrual period?
  - Describe your "normal flow."
- Pain (dysmenorrhea)
  - Describe the pain: Is it dull, sharp, radiating, intermittent, continuous?
  - When did the pain start?
  - Are you having any pain in the area now?
  - What makes the pain better or worse?
  - Do you have any associated symptoms of headache, vomiting, or diarrhea?
- Amenorrhea
  - What is your menstrual history?
  - What is your pregnancy history?
  - What is your sexual history?
  - Do you use prescription or over-the-counter (OTC) drugs? If so, what?
  - Do you exercise every day? What type of exercise and what is the duration of the activity?
  - Can you describe any emotional stresses you have?
  - What are your eating habits?
- Urinary symptoms
  - Do you have pain when voiding?
  - Describe the pain.
  - How often do you void and how much at one time?
  - Do you take showers or tub baths (bubble baths)?
  - How many times do you get up at night to void?
  - How long have you had the symptoms?
  - Do you have pain in any other area?

SEXUAL HISTORY
- Have you ever been sexually active?
- Are you currently sexually active? That is, have you had

sex with anyone in the past few months? If the answer is yes, answer next question.
- Do you have sex with men, women, or both (heterosexual, homosexual, or bisexual)?
- Type of sexual activity (oral or anal)?
- Do you have more than one partner? How many partners have you had in the last 6 months? Number of lifetime partners? Do you trade sexual favors for drugs or money?
- Are you using birth control? What kind? How often?
- Are you worried about the AIDS virus or other STDs?
- Do you take any precautions to avoid infections? If so what?
- Do you have any problems or concerns about your sexual function?
- Have you had surgery on any of your reproductive organs? If so, what and when?
- Are you taking any medications, prescribed or OTC (Table 10–1)?

Table 10–1. *Drugs That Adversely Affect the Female Reproductive System*

DRUG CLASS	DRUG	POSSIBLE ADVERSE REACTIONS
Androgens	danazol	Vaginitis with itching, dryness, burning, or bleeding; amenorrhea
	fluoxymesterone, methyltestosterone, testosterone	Amenorrhea and other menstrual irregularities; virilization, including clitoral enlargement
Antidepressants	tricyclic anti-depressants	Changed libido, menstrual irregularity
	selective serotonin reuptake inhibitors	Decreased libido, anorgasmia
Antihypertensives	clonidine hydrochloride, reserpine	Decreased libido
	methyldopa	Decreased libido, amenorrhea

(continued)

Table 10–1. *Drugs That Adversely Affect the Female Reproductive System (Continued)*

DRUG CLASS	DRUG	POSSIBLE ADVERSE REACTIONS
Antipsychotics	chlorpromazine hydrochloride, perphenazine, prochlorperazine, promazine hydrochloride, thioridazine hydrochloride, trifluoperazine hydrochloride, haloperidol	Inhibition of ovulation (chlorpromazine only), menstrual irregularities, amenorrhea, changed libido
Beta blockers	atenolol, labetalol hydrochloride, nadolol, propranolol hydrochloride, metoprolol	Decreased libido
Cardiac glycosides	digoxin, digitoxin	Changes in cellular level of vaginal walls in postmenopausal women
Cytotoxics	busulfan	Amenorrhea with menopausal symptoms in postmenopausal women, ovarian suppression, ovarian fibrosis and atrophy
	chlorambucil	Amenorrhea
	cyclophosphamide	Gonadal suppression (possibly irreversible), amenorrhea, ovarian fibrosis
	methotrexate	Menstrual dysfunction, infertility
	tamoxifen	Vaginal discharge or bleeding, menstrual irregularities, pruritus vulvae
	thiotepa	Amenorrhea

(continued)

Table 10–1. *Drugs That Adversely Affect the Female Reproductive System (Continued)*

DRUG CLASS	DRUG	POSSIBLE ADVERSE REACTIONS
Estrogens	chlorotrianisene, conjugated estrogens, esterified estrogens, estradiol, estrone, ethinyl estradiol	Altered menstrual flow, dysmenorrhea, amenorrhea, cervical erosion or abnormal secretions, enlargement of uterine fibromas, vaginal candidiasis
	dienestrol	Vaginal discharge, uterine bleeding with excessive use
	diethylstilbestrol	Breakthrough bleeding, altered menstrual flow, dysmenorrhea, amenorrhea, cervical erosion, altered cervical secretions, enlargement of uterine fibromas, vaginal candidiasis, change in libido, increased risk of vaginal cancer in female offspring
Progestins	hydroxyprogesterone caproate, medroxyprogesterone acetate, norgestrel, progesterone	Breakthrough bleeding, dysmenorrhea, amenorrhea, cervical erosion and abnormal secretions
Steroids	dexamethasone, hydrocortisone, prednisone	Amenorrhea and menstrual irregularities
Thyroid hormones	levothyroxine sodium, thyroid USP, thyrotropin, and others	Menstrual irregularities with excessive doses
Miscellaneous	lithium carbonate, L-tryptophan	Decreased libido
	spironolactone	Menstrual irregularities, amenorrhea, postmenopausal bleeding
	valproate	Menstrual irregularities, amenorrhea, possible polycystic ovarian syndrome

AREAS TO INVESTIGATE	RATIONALE/SIGNIFICANCE
Menstrual Period Age of menarche, last menstrual period (LMP), length of cycle, regularity of cycle, duration of menses, character and amount of flow, amenorrhea, menorrhagia, dysmenorrhea, spotting	Late onset of menarche (by age 16–18) can result from inadequate nutrition caused by eating disorders, chronic diseases such as Crohn's disease, environmental stresses, intensive athletic training, hypothyroidism, or the use of opiates or steroids.
Premenstrual Syndrome Breast tenderness; bloating; moodiness; cravings for salt, sugar, or chocolate; fatigue; weight gain; headaches; joint pain	Uncomfortable signs and symptoms may be alleviated by offering instruction about stress-reducing techniques and avoidance of certain foods.
Obstetric History LMP, use of fertility drugs, previous pregnancies, number of living children, number of abortions or miscarriages, complications with pregnancy, duration of labor, postpartum complications	Past obstetric health is a predictor of future reproductive health.
Perimenopause Spotting, hot flashes, palpitations, numbness, tingling, drenching sweats, mood swings, vaginal dryness, itching, use of estrogen replacement therapy, feelings about menopause	Women may have various discomforting signs and symptoms associated with menopause. Hormonal and physical changes relate to changes in self-concept. Identifying symptoms can help plan appropriate interventions for your client.
Sexual Functioning History Frequency of intercourse; number of sexual partners; ability to achieve orgasm; heterosexual, bisexual, homosexual; sexual practices; trading of sex for drugs or money	Changes in sexual functioning may indicate pain, infection, hormonal changes, disease, change in mental status, or altered role and relationship patterns. Sexual preferences and practices may increase risk for certain diseases or cross-contamination to other areas.

(continued)

AREAS TO INVESTIGATE	RATIONALE/SIGNIFICANCE
	Risk of STDs, HIV/AIDS, hepatitis, cervical carcinoma, and dysplasias increases with increase in number of partners.
Contraceptive History Use of contraceptives (if used, types used, frequency, methods used to prevent STDs, problems with contraceptive use, smoking history)	Intrauterine devices increase the risk of pelvic inflammatory disease (PID). Diaphragms may cause urinary discomfort. A client may be allergic to spermicides or latex. Oral contraceptives have a variety of side effects. Smokers' use of oral contraceptives increases the risk for cardiovascular problems. Obtaining this history is an opportunity to provide the client with education about the methods used for contraception.

Assessment of Female Genitourinary System's Relationship to Other Systems

Remember, all systems are related! As you assess the female genitourinary system, look at the relationship between it and all other systems.

SUBJECTIVE DATA	OBJECTIVE DATA
Area/System: General *Ask about:* Changes in energy level Weight changes Fevers	*Measure:* Height and weight Vital signs, checking for temperature elevations, hypertension (HTN) *Inspect:* Signs of discomfort Affect

(continued)

SUBJECTIVE DATA	OBJECTIVE DATA
Area/System: Integumentary	
Ask about:	*Inspect for:*
Changes in hair growth	Skin lesions
Rashes, lesions	Hair distribution
Area/System: HEENT	
Head and Neck	
Ask about:	*Palpate:*
Headaches	Lymph node enlargement
Swollen glands, nodes	Thyroid enlargement
Eyes, Mouth, and Throat	
Ask about:	*Inspect:*
Eye drainage	Oral mucosa for redness and
Oral lesions	lesions
Sore throat	Conjunctiva for drainage
Area/System: Respiratory	
Ask about:	*Inspect:*
History of respiratory disease	Signs of respiratory distress
	Auscultate:
	Abnormal breath sounds
Area/System: Cardiovascular	
Ask about:	*Inspect:*
History of cardiovascular disease,	Signs of impaired circulation
HTN, thrombophlebitis, heart	Skin changes
murmurs	*Palpate:*
	Pulses, edema, presence of
	Homans' sign
	Auscultate:
	Extra heart sounds
Area/System: Gastrointestinal	
Ask about:	*Inspect:*
History of liver disease	Ascites
Loss of appetite	*Palpate/percuss:*
Abdominal pain	Liver enlargement
	Masses
Area/System: Musculoskeletal	
Ask about:	*Test:*
Weakness/limitations	Muscle strength
Joint pain, swelling	*Inspect:*
Unexplained fracture	Joint swelling and deformity
	Spinal deformities
Area/System: Neurological	
Ask *about:*	*Test:*
History of neurological problems	Changes in mental status and
Paralysis	affect
Tremors	Sensory deficits
Personality changes	
Depression	*(continued)*

SUBJECTIVE DATA	OBJECTIVE DATA
Area/System: Endocrine	
Ask about:	*Palpate:*
History of diabetes and thyroid disease	Thyroid
Area/System: Lymphatic/Hematological	
Ask about:	*Palpate:*
History of malignancies, HIV, AIDS	Lymph nodes
Abnormal menses	

HEENT = head, eyes, ears, nose, and throat

Physical Assessment

APPROACH: Inspection, palpation; external and internal exam

POSITION: Lithotomy

TOOLBOX: Large hand mirror, gooseneck lamp, disposable exam gloves, drape, vaginal specula (Graves' size medium and large are adequate for most sexually active adult women; Pederson size small and medium are useful for non-sexually active women and children), cytological materials (Ayre spatula, cytobrush, cotton tipped applicators, OB swabs, microscope slides), Thayer-Martin culture plate labeled, cytology fixative spray, reagents (normal saline solution, potassium hydroxide or KOH), Hemoccult slide and developer, acetic acid, warm water, and water-soluble lubricant.

AREA/PA SKILL	NORMAL FINDINGS	ABNORMAL FINDINGS
Inspection (Have client void before the examination.)		

(continued)

AREA/PA SKILL	NORMAL FINDINGS	ABNORMAL FINDINGS
Inspection *External Genitalia*		
Note color, hair distribution, condition of skin, swelling, lesions, polyps, discharge or odor, prolapse, and pediculosis.	External genitalia intact, pink and moist; color depends on client's pigmentation. Hair distribution depends on age and development of client No lesions, edema, discharge , odor, or prolapse (bladder, uterus, or rectum) Normal cervical discharge depends on menstrual cycle: Clear and stretchy before ovulation, white and opaque after, bloody during menstruation	Diamond-shaped hair distribution pattern is abnormal if not associated with cultural or familial differences. May be hirsutism, indicating an endocrine disorder Pubic lice, nits, or flecks of residual blood on skin: Pediculosis pubis Ecchymosis over mons pubis: Blunt trauma Labial varicosities: Pregnancy or uterine tumor Edema: Hematoma formation, obstruction of lymphatic system, or Bartholin's cyst Broken areas of skin surface: Ulcerations or abrasions from infection or trauma Rash over mons pubis and labia is abnormal Painless, reddish, round ulcer with depressed center, raised with indurated edges (chancre): Primary stage of syphilis White, dry, painless growths with narrow bases: Condylomata acuminata (venereal warts) caused by human papillomavirus (HPV) *(continued)*

AREA/PA SKILL	NORMAL FINDINGS	ABNORMAL FINDINGS
Inspection *External Genitalia (Continued)*		
Examine clitoris.	Clitoris about 2 cm long and 0.5 cm in diameter. No redness or lesions	Small, red, painful vesicles that progress to the ulcer stage: Herpes simplex. Pruritus may be present Hypertrophy of clitoris: Female pseudohermaphroditism from androgen excess Female circumcision is widespread in many African countries and among some Muslim groups
Inspect urethral meatus for shape, color, and size.	Urethral opening is slitlike, midline, and free of discharge, swelling, redness, or lesions.	Discharge of any color from urethral meatus: Urinary tract infection Swelling or redness around meatus: Infection of Skene's glands, urethral caruncle, urethral carcinoma, or prolapse of urethral mucosa
Inspect introitus for color and moistness of mucosa, discharge or odor, patency, bulging, or tenderness.	Introitus mucosa is pink, moist. Normal discharge is clear to white with no foul odors. Introitus is patent, with no bulging or tenderness.	Pale color and dryness of introitus mucosa: Atrophy from topical steroids and aging Foul-smelling discharge that is not clear to slightly pale white is abnormal

(continued)

AREA/PA SKILL	NORMAL FINDINGS	ABNORMAL FINDINGS

Inspection
External Genitalia (Continued)

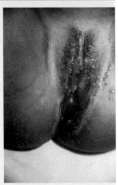

Herpes vulvovaginitis

Gonorrhea, chlamydia, *Candida, Trichomonas,* bacterial vaginosis, atrophic vaginitis, and cervicitis are possible infectious processes that produce an abnormal vaginal discharge

External tear: Trauma from sexual activity or abuse

Fissure: Congenital malformation or childbirth trauma

Bulging of anterior vaginal wall: Cystocele

Bulging of anterior vaginal wall, bladder, and urethra into vaginal introitus: Cystourethrocele

(continued)

AREA/PA SKILL	NORMAL FINDINGS	ABNORMAL FINDINGS
Inspection *External Genitalia (Continued)*		
		Bulging of posterior vaginal wall: Rectocele
Rectal Area		
Note condition of skin, inflammation, rashes, excoriation, rectal prolapse, external hemorrhoids, polyps, lesions, fissures, bleeding, discharge.	Rectal area intact, no inflammation, lesions, prolapse, hemorrhoids, discharge, or bleeding.	Fissure or tear of perineum: Trauma, abscess, or unhealed episiotomy. Venous prominences around anal area: External hemorrhoids
Pelvic Examination with Speculum (Use warm speculum)		
Note color, lesions, discharge, bleeding, position, size, shape and symmetry of cervix, shape and patency of os. Obtain specimens as indicated.	Cervix round, midline, pink, no lesions or discharge; os is slit in parous women, round and closed in nulliparous women. Bluish color seen with pregnancy, paler color seen in postmenopausal women	Cyanosis without pregnancy: Venous congestion or systemic hypoxia as in congestive heart failure (CHF) Redness or a friable cervix: Infection and inflammation (e.g., chlamydia or gonorrhea) Lateral positioning of cervix: Tumor or adhesions Projection of cervix into vaginal vault >2.5 cm: Uterine prolapse Cervical size >4 cm: Hypertrophy from inflammation or tumor A reddish circle around the os may be abnormal Ectropion or eversion: Lacerations during childbirth or congenital variation

(continued)

AREA/PA SKILL	NORMAL FINDINGS	ABNORMAL FINDINGS

Inspection
Pelvic Examination with Speculum (Use warm speculum)
(Continued)

Small, round, yellow lesions: Nabothian cysts, benign cysts from obstruction of cervical glands

Bright red, soft protrusions through the cervical os: Polyps; they are abnormal

Hemorrhages over the surface: Strawberry spots, associated with trichomonal infection

Unilateral transverse, bilateral transverse, stellate, or irregular cervical os: Caused by cervical tears occurring during rapid second-stage childbirth delivery, forceps delivery, or trauma

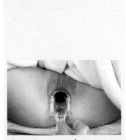

Inserting speculum

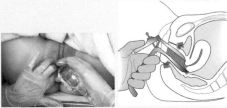

Proper position of speculum in vagina

Greenish yellow mucopurulent discharge that adheres to vaginal walls, with pus in os: Gonococcal infection

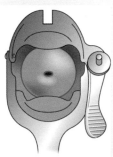

View through speculum

Opening speculum

White, cottage-cheeselike discharge that adheres to vaginal walls, with patches of discharge on os: *Candida* infection

(continued)

AREA/PA SKILL	NORMAL FINDINGS	ABNORMAL FINDINGS
Inspection *Pelvic Examination with Speculum (Use warm speculum)* *(Continued)*		
Inspect the vaginal walls while withdrawing the speculum.	Vaginal walls pink with rugae, no lesions	Grayish-yellow, purulent, often bubbly discharge that smells fishy and often pools in fornix: *Trichomonas;* cervix may show red spots
		White spots on vaginal wall: Leukoplakia from *Candida albicans.* Repeated occurrences may indicate HIV infection
		Pallor of vaginal walls: Anemia or menopause
		Redness of vaginal walls: Inflammation, hyperemia, or trauma from tampon insertion or removal
		Vaginal lesions or masses: Carcinoma, tumors, and diethylstilbestrol (DES) exposure

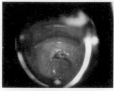

Chadwick's sign

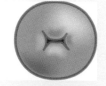

A   B
(A) Nulliparous cervical os; (B) Parous cervical os

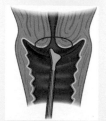

Taking an endocervical smear   *Taking a cervical smear*

(continued)

AREA/PA SKILL	NORMAL FINDINGS	ABNORMAL FINDINGS
Palpation (Lubricate index and middle fingers of gloved hand. Vaginal exam performed first, then rectovaginal exam can be performed.) *Skene's Glands and Bartholin's Glands Usually performed before speculum insertion. Insert index finger into vagina with finger pad upward, milk urethra and Skene's gland.*		
Note any masses, swelling, discharge, or tenderness.	Area smooth, no swelling, discharge, masses, or tenderness.	Swelling, redness, induration, or purulent discharge from labial folds with hot, tender areas: Bartholin's gland infection from gonococci and *Chlamydia trachomatis* Pain and discharge from urethra: Skene's gland infection or urinary tract infection
Vaginal Walls		
Note texture, swelling, lesions, tenderness.	Vaginal walls have rugae; no swelling, lesions, nodules, or tenderness. Fewer rugae in postmenopausal women.	Significantly diminished or absent vaginal muscle tone and bulging of vagina: Injury, age, childbirth, medication Bulging: Cystocele, rectocele, or uterine prolapse Lesions, masses, scarring, or cysts: Benign lesions (e.g., inclusion cysts, myomas, or fibromas) or malignant ones. Most common site for malignant lesions of vagina in upper one third of posterior wall

(continued)

AREA/PA SKILL	NORMAL FINDINGS	ABNORMAL FINDINGS
Palpation *Perineum*		
Assess tone and texture.	Perineum is smooth, firm, and homogeneous in nulliparous women; thinner in parous women	Thin perineum, fissures, or tears: Atrophy, trauma, or unhealed episiotomy
Cervix		
Note size, shape, consistency, position, mobility, tenderness.	Cervix round, smooth, firm, midline, mobile, and nontender Cervix smaller in older women. Cervix softer and enlarged during pregnancy. Softening of cervix (Goodell's sign) seen at the fifth to sixth week of pregnancy	Pain on palpation or when assessing mobility (presence of chandelier sign or cervical motion tenderness): PID or ectopic pregnancy Irregular surface, immobility, or nodular surface of cervix: Malignancy, nabothian cysts, or polyps Nodules or irregularities on fornices: Malignancy, polyps, herniations
Uterus		
Note size, shape, symmetry, position, masses, tenderness. *Palpating the uterus*	Uterus midline; may be anteflexed or anteverted, midplane, retroflexed or retroverted. Size and shape depend on parity: pear-shaped in nongravid, more rounded in parous women; size increases with pregnancy. Firm, mobile, slightly tender. No masses	Enlargement and changes in uterine shape: Intrauterine pregnancy or tumor Nodule: Myomas, tumors containing muscle tissue A retroverted and retroflexed uterus can only be assessed rectovaginally

(continued)

AREA/PA SKILL	NORMAL FINDINGS	ABNORMAL FINDINGS
Palpation *Ovaries*		
Note size, shape, symmetry, tenderness. 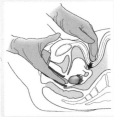 *Palpating the ovaries*	Ovaries nonpalpable; or if palpable, almond shape, firm, smooth, about 3 × 2 × 1 cm, mobile, sensitive to palpation. Ovaries are not palpable in postmenopausal women or prepubertal girls.	Enlarged, irregular, nodular, painful, immobile ovaries: Ectopic pregnancy, ovarian cyst, PID, or malignancy

Anus and Rectum (Vaginal examination performed first, then rectovaginal examination. Remember to change gloves before rectovaginal examination to prevent cross-contamination.)

Perform rectal examination and note sphincter tone, pain, tenderness, nodules, lesions, masses, hemorrhoids, polyps, bleeding.	+ sphincter tone, nontender, no masses, polyps, lesions, hemorrhoids, or bleeding	Masses or lesions: Malignancy or internal hemorrhoids Lax sphincter tone: Perineal trauma from childbirth or anal intercourse, or neurological disorders
Note color of stool; test for occult blood.	Stool brown; negative for occult blood	

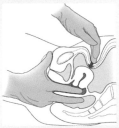

Proper position of hands

PA = physical assessment

CHAPTER 11

ASSESSING THE MALE GENITOURINARY SYSTEM

Primary Functions

- Manufacturing and protecting sperm for fertilization
- Transporting sperm
- Regulating hormonal production and secretion of male sex hormones
- Providing sexual pleasure
- Excreting urine

Developmental Considerations

Infants

- Premature infants may have undescended testes and few rugae.
- Breech-delivered infants may have scrotal edema and ecchymoses.
- Hydroceles and hernias are common findings in boys younger than age 2.
- Decision to circumcise is culturally based.

Children and Adolescents

- Tanner staging, characterizing pubic hair distribution and penile and testicular size, is used to track sexual maturation during puberty.

MATURATION STATES IN BOYS

STAGE	PUBIC HAIR	PENIS	TESTES AND SCROTUM
Stage 1: Preadolescent	No pubic hair except for fine body hair similar to that on abdomen.	Same size and proportions as in childhood.	Same size and proportions as in childhood.
Stage 2	Sparse growth of long, slightly pigmented, downy hair, straight or only slightly curled, chiefly at base of penis.	Slight or no enlargement.	Testes larger; scrotum larger, somewhat reddened, and altered in texture.
Stage 3	Darker, coarser, curlier hair spreading sparsely over pubic symphysis.	Larger, especially in length	Further enlarged
Stage 4	Coarse and curly hair, as in adult; area covered greater than in stage 3 but not as great as in adult.	Further enlarged in length and breadth, with development of glans.	Further enlarged; scrotal skin darkened.
Stage 5	Hair same as adult in quantity and quality, spread to medial surfaces of thighs but not up over abdomen.	Adult in size and shape.	Adult in size and shape.

Older Adults

- Pubic hair thins on the external genitalia.
- Penis appears atrophic and testicles smaller and slightly softer than in a younger man.
- Prostate may feel larger than in a younger client.
- Scrotal sac loses its elasticity.
- Reduction in testosterone levels occurs by age 50 years.
- Although sperm output may be decreased, normal spermatogenesis is present in most men until age 70.
- Prevalence of impotence increases markedly with aging.

Cultural Considerations

- Decision to circumcise is culturally based.
- United States has a higher rate of newborn male circumcisions than Canada, England, or Sweden, where circumcision is considered unnecessary.
- Native Americans and Hispanics have no tradition to practice circumcision.
- Jews and Muslims practice circumcision as part of their religious value system.

Assessment

History

SYMPTOMS ("PQRST" ANY + SYMPTOM)
- Pain
  - Do you have pain in your penis, scrotum, testes, or groin? If so, please describe the pain (pain assessment pattern).
  - Have you noticed any pain or burning when urinating?
  - When did the pain first begin?
- Lesions
  - Have you noticed any blisters, ulcers, sores, warts, or rashes on your penis, scrotum, or surrounding areas? If so, please describe them.
  - When did you first notice the lesion?
  - Has the appearance of the lesion changed?
  - Is the lesion painful?
  - Did you have a painful lesion that healed?

- Has anyone you have been intimate with told you they had a sexually transmitted disease (STD)?
- Swelling
  - Have you felt any lumps, swelling, or masses in the scrotum, genital, or groin area? If so, describe it and its location. Was the onset gradual or sudden?
  - Have you noticed any heaviness or dragging feeling in the scrotum?
  - When did you first notice the lumps, swelling, or masses?
  - Is tenderness present?
  - If you exert pressure on the lumps or masses, do they disappear?
- Discharge
  - Have you noticed any unusual discharge from your penis? If so, what color is the discharge?
  - Is there any odor to the discharge?
  - Is it a small, moderate, or large amount?
  - Is there any burning or pain with the discharge?
- Genitourinary symptoms
  - Do you ever have blood in your urine? If so, when or how often?
  - Describe the color of your urine.
  - How many times do you wake during the night to urinate?
  - Have you had any changes in your voiding pattern (i.e., frequency)?
  - Have you ever had kidney stones?

SEXUAL HISTORY
- Have you ever been sexually active?
- Are you currently sexually active? That is, have you had sex with anyone in the past few months? If the answer is yes, answer next question.
- Do you have sex with men, women, or both (heterosexual, homosexual, or bisexual)?
- Type of sexual activity (oral or anal)?
- Do you have more than one partner? How many partners have you had in the last 6 months?
- Are you using birth control? What kind? How often?
- Are you worried about the AIDS virus or other sexually transmitted diseases (STDs)?

- Do you take any precautions to avoid infections? If so, what?
- Do you have any problems or concerns about your sexual function?
- Have you had surgery on any of your reproductive organs? If so, what and when?
- Have you been taught to examine your testes?
- Are you taking any medications, prescribed or over the counter (Table 11–1)?

Table 11–1. *Drugs That Adversely Affect the Male Genitourinary System*

DRUG CLASS	DRUG	POSSIBLE ADVERSE REACTIONS
Antiandrogen	finasteride	Impotence
Antianxiety/ sedative	benzodiazepines, chlordiazepoxide	Changes in libido
Anticholinergic	atropine	Impotence
Antidepressants	tricyclic anti- depressants (e.g., amitriptyline)	Increased/decreased libido and impotence
	trazodone	Decreased libido, impotence, priapism, retrograde ejaculation
	selective serotonin reuptake inhibitors (e.g., fluoxetine)	Decreased libido, delayed orgasm, anorgasmia, ejaculatory dysfunction
Antiepileptic	primidone	Impotence
Antihypertensive	methyldopa	Ejaculatory failure
	prazosin	Impotence
	clonidine	Impotence, decreased sexual activity, decreased libido
Antihypertensives/ antianginal	beta blockers, atenolol, labetalol, propranolol, nadolol	Impotence, decreased libido
Antihyper- lipidemics	simvastatin	Impotence
Antipsychotics	all antipsychotics	Priapism, impotence, ejaculatory inhibition
Diuretics	chlorothiazide, spironolactone	Impotence
Estrogen	conjugated estrogen	Impotence, testicular atrophy
Tranquilizers	diazepam, alprazolam	Changes in libido

ERECTILE DYSFUNCTION
- Have you maintained an interest in sex?
- Are you able to achieve and maintain an erection?
- Do you have morning erections?
- Were there any changes in your relationship with your partner or in your life situation when the problem began?
- How long does intercourse last?
- Do you sometimes feel that you cannot ejaculate?
- Are you satisfied with your sex life as it is now?

Assessment of Male Genitourinary System's Relationship to Other Systems

Remember, all systems are related! As you assess the male genitourinary system, look at the relationship between it and all other systems.

SUBJECTIVE DATA	OBJECTIVE DATA
Area/System: General	
Ask about:	*Measure:*
Changes in energy level, weight	Vital signs, checking for
Fevers	temperature elevations, hypertension (HTN)
	Note:
	Signs of discomfort
	Affect
Area/System: Integumentary	
Ask about:	*Inspect for:*
Changes in hair growth	Skin lesions
Rashes, lesions	Hair distribution
	Areas of alopecia
HEENT	
Ask about:	*Palpate:*
Swollen glands/nodes	Lymph node enlargement
Eye drainage	Thyroid enlargement
Sore throat	*Inspect:*
Oral lesions	Conjunctiva for drainage
	Oral mucosa for redness and lesions
Area/System: Respiratory	
Ask about:	*Inspect for:*
History of respiratory disease	Signs of respiratory distress
	Auscultate:
	Abnormal breath sounds

(continued)

SUBJECTIVE DATA	OBJECTIVE DATA
Area/System: Cardiovascular	
Ask about:	*Inspect for:*
History of cardiovascular disease (CVD), HTN, congestive heart failure (CHF)	Signs of impaired circulation Skin changes
	Palpate:
	Pulses, edema
	Auscultate:
	Extra heart sounds
Area/System: Gastrointestinal	
Ask about:	*Inspect for:*
History of liver disease	Ascites
	Palpate/percuss:
	Liver enlargement
Area/System: Breasts	
	Inspect :
	Gynecomastia
Area/System: Musculoskeletal	
Ask about:	*Test:*
Weakness, limitations	Muscle strength
Joint pain, swelling	*Inspect:*
	Joint swelling and deformity
Area/System: Neurological	
Ask about:	*Test for:*
History of neurological problems	Changes in mental status, affect
Paralysis	Sensory deficits
Tremors	
Personality changes	
Depression	
Area/System: Endocrine	
Ask about:	
History of thyroid disease and diabetes	
Area/System: Lymphatic/Hematological	
Ask about:	
History of HIV, AIDS, sickle cell anemia	

HEENT = head, eyes, ears, nose, and throat

Physical Assessment

APPROACH: Inspection, palpation, auscultation; external and rectal exam

POSITION: Standing

TOOLBOX: Nonsterile gloves, water-soluble lubricant, penlight, stethoscope, Culturette tube, sterile cotton swabs,

1½-2″ gauze wrap, 5% acetic acid solution in a spray bottle, and Thayer-Martin plate.

AREA/PA SKILL	NORMAL FINDINGS	ABNORMAL FINDINGS
Inspection *Have client void before examination.* **Penis**		
Inspect dorsal, lateral, and ventral sides. Note condition of skin, color lesions, discharge. Note size in relation to physical development and age. Note position of urinary meatus. Note presence of foreskin or circumcised. If uncircumcised, retract foreskin; note ease of retraction and presence of lesions.	Skin intact, color pink to light brown in Caucasians, light to dark brown in Blacks; no lesions or discharge Urinary meatus midline at tip of glans Foreskin retracts easily	Sparse or absent hair in genital area: Genetic factors (e.g., developmental defects and hereditary disorders), aging, local or systemic disease (e.g., infection, neoplasms, endocrine diseases, nutritional or metabolic deficiencies), physical or chemical agents, destruction of or damage to hair follicles Painless, ulcerated, exudative, papular lesion with an erythematous halo, surrounding edema, and a friable base: Chancre, the lesion of primary syphilis Pinhead papules to cauliflower-like groupings of painful, filiform, skin-colored, pink, or red lesions: Chancroid; caused by *Haemophilus* through small breaks in epidermal tissue *(continued)*

AREA/PA SKILL	NORMAL FINDINGS	ABNORMAL FINDINGS

Inspection
Penis (Continued)

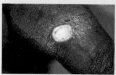
Chancre

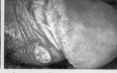
Chancroid

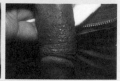
Genital warts on penis

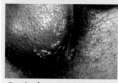
Genital warts on scrotum

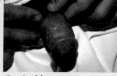
Genital herpes

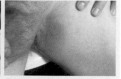
Tinea cruris

Multifocal, wartlike, maculopapular lesions—tan, brown, pink, violet, or white: Condylomata acuminatum (genital warts); caused by HPV infection

Erythematous plaques with scaling, papular lesions with sharp margins and occasionally clear centers and pustules: *Candida* infection

Painful eruptions of pustules and vesicles that rupture: Herpes simplex virus I and II (accompanying symptoms: Fever, headache, dysuria, dyspareunia, and urinary retention)

(continued)

AREA/PA SKILL	NORMAL FINDINGS	ABNORMAL FINDINGS
Inspection *Penis (Continued)*		
		Tinea cruris ("jock itch"): Fungal infection of groin
		Foreskin unable to retract; may become swollen: Phimosis
		Priapism: Leukemia, metastatic carcinoma, or sickling hemoglobinopathies
		Ventral or dorsal curvature of penis: Chordee (ventral chordee seen mostly with epispadias)
		Urethral meatus opens on dorsal side of glans on shaft of penis: Epispadias
		Urethral meatus opens on ventral side of glans on shaft of penis: Hypospadias
Scrotum		
Note color, hair distribution, lesions, swelling, size, and position.	Skin color darker than rest of body. Hair distribution appropriate for age of client	Scrotal swelling: Inguinal hernia, hydrocele, varicocele, spermatocele, tumor, edema
	Testes hang freely, left testis slightly lower than right	Erythema and swelling are abnormal
Note pubic pediculosis.	No lesions, pediculosis	Nontender accumulation of fluid between two layers of tunica vaginalis: Hydrocele; idiopathic or from

(continued)

AREA/PA SKILL	NORMAL FINDINGS	ABNORMAL FINDINGS
Inspection *Scrotum (Continued)*		
		trauma, inguinal surgery, epididymitis, or tumor. Mass transilluminate Nontender, well-defined cystic mass on superior testis or epididymis: Spermatocele; from blockage of efferent ductules of rete testis Varicose veins of spermatic cord that feel like a "bag of worms" and slowly collapse when scrotum is elevated: Varicocele, caused by dilated veins in pampiniform plexus of spermatic cord. Right-sided may indicate obstruction at vena cava Round, firm, nontender cutaneous cyst confined to scrotal skin: Sebaceous cyst from decrease in localized circulation and closure of sebaceous glands or ducts
Inguinal Area		
Note condition of skin, bulges. Have client bear down, and inspect again for any bulges. Note enlarged lymph nodes.	Skin intact, no bulges, no palpable lymph nodes	Bulge: Hernia or enlarged lymph node

(continued)

AREA/PA SKILL	NORMAL FINDINGS	ABNORMAL FINDINGS

Inspection
Inguinal Area (Continued)

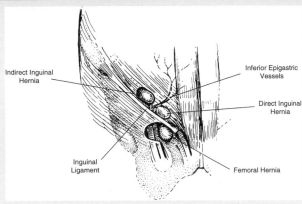

Location of indirect and direct femoral and inguinal hernias

Rectal Area

Note condition of skin, inflammation, rashes, excoriation, rectal prolapse, external hemorrhoids, polyps, lesions, fissures, bleeding, discharge.	Rectal area intact; no inflammation, lesions, prolapse, hemorrhoids, discharge, or bleeding	STD lesions, warts, hemorrhoids, fissures, bleeding, rectal prolapse

Palpation
Maintain standard precautions; wear gloves.

Penis

Use thumb and two fingers to palpate shaft		
Note consistency, tenderness, induration, masses, or nodules.	Nonerect penis soft, nontender, no nodules	Diminished/absent palpable pulse or pulsations: Possible vascular insufficiency. Normal blood flow may be affected by systemic disease or localized trauma or disease

(continued)

AREA/PA SKILL	NORMAL FINDINGS	ABNORMAL FINDINGS
Palpation *Penis (Continued)*		
		Priapism: Spinal cord lesions or sickle cell anemia
		Phimosis or paraphimosis (foreskin retracts but does not return). ***Seek immediate assistance if foreskin cannot be retracted. Prolonged constriction of vessels can constrict blood flow and lead to necrosis***
		Purulent discharge or mucus shreds: Bacterial infection of genitourinary tract; causes inflammation with leukocytes, shedding tissue cells, and bacteria
Scrotum, Testes, and Epididymis		
Use thumb and two fingers to palpate scrotum.		
Palpate surface characteristics of scrotum. Note size, shape, consistency, mobility, masses, nodules, tenderness of testes.	Scrotal skin rough without lesions. Testes rubbery, round, movable, smooth, 2 cm × 5 cm in size, slight tenderness with compression	Unilateral mass within or about testicle is abnormal. Intratesticular masses are nodular and painless. They should be considered malignant until proven otherwise. Testicle enlarged, retracted, in a lateral position, and extremely sensitive: Testicular torsion

(continued)

AREA/PA SKILL	NORMAL FINDINGS	ABNORMAL FINDINGS
Palpation *Scrotum, Testes, and Epididymis (Continued)*		
		Abnormal for one or both testes to be undescended. Absence of testes and epididymis in scrotal sac: Cryptorchidism; related to testicular failure, deficient gonadotrophic stimulation, mechanical obstruction, or gubernacular defects. Because undescended testes have a histologic change by age 6, referral should take place as early as possible. Acute, painful onset of swelling of testicle, with warm scrotal skin: Orchitis. Testes may feel heavy in the scrotum Atrophic testicle and scrotal edema are abnormal Red glow with transillumination: Serous fluid within scrotal sac; seen in hydrocele and spermatocele
Palpate epididymis and vas deferens on the posterolateral surface. Note swelling or nodules. Transilluminate any lumps, nodules, or edematous areas.	Ridge of epididymis noted, and vas deferens smooth and movable. No swelling or nodules	Abnormal to palpate indurated, swollen, tender epididymis

(continued)

AREA/PA SKILL	NORMAL FINDINGS	ABNORMAL FINDINGS
Palpation *Inguinal Area*		
Palpate for inguinal and femoral hernias or masses. Have client bear down or cough as you palpate for a bulge or hernia.	No inguinal or femoral hernias or masses	Mass that comes down inguinal canal and is palpable at inguinal ring or in scrotum: Indirect inguinal hernia Mass that enlarges with coughing: Direct inguinal hernia Mass palpated in medial to femoral vessels and inferior to inguinal ligament: Femoral hernia *A strangulated hernia is a surgical emergency*
Palpate inguinal lymph nodes.	No palpable nodes	Unilateral enlargement of lymph nodes along with erythematous skin: Bacterial infections Unilateral or bilateral enlargement of inguinal lymph nodes, tender or painless: Bacterial infections or malignancy

Internal inguinal ring   Inguinal canal

Inguinal ligament   External inguinal ring   Femoral artery   Femoral vein

Palpating for inguinal and femoral hernias

(continued)

AREA/PA SKILL	NORMAL FINDINGS	ABNORMAL FINDINGS
Palpation *Anus and Rectum*		
Have client bend over exam table or assume side-lying position. Note sphincter tone, pain, tenderness, nodules, lesions, masses, hemorrhoids, polyps, bleeding. Note color of stool; test for occult blood.	+ Sphincter tone, nontender, no masses, polyps, lesions, hemorrhoids, or bleeding. Stool brown; negative for occult blood.	Fissure, warts, hemorrhoids, bleeding, rectal prolapse
Prostate		
Note size, shape, symmetry, mobility, consistency, nodules, tenderness. Grading scale for prostate gland: Grade I: <1-cm protrusion into rectum Grade II: 1- to 2-cm protrusion into rectum Grade III: 2- to 3-cm protrusion into rectum Grade IV: >3 cm protrusion into rectum	Prostate is shape and size of walnut, smooth, rubbery, nontender	Soft, nontender, enlarged prostate: Benign prostatic hypertrophy; related to aging and presence of dihydroxytestosterone Firm, tender, or fluctuant mass on prostate: Acute bacterial prostatitis or urinary tract infection; client at risk for prostatic abscess Firm, hard, or indurated nodule(s) on prostate: Possible prostate cancer Extremely tender, warm prostate: Bacterial prostatitis. If suspected, do not vigorously palpate, because of possibility of bacteremia

(continued)

AREA/PA SKILL	NORMAL FINDINGS	ABNORMAL FINDINGS
Palpation *Prostate (Continued)*		

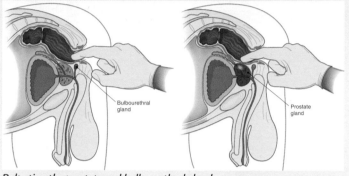

Palpating the prostate and bulbourethral glands

Auscultation *Scrotum*		
If scrotal mass detected, auscultate the scrotum for bowel sounds.	No bowel sounds	Bowel sounds in scrotum: Indirect inguinal hernia

PA = physical assessment

CHAPTER 12

ASSESSING THE MOTOR-MUSCULOSKELETAL SYSTEM

Primary Functions

- Provides shape and support to the body
- Allows for movement
- Protects the internal organs
- Produces red blood cells (hematopoiesis)
- Stores calcium and phosphorus in the bones

Developmental Considerations

Infants and Children

- Rapid growth periods occur during infancy and adolescence.
- Longitudinal bone growth continues until closure of the epiphyses, at age 20.
- Infant has C-shaped spine.
- Toddler has wide base of support while learning to walk.
- Toddlers with "potbellies" often have a postural lordosis.
- Common knee deviations include genu valgum (knock knees) and genu varum (bowlegs).
- Scoliosis often becomes apparent during adolescence; more common in girls than in boys

Pregnant Clients

- Postural lordosis with anterior cervical flexion (kyphosis) occurs in latter part of pregnancy.
- Wide base of support compensates for shifting center of gravity.
- Low back pain is common late in pregnancy.
- Increased mobility of the sacroiliac, sacrococcygeal, and symphysis pubis joints in preparation for delivery contributes to "waddling" gait.

Older Adults

- Muscle changes cause a wider base of support.
- Older adults have increased risk for osteoporosis, especially women.
- Kyphosis occurs with aging.
- Height decreases.
- Body fat is redistributed to abdomen and hips.
- Loss of muscle mass occurs.
- Older adults have a high incidence of degenerative joint disease (DJD).

Cultural Considerations

- African-Americans
  - Tendency toward hyperplasia of connective tissue accounts for increased incidence of lupus erythematosus.
  - Greater bone density than Europeans, Asians, and Hispanics accounts for decreased incidence of osteoporosis.
- Amish
  - Dwarfism syndrome found in nearly all Amish communities
- Chinese-Americans
  - Generally shorter than Westerners
  - Bone structure also differs from that of Westerners:
    - *Ulna longer than radius*
    - *Hip measurements smaller (women 4.14 cm smaller; men 7.6 cm smaller)*

- *Bone length shorter*
- *Bone density less*
- Egyptian-Americans
  - Relatively short in stature. Average height for men 5′ 10″; for women 5′4″
- Filipino-Americans
  - Short in stature. Average height ranges from 5″ to average American size
- Irish-Americans
  - Taller and broader than average European-American and Asian
  - Hip width greater
  - Bone density less than African-Americans
- Navajo Native Americans
  - Taller and thinner than other American tribes
  - Noted for being good runners
- Vietnamese-Americans
  - Small in stature. Average height 5′ for women, with men being a few inches taller

Assessment

History

SYMPTOMS ("PQRST" ANY + SYMPTOM)
- Pain
  - When did you first become aware of the pain?
  - Where do you feel the pain? Point to the area where you feel the pain.
  - How would you describe the pain—for instance, dull, aching, burning, stabbing, or throbbing?
  - When you have this pain, do you also have pain in any other location?
  - When did the pain begin? What were you doing at the time it began?
  - Did the pain occur suddenly?
  - Does the pain occur daily?
  - During what part of the day is your pain worse: morning, afternoon, or evening?
  - Did a recent illness precede the pain?
  - What makes the pain worse?
  - What do you do to relieve the pain?

- What kind of medications have you taken to help with the pain?
- Does the pain change according to the weather?
- Do you have difficulty dressing?
- Does the pain interfere with your sleep?
- Does the pain move from one joint to another?
- Has there been an injury, strain, overuse?
- Have you noticed any swelling?
- Do you have any other unusual sensations, such as tingling, with the pain?
- Weakness
  - When did you first notice muscle weakness?
  - Do you have difficulty lifting objects?
  - Do you have difficulty writing with a pen or pencil?
  - Do you have trouble standing up after sitting in a chair?
  - Does the weakness worsen or improve as the day progresses?
  - Have your muscles decreased in size?
  - Is there any pain or stiffness with your weak muscles?
  - Do you have trouble with double vision, swallowing, or chewing?
- Stiffness
  - When did the stiffness begin?
  - Has the stiffness increased since it began?
  - Do you feel stiff only on awakening or all the time?
  - Is pain associated with the stiffness?
  - What methods have you tried to reduce the stiffness?

FOCUSED MUSCULOSKELETAL HISTORY
- Do you have a history of musculoskeletal problems, pain, or disease? If yes, are you taking any medications or undergoing any treatments for these problems?
- Do you have any other medical problems?
- Have any accidents or trauma ever affected your bones or joints?
- Do your joint, muscle, or bone problems limit your usual activities?
- Do you have any occupational hazards that could affect your muscles and joints?
- Have you been immunized for tetanus and polio?

- Do you smoke or consume alcohol or caffeine? If yes, how much and how often?
- Are you taking any medications, prescribed or over the counter (Table 12–1)?

Table 12-1. *Drugs That Adversely Affect the Musculoskeletal System*

DRUG CLASS	DRUG	POSSIBLE ADVERSE REACTIONS
Adrenocorticosteroids	prednisone	Muscle weakness, muscle wasting, osteoporosis, vertebral compression fractures, aseptic necrosis of humeral or femoral heads
Adrenocorticotropic hormone (ACTH)	corticotropin	Muscle weakness, muscle wasting, osteoporosis, vertebral compression fractures, aseptic necrosis of humeral or femoral heads
Anticoagulants	heparin sodium	Bleeding into joints with high dosages
Anticonvulsants	phenytoin sodium	Ataxia, osteomalacia, rickets
Antidepressants	trazodone hydrochloride	Musculoskeletal aches and pains
Antigout agents	colchicine	Myopathy with prolonged administration
Antilipemic agents	clofibrate	Acute flulike muscular syndrome characterized by myalgia or myositis with symptoms of muscle cramps, weakness, and arthralgia
Benzodiazepines	diazepam	Ataxia
Central nervous system stimulants	amphetamine sulfate	Increased motor activity
Diuretics	bumetanide, furosemide	Muscle cramps
Phenothiazines	chlorpromazine hydrochloride	Extrapyramidal symptoms (dystonic reactions, motor restlessness, and Parkinsonian signs and symptoms)
Miscellaneous skin agents	isotretinoin	Bone or joint pain, general muscle aches

Assessment of Musculoskeletal System's Relationship to Other Systems

Remember, all systems are related! As you assess the musculoskeletal system, look at the relationship between it and all other systems.

SUBJECTIVE DATA	OBJECTIVE DATA
Area/System: General	
Ask about:	*Measure:*
General health	Vital signs
Weight gain	Height and weight
Height loss	
Fever	
Area/System: Integumentary	
Ask about:	*Inspect for:*
Rashes	Rashes, lesions, alopecia
Hair loss	
HEENT	
Ask about:	*Inspect:*
Swollen glands	Eyes for redness
Dry, red eyes	*Palpate:*
	Lymph nodes, thyroid
Area/System: Respiratory	
Ask about:	*Auscultate:*
Breathing difficulty	Lungs
Area/System: Cardiovascular	
Ask about:	*Auscultate:*
History of cardiovascular	Heart sounds
problems	
Area/System: Gastrointestinal	
Ask about:	*Auscultate:*
Nausea, vomiting, diarrhea	Bowel sounds
Area/System: Genitourinary/Reproductive	
Ask about:	*Inspect for:*
History of sexually transmitted	Lesions
diseases	
Menopausal women:	
Hormone replacement therapy	
Area/System: Neurological	
Ask about:	*Test:*
Changes in sensation	Sensory deficits, paralysis
Numbness, tingling	
Area/System: Endocrine	
Ask about:	
History of diabetes mellitus,	
thyroid disease	

SUBJECTIVE DATA	OBJECTIVE DATA
Area/System: Lymphatic/Hematological	
Ask about:	
Bruising	

HEENT = head, eyes, ears, nose, and throat

Physical Assessment

ANATOMICAL LANDMARKS: Types of joints (Table 12–2).

APPROACH: Inspection, palpation

POSITION: Standing, sitting, supine

TOOLBOX: Tape measure and goniometer

Table 12-2. *Types of Synovial Joints*

DESCRIPTION	EXAMPLE/MOVEMENT
Pivot	
Permits rotation in one axis. Axis is longitudinal, with bone moving around a central axis without any displacement from that axis.	*Proximal radioulnar joint* Supination, pronation, and rotation
Hinge	
Allows movement in only one axis, namely flexion or extension, with axis situated transversely.	*Elbow, knee* Flexion and extension
Condyloid	
Permits movement in two axes. Described as an "egg-in-spoon joint," with long diameter of oval serving as one axis, and short diameter of oval serving as other axis.	*Wrist* Flexion, extension, abduction, adduction, and circumduction
Saddle	
Has two axislike condyloid joints. Articular surfaces are saddle shaped and move in similar fashion to condyloid joint.	*Thumb* Abduction, adduction, opposition, and reposition

(continued)

Table 12–2. *Types of Synovial Joints (Continued)*	
DESCRIPTION	**EXAMPLE/MOVEMENT**
Ball and Socket Moves across many possible axes. Articular surfaces are reciprocal segments of a sphere.	*Shoulder and hip* Flexion, extension, internal rotation, external rotation, abduction, adduction, and circumduction
Plane/Gliding Moves across many axes. Articular surfaces are flat, and one bone rides over the other in many directions.	*Patellofemoral and acromioclavicular joints, some carpal and tarsal bones, and articular vertebral processes* Limited movement in many directions

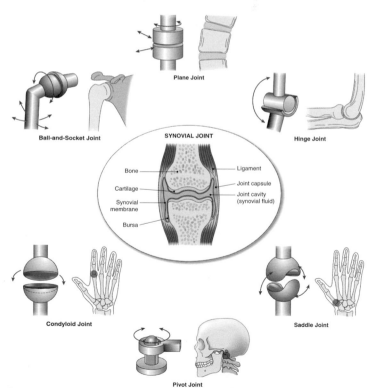

Types of synovial joints

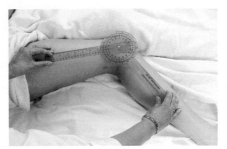

Using a goniometer

AREA/PA SKILL	NORMAL FINDINGS	ABNORMAL FINDINGS
Inspection *Posture and Spinal Curves*		
Note posture in relation to environment, head position, body alignment.	Posture erect, head midline	
Note knee position, draw imaginary line from anterior superior iliac crest through knee to feet.	Knees aligned with no valgus or varus deviation	Knees touch and medial malleoli are 2–3 cm or more apart: Genu valgum Knees are >2.5 cm (1″) apart and medial malleoli touch: Genu varum
Inspect normal curves of the spine (cervical, thoracic, lumbar, and sacral). **Determine if spinal deformities are structural or functional (postural).** Test for kyphosis and scoliosis by having client bend from waist. **In true structural scoliosis, deviation is apparent when client bends at waist. In functional scoliosis, deviation disappears.**	Normal spinal curves noted; no kyphosis, scoliosis, or lordosis 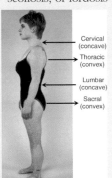 Cervical (concave) Thoracic (convex) Lumbar (concave) Sacral (convex) *Assessing for normal curves*	Spinal deformities include: • Kyphosis: Accentuated thoracic curve • Scoliosis: Lateral "S" spinal deviation • Lordosis: Accentuated lumbar curve

(continued)

AREA/PA SKILL	NORMAL FINDINGS	ABNORMAL FINDINGS

Inspection
Posture and Spinal Curves (Continued)

Test for lordosis by having client flatten back against wall.

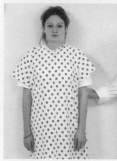

Assessing for lordosis

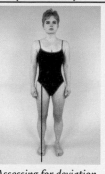

Assessing for deviation of knees

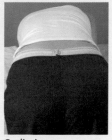

Scoliosis

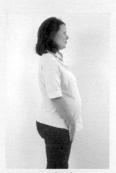

Pregnancy lordosis

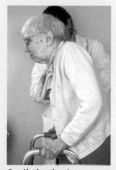

Senile kyphosis

(continued)

AREA/PA SKILL	NORMAL FINDINGS	ABNORMAL FINDINGS
Inspection *Gait*		
(Inspect gait as client walks. See Table 12–3.) Note wear of shoes. Note phases of gait, arm swing, cadence, base of support, stride length, toeing. **Wider base of support and shorter stride length often reflect balance problem.**	Shoes worn evenly Phases of gait conform; gait smooth, fluid, rhythmic; arms swing in opposition; no toeing in or out; 2–4″ base of support; 12–14″ stride length Toddler, older adult, obese, or pregnant client may have a wider base of support, shorter stride length, and uneven rhythm	Uneven weight bearing: Associated with joint pain Wide base of support: Cerebellar dysfunction Ataxia, spasticity, and tremors: Parkinson's disease, multiple sclerosis (MS), cerebral palsy (CP) Scissors gait: Disorders of motor cortex or corticospinal tracts (e.g., bilateral spastic paresis) Spastic movements: Upper motor neuron disorders Flaccidity: Lower motor neuron disorders Flaccidity and foot drop: Peripheral nerve disorders
Cerebellar Function		
Balance		
Observe gait, tandem walk (heel to toe), heel-and-toe walk, deep knee bend. Perform Romberg's test. Stand close to client when performing	Coordinated, balanced gait; + tandem walk, heel-and-toe walk, deep knee bend Negative results on Romberg's test	Balance problems: Cerebellar disorder Positive results on Romberg's test: Cerebellar disorder if client has *(continued)*

AREA/PA SKILL	NORMAL FINDINGS	ABNORMAL FINDINGS
Inspection *Cerebellar Function*		
Balance (Continued)		
Romberg's test; client's feet together, eyes opened then closed. Note swaying.		difficulty maintaining balance with eyes open or closed. If client loses balance only when eyes are closed, damage to the dorsal column should be suspected
Coordination		
Test upper extremities using finger-thumb opposition and rapid alternating movements (RAM). Test lower extremities using toe tapping and running heel down shin. **Note dominant side; usually more coordinated.**	Coordination intact. RAM intact bilaterally; + finger-thumb opposition + toe tapping; able to run heel down shin bilaterally	Slowness and awkwardness in performing movements: Cerebellar disorder or motor weakness associated with extrapyramidal disease
Accuracy of Movements		
Assess point-to-point localization with eyes open, then closed.	Point-to-point localization intact bilaterally	Inaccurate movements: Cerebellar disorder
Pronator Drift		
Test with eyes open then closed. Note drifting.	Negative pronator drift	+ pronator drift: Weakness (e.g., hemiparesis, cerebrovascular accident [CVA])

Assessing pronator drift

(continued)

AREA/PA SKILL	NORMAL FINDINGS	ABNORMAL FINDINGS
Inspection ***Cerebellar Function (Continued)***		
Measurements		
Measure arm and leg lengths and circumferences in cm.	Equal arm and leg lengths, or differences not >1 cm	Leg length discrepancies can cause back and hip pain, gait problems, and pseudoscoliosis
Arm lengths: Measure from the acromion process to tip of middle finger. Leg lengths: Measure from anterosuperior iliac crest to medial malleolus. **To ensure accurate circumference measurements, determine midpoint of extremity.**	Equal arm and leg circumferences; note that dominant side may be greater, but not >1 cm difference 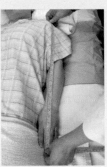 *Measuring arm length*	Equal true leg lengths but unequal apparent leg lengths: Hip and pelvic-area abnormalities Circumference differences >1 cm: Muscular atrophy or hypertrophy

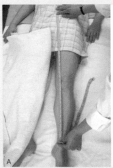 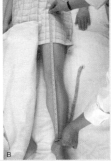

Measuring leg length. A. Apparent, B. True

(continued)

AREA/PA SKILL	NORMAL FINDINGS	ABNORMAL FINDINGS
Palpation *Muscle Tone*		
Palpate muscles of upper and lower extremities in relaxed and contracted state. Note any involuntary movement or tenderness. Note atony, hypotony, or hypertony of muscles.	Muscles at rest soft and pliable; contracted, +muscle tone and firm No involuntary movements or tenderness No atony, hypotony, or unexplained hypertony	Atrophy, unexplained hypertrophy, atony, weakness, fasciculations, tremors
Muscle Strength		
Screen strength with hand grip and foot push/leg raise. Test muscle strength by noting ability to perform active range of motion (AROM) against resistance for face, neck, shoulders, arms, elbows, hands, wrists, hips, knees, ankles, and feet. Grade strength on 0–5 scale (Table 12–4). **Compare side to side. Note that dominant side may be stronger.** **Inspection/Palpation of Joints** Test muscle strength as you assess range of motion (ROM) of joints. Assess all joints for ROM, condition of skin, erythema, edema, heat, deformity, crepitus, tenderness, and stability.	All muscle groups 4/5–5/5 muscle strength. Hand grip strong and equal. Foot push and leg raise against resistance strong and equal	Weakness: Paralysis, CVA, muscle disease, myasthenia gravis, Guillain-Barré syndrome

(continued)

AREA/PA SKILL	NORMAL FINDINGS	ABNORMAL FINDINGS

Inspection/Palpation of Joints

Depression: Lowering a body part
Elevation: Raising a body part

Retraction: moving backward
Protraction: moving forward

Circumduction: moving in a circular fashion

Opposition   Reposition

Extension: straightening, increasing the joint angle

Flexion: bending, decreasing the joint angle

Abduction: moving away from midline
Adduction: moving toward midline

Internal rotation: turning toward midline

External rotation: turning away from midline

Pronation: turning downward

Supination: turning upward

Eversion: turning outward

Inversion: turning inward

Body movement

Temporomandibular Joint (TMJ)

Assess as for all joints, with attention to crepitus or clicks.	Full AROM (flexion, extension, side to side, protraction, retraction). No tenderness, deformity, crepitus, edema, or erythema	Decreased ROM, tenderness, swelling, crepitus: Arthritis Pain, swelling, popping, clicking, or grating sounds: TMJ dysfunction ***TMJ dysfunction may present as ear pain and headache***

(continued)

AREA/PA SKILL	NORMAL FINDINGS	ABNORMAL FINDINGS
Inspection/Palpation of Joints *Temporomandibular Joint (TMJ) (Continued)*		
		Decreased muscle strength: Muscle and joint disease Pain and spasms: Myofacial pain syndrome Less-than-full contraction: Lesion to cranial nerve V
Cervical Spine (Neck)		
Assess as for all joints.

Note cervical curve. | Full AROM (flexion, extension, hyperextension, rotation, lateral bend). No tenderness, crepitus, erythema, or deformity
Normal cervical curve | A neck not straight and erect is abnormal
Inability to perform ROM because of pain: Cervical disc degenerative disease, spinal cord tumor. Pain may radiate to back, shoulder, or arms
Neck pain associated with weakness/loss of sensation in legs: Cervical spinal cord compression
Inability to perform ROM against resistance: Muscle and joint disease |
| **Scapulae** | | |
| Assess as for all joints.
Note location and symmetry and winging. | Scapula equal over 2nd–7th ribs, no winging | Winging |
| **Ribs** | | |
| Assess as for all joints.
Note condition of ribs. | Ribs firm, continuous, and nontender | Swelling, redness, enlargement, tenderness: Inflammation |

(continued)

AREA/PA SKILL	NORMAL FINDINGS	ABNORMAL FINDINGS
Inspection/Palpation of Joints *Shoulders*		
Assess as for all joints, with attention to stability.	Full AROM (flexion, extension, adduction, abduction, internal/external rotation, circumduction). Joint stable, no deformity, crepitus, or tenderness	Weakness and limited ROM: Torn rotator cuff
Elbows		
Assess as for all joints, with attention to nodules.	Full AROM (flexion, extension, supination, pronation). No nodules, crepitus, tenderness, or swelling	Redness, swelling and tenderness at elbow (olecranon process): Bursitis

Bursitis of elbow

Tennis elbow (lateral epicondylitis): Inflammation of forearm extensors or supinator muscles of fingers and wrist, or tendon attachment to lateral epicondyle or lateral collateral ligament caused by repetitive supination of forearm against resistance

Golf elbow (medial epicondylitis): Same as tennis elbow, except flexor and pronator muscles and tendons are affected

(continued)

AREA/PA SKILL	NORMAL FINDINGS	ABNORMAL FINDINGS
Inspection/Palpation of Joints *Wrists*		
Assess as for all joints.	Full AROM (flexion, extension, hyperextension, radial/ulnar deviation). Joint stable, no crepitus or tenderness	Swelling, tenderness, nodules, ulnar deviation, limited ROM: Rheumatoid arthritis (RA) Nontender, round, enlarged, swollen, fluid-filled cysts on wrists: Ganglion cyst Pain with movement: Tendonitis Pain on extension of wrist against resistance: Epicondylitis Pain on flexion of wrist against resistance: Medial epicondylitis Decreased muscle strength: Muscle and joint disease
If indicated, assess for carpal tunnel syndrome with Tinel sign or Phalen test.	Negative Tinel and Phalen tests	+ Tinel's or Phalen's test: Carpal tunnel syndrome

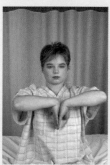
Phalen's test

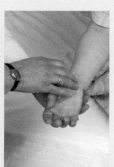
Tinel's test

(continued)

AREA/PA SKILL	NORMAL FINDINGS	ABNORMAL FINDINGS
Inspection/Palpation of Joints *Fingers and Thumbs*		
Assess as for all joints, with attention to deformities. Inspect palmar surface for shape and symmetry.	Full AROM (flexion, extension, hyperextension, abduction, adduction) Nontender, no deformities Palms concave and symmetrical	*Swollen, stiff, tender finger joints:* Acute RA Boutonnière deformity and swan-neck deformity: Long- term RA 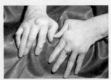 *Rheumatoid arthritis* Atrophy of thenar prominence: Carpal tunnel syndrome Hard, painless nodules over distal interphalangeal joints: Heberden's nodes 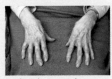 *Heberden's nodes* Hard, painless nodules over proximal interphalangeal joints: Bouchard's nodes Both types of nodes seen in osteoarthritis and RA. Gouty arthritis: Deformities and nodules of hands

(continued)

AREA/PA SKILL	NORMAL FINDINGS	ABNORMAL FINDINGS
Inspection/Palpation of Joints *Fingers and Thumbs (Continued)*		
		Gouty arthritis Pain on extension of a finger: Tenosynovitis Inability to extend ring finger: Dupuytren's contracture Decreased muscle strength: Muscle and joint disease
Thoracic and Lumbar Curves		
Assess as for all joints. Note thoracic and lumbar curves.	Full AROM (flexion, extension, hyperextension, lateral bends, rotation)	Limited ROM related to arthritis, DJD, disc disease of spine
Hips		
Assess as for all joints, with attention to stability.	Full AROM (flexion, extension, hyperextension, internal/external rotation, abduction, adduction) Joint stable, no crepitus, nontender	Unequal gluteal folds: Dislocated hip Inability to abduct hip: Common sign of hip disease Decrease in internal hip rotation: Early sign of hip disease Decreased muscle strength against resistance: Muscle and joint disease + Trendelenburg: Hip dislocation
If indicated, perform Trendelenburg's test for hip dislocation.		

(continued)

AREA/PA SKILL	NORMAL FINDINGS	ABNORMAL FINDINGS

Inspection/Palpation of Joints
Hips (Continued)

If indicated, do Thomas test for hip flexure contraction.	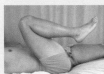 *Straight leg raising*	+ Thomas test: Hip flexure contraction may be hidden by excessive lumbar lordosis
In newborn, do Ortolani's maneuver to test for hip dislocation.		+ Ortolani's maneuver: Hip dislocation
If sciatica is present, do straight leg raise.	*Thomas test*	+ Straight leg: Herniated disc

Knees

Assess as for all joints, with attention to crepitus and swelling.	Full AROM (flexion, extension). Knee stable. No swelling, tenderness, crepitus, nodules	Tenderness, warmth, boggy consistency: Synovitis Crepitation: Osteoarthritis Decreased ROM: Synovial thickening Inability to extend knee fully: Flexion contracture of knee Decreased muscle strength against resistance: Muscle and joint disease
If indicated, do McMurray's and Apley's tests for foreign body, torn meniscus.		+ Apley's and McMurray's tests: Meniscus tear
If indicated, do Lachman test for anterior cruciate ligament (ACL)/posterior cruciate ligament (PCL) tears.		+ Lachman: ACL or PCL tear
If indicated, do bulge sign or patellar tap for fluid.		+ Bulge sign and patellar tap: Fluid

(continued)

AREA/PA SKILL	NORMAL FINDINGS	ABNORMAL FINDINGS

Inspection/Palpation of Joints
Knees (Continued)

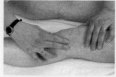
Bulge test

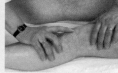
Patellar ballottement

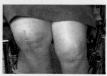
Degenerative joint disease of knees

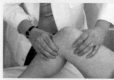
Lachman test

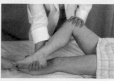
McMurray's test

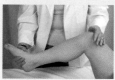
Apley's test

Ankles

Assess as for all joints, with attention to tenderness.	Full AROM (plantarflexion, dorsiflexion, eversion, inversion). No tenderness or crepitus	Nodules on posterior ankle: RA

Feet and Toes

Assess as for all joints, with attention to deformities, corns, bunions, hammer toes, hallux valgus. Note flat feet or high arches. **Look at type of shoes client wears! Many foot problems are**	Full AROM (flexion, extension, hyperextension, dorsiflexion, abduction, adduction). No deformities; longitudinal arch; weight bearing on foot at midline	Hallux valgus often on medial side, may present with laterally deviated great toe with overlapping of second toe Bunion: Enlarged, painful, inflamed bursa, often occurs with hammer toe *(continued)*

AREA/PA SKILL	NORMAL FINDINGS	ABNORMAL FINDINGS
Inspection/Palpation of Joints *Feet and Toes (Continued)*		
caused by poorly fitting shoes.		Hammer toe: Hyperextension of metatarsophalangeal joint and flexion of proximal interphalangeal joint

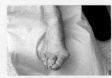

Hallux valgus, bunion, and hammer toe

Flat feet (pes planus): No arches
High arches (pes cavus)
Corns: Painful, thickened skin over bony prominences and pressure points

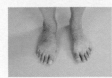

Corns and bunions

Callus: Nonpainful, thickened skin over pressure points

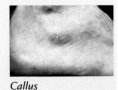

Callus

(continued)

AREA/PA SKILL	NORMAL FINDINGS	ABNORMAL FINDINGS
Inspection/Palpation of Joints *Feet and Toes (Continued)*		
		Plantar warts (verruca vulgaris): Painful warts that occur under a callus
		Tender, painful, reddened, hot, swollen metatarsophalangeal joint of great toe: Gouty arthritis
		Pain and tenderness of metatarsophalangeal joints: DJD, RA, joint inflammation

PA = physical assessment

Table 12–3. *Abnormal Gaits*

TYPE OF GAIT	DESCRIPTION/CAUSE
Propulsive gait	Rigid, stooped posture with head leaning forward and arms, knees, and hips stiffly flexed. Rapid, short, shuffling steps. *Causes:* Classic gait of Parkinson's disease.
Scissors gait	Bilateral spastic paresis of legs; arms not involved. Legs flexed at hip and knees. Knees adduct and meet or cross like scissors. Short steps, foot plantarflexed, walks on toes *Causes:* CP, MS, spinal cord tumors

(continued)

Table 12–3. *Abnormal Gaits (Continued)*

TYPE OF GAIT	DESCRIPTION/CAUSE
Spastic gait (hemiplegic) 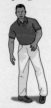	Unilateral stiff, dragging leg from leg, muscle hypertonicity *Causes:* CVA, MS, brain tumor
Steppage gait (equine, prancing, paretic, or weak) 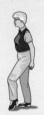	Foot drop with external rotation of hip and hip and knee flexion. Foot slaps when it hits ground *Causes:* MS, herniated lumbar disk, Guillain-Barré syndrome, perineal muscle atrophy, or nerve damage
Waddling gait 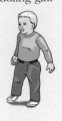	Ducklike walk with wide base of support, chest thrown back, exaggerated lumbar curve (lordosis), and protruding abdomen *Causes:* Normal in toddlers and late stages of pregnancy Weak pelvic girdle muscles (gluteus medius, hip flexors, and extensors) *Causes:* MS, hip dislocation

Table 12-4. *Rating Scale for Muscle Strength*

RATING SCALE	EXPLANATION	CLASSIFICATION
5	Active motion against full resistance	Normal
4	Active motion against some resistance	Slight weakness
3	Active motion against gravity	Average weakness
2	Passive ROM (gravity removed and assisted by examiner)	Poor ROM
1	Slight flicker of contraction	Severe weakness
0	No muscular contraction	Paralysis

CHAPTER 13

ASSESSING THE SENSORY-NEUROLOGICAL SYSTEM

Primary Functions

- Acts as main "circuit board" of the body.
- Allows interaction with the external environment.
- Maintains activities of internal organs.

Developmental Considerations

Newborns and Infants

- Reflexes are primitive because of immature neurological system.
- Injury to the facial nerve during vaginal birth can cause a transient palsy.
- Down syndrome is a genetic disorder that causes mental retardation ranging from mild to severe.
- Maternal use of drugs (including alcohol) during pregnancy, dietary deficiencies, antepartal infections, systemic diseases, and birth trauma can result in neurological disorders such as mental retardation, blindness, deafness, seizures, neuromuscular impairments, and other deficits.

Children and Adolescents

- Later-onset disorders, such as obsessive-compulsive disorder and hyperactivity, may become apparent only during the preschool years.
- Changes in behavior may also signal abuse.
- If the parent reports seizure activity, assess whether or not it is associated with signs of infection, such as a runny nose, high temperature, or recent immunizations. Fevers in toddlers and preschoolers occasionally cause seizures. Repeated episodes of seizure activity may indicate epilepsy.
- Lead poisoning can cause neurological problems in children.
- Diets high in caffeine and sugar may contribute to hyperactivity.

Pregnant Clients

- Folic acid deficiency, especially in the first trimester of pregnancy, is closely linked to neural tube defects, such as spina bifida, in the newborn.
- Transient episodes of neurological pain occur, including carpal tunnel syndrome, foot and leg cramps, numbness or tingling in the thigh, and frequent headaches. They usually resolve after delivery.
- Hyperactive reflexes during pregnancy may suggest the presence of preeclampsia, a hypertensive disorder that can be accompanied by seizures.

Older Adults

- Neural impulses slow.
- Creative, critical, and abstract thinking, as well as problem-solving ability, is more typically *increased* in older adults.
- Neurological deficits in older adults are commonly caused by:
  - Adverse effects of medications or medication interactions
  - Nutritional deficiencies
  - Dehydration

- Cardiovascular disease affecting cerebral perfusion
- Diabetes and other endocrine disorders
- Neurological trauma
- Degenerative neurological diseases, such as Alzheimer's disease and Parkinson's disease
- Alcohol or drug abuse
- Stress, grief, isolation
- Psychiatric disorders
- Abuse or neglect

- The number and sensitivity of sensory neurons decreases in older adults, leading to a diminished sense of touch.
- Reflexes are also diminished: the Achilles tendon reflex may be totally lost in older adults; other deep tendon reflexes should be present, but may be less brisk.

Cultural Considerations

- African-Americans have a higher incidence of hypertension and, subsequently, a higher incidence of stroke.
- Irish-Americans have a high incidence of neural tube defects.
- Navajo Native Americans have a unique neuropathy that causes death by age 24.

Assessment

History

SYMPTOMS ("PQRST" ANY + SYMPTOM)
- Headache
    - Any recent trauma?
    - Stress?
    - When does it occur; how long does it last?
    - Any medical problems?
    - Where does it hurt?
    - What does it feel like?
    - Any vision changes, nausea, vomiting, or numbness?
    - Recent infections?
- Change in mental status
    - Any medical problems?
    - Recent head trauma?
    - Psychiatric problems?

- Are you taking any medications?
- Alcohol or drug use?
- Dizziness, vertigo, syncope
  - Any cardiovascular (CV) problems? Hypertension (HTN)?
  - Are you taking any medications?
- Numbness, loss of sensation
  - Do you have any vascular problems? Diabetes? Neurological problems?
  - Any recent injury?
- Change in any of the five senses
  - Any changes in sense of sight, smell, touch, taste, or hearing?
  - Any other medical problems?
  - Are you taking any medications?
  - Drug and alcohol use?

FOCUSED SENSORY-NEUROLOGICAL HISTORY

- Do you have any neurological problems?
- Do you have any other medical problems?
- Are you taking any medications, prescribed or over the counter (Table 13–1)?

Table 13–1. *Drugs That Adversely Affect the Sensory-Neurological System*

DRUG CLASS	DRUG	POSSIBLE ADVERSE REACTIONS
Adrenergics	albuterol sulfate, epinephrine, isoproterenol hydrochloride, terbutaline sulfate	Nervousness, tremors, dizziness, restlessness, insomnia
Adrenergic blockers	ergotamine tartrate, methysergide maleate	Lightheadedness, vertigo, insomnia, euphoria, confusion, hallucinations, numbness and tingling of fingers and toes
Antianginals	diltiazem hydrochloride	Headache, fatigue

(continued)

Table 13–1. *Drugs That Adversely Affect the Sensory-Neurological System (Continued)*

DRUG CLASS	DRUG	POSSIBLE ADVERSE REACTIONS
	isosorbide dinitrate, nitroglycerin	Throbbing headache, dizziness, weakness, orthostatic hypotension
	nifedipine	Headache, dizziness, light-headedness, flushing
	verapamil hydrochloride	Headache, dizziness
Antiarrhythmics	lidocaine hydrochloride	Lightheadedness, dizziness, paresthesias, tremors, restlessness, confusion, hallucinations, headache
Antimicrobials	aminoglycosides	Neuromuscular blockade; ototoxicity causing vertigo, hearing impairment, or both.
	acyclovir	Myoclonus, seizures
	isoniazid, nitrofurantoin	Peripheral neuropathy
	penicillin G	Delirium, headaches, mania, coma
Anticonvulsants	carbamazepine	Dizziness, drowsiness, ataxia, confusion, speech disturbances, involuntary movements
	phenytoin sodium	Dose-related headache, confusion, ataxia, slurred speech, lethargy, drowsiness, nervousness, insomnia, blurred vision, diplopia, nystagmus
Antidepressants	tricyclic antidepressants	Drowsiness, weakness, lethargy, fatigue, agitation, nightmares, restlessness, confusion, disorientation (especially in older clients)
	monoamine oxidase inhibitors	Restlessness, insomnia, drowsiness, headache, orthostatic hypotension, hypertension

(continued)

Table 13-1. *Drugs That Adversely Affect the Sensory-Neurological System (Continued)*

DRUG CLASS	DRUG	POSSIBLE ADVERSE REACTIONS
Antihypertensives	clonidine hydrochloride	Drowsiness, sedation, dizziness, headache, nightmares, depression, hallucinations
	hydralazine hydrochloride	Headache
	methyldopa	Drowsiness, sedation, decreased mental acuity, vertigo, headache, psychic disturbances, nightmares, depression
	propranolol hydrochloride	Fatigue, lethargy, vivid dreams, hallucinations, depression
Antineoplastic agents	fludarabine	Dysarthrias, paresthesias, weakness, seizures, paralysis
	procarbazine hydrochloride	Paresthesias, neuropathy, confusion
	vinblastine sulfate	Paresthesias, numbness
	vincristine sulfate	Peripheral neuropathy, loss of deep tendon reflexes, jaw pain
Antiparkinsonian agents	amantadine hydrochloride	Psychic disturbances, nervousness, irritability, fatigue, depression, insomnia, confusion, hallucinations, difficulty concentrating
	levodopa, pramipexole, ropinirole	Psychic disturbances, decreased attention span, memory loss, nervousness, vivid dreams, involuntary muscle movements
Antipsychotics	haloperidol, phenothiazines	Extrapyramidal reactions, tardive dyskinesia, headache, lethargy, confusion, agitation, hallucinations

(continued)

Table 13-1. *Drugs That Adversely Affect the Sensory-Neurological System (Continued)*

DRUG CLASS	DRUG	POSSIBLE ADVERSE REACTIONS
Cholinergic blockers	atropine sulfate, benztropine mesylate, glycopyrrolate	Blurred vision, headache, nervousness, drowsiness, weakness, dizziness, insomnia, disorientation
Corticosteroids	dexamethasone, hydrocortisone, methylprednisolone, prednisone	Mood swings, euphoria, insomnia, headache, vertigo, psychotic behavior
Gastrointestinal agents	cimetidine	Confusion (especially in older clients), depression
	metoclopramide hydrochloride	Restlessness, anxiety, drowsiness, lassitude, extrapyramidal reactions, tardive dyskinesia
Narcotic analgesics	morphine sulfate, hydromorphone hydrochloride, meperidine hydrochloride, methadone hydrochloride, oxycodone hydrochloride	Sedation, dizziness, visual disturbances, clouded sensorium
	butorphanol tartrate, nalbuphine hydrochloride, pentazocine hydrochloride	Sedation, headache, dizziness, vertigo, lightheadedness, euphoria
Nonsteroidal anti-inflammatory agents	ibuprofen, indomethacin	Headache, drowsiness, dizziness
Sedatives and hypnotics	barbiturates	Drowsiness, lethargy, vertigo, headache, depression, "hangover," paradoxical excitement in older clients, hyperactivity in children
	benzodiazepines	Drowsiness, dizziness, ataxia, daytime sedation, headache, confusion

(continued)

Table 13-1. *Drugs That Adversely Affect the Sensory-Neurological System (Continued)*

DRUG CLASS	DRUG	POSSIBLE ADVERSE REACTIONS
Skeletal muscle relaxants	baclofen	Drowsiness
	chlorzoxazone	Drowsiness, dizziness
	cyclobenzaprine hydrochloride	Drowsiness, dizziness, headache, nervousness, confusion
Miscellaneous agents	lithium carbonate	Lethargy, tremors, headache, mental confusion, dizziness, seizures, difficulty concentrating

- History of head trauma, loss of consciousness, dizziness, headaches?
- History of seizures?
- Memory problems, changes in senses?
- Weakness, numbness, paralysis?
- Problems walking or performing activities of daily living (ADLs)?
- Mood problems, depression?
- Drug and alcohol use?
- Allergies?
- Ever treated for neurological or psychiatric problem?
- Time of onset of symptoms?

Assessment of Sensory-Neurological System's Relationship to Other Systems

Remember, all systems are related! As you assess the sensory-neurological system, look at the relationship between it and all other systems.

SUBJECTIVE DATA	OBJECTIVE DATA
Area/System: General	
Ask about:	*Measure:*
General health	Vital signs

(continued)

SUBJECTIVE DATA	OBJECTIVE DATA
Fever	*Observe:* Mental status, grooming, affect, behavior, symmetry
Area/System: Integumentary	
Ask about:	*Inspect for:*
Rashes	Rashes or petechiae
Changes in sensations	*Test:* Superficial sensations
Area/System: HEENT	
Ask about:	*Inspect:*
Changes in sense of smell, taste, sight, hearing, touch	Symmetry of facial features *Palpate:*
Headaches	Lymph nodes, thyroid
Changes in speech or swallowing	*Examine:* Optic disk *Test:* Cranial nerves
Area/System: Respiratory	
Ask about:	*Auscultate:*
Breathing difficulty	Lungs
Area/System: Cardiovascular	
Ask about:	*Auscultate:*
History of CV problems	Heart sounds, noting rhythm Carotids for bruits and thrills
Area/System: Gastrointestinal	
Ask about:	*Auscultate:*
Nausea, vomiting	Bowel sounds
Changes in bowel function	
Difficulty swallowing	
Area/System: Genitourinary/Reproductive	
Ask about:	*Inspect for:*
History of STDs	Lesions
Changes in sexual activity, desire, ability	*Palpate:* Bladder distention
Changes in bladder function	
Area/System: Musculoskeletal	
Ask about:	*Inspect:*
Muscle weakness	Gait
Paralysis	*Test:*
Problems walking	Muscle strength
Balance problems	Range of motion (ROM) Cerebellar function
Area/System: Endocrine	
Ask about:	
History of diabetes mellitus and thyroid disease	

(continued)

SUBJECTIVE DATA	OBJECTIVE DATA
Area/System: Lymphatic/Hematological *Ask about:* Fever Bruising	
HEENT = head, eyes, ears, nose, and throat	

Physical Assessment

APPROACH: Inspection, palpation; cerebral function, cranial nerves, sensory function, reflexes

POSITION: Sitting

TOOLBOX: Stethoscope, blood pressure (BP) cuff, penlight, nonsterile gloves, wisp of cotton, sharp object (e.g., toothpicks or sterile needle), objects to touch (e.g., a coin, button, key, or paper clip), something fragrant (e.g., rubbing alcohol or coffee), things to taste (e.g., lemon juice, for sour; sugar; salt; and quinine, for bitter), tongue blade, two test tubes or other vials, reflex hammer, ophthalmoscope. **Remember, if the right side of the brain has a problem, the clinical manifestations will be on the left side, and vice versa.**

If your client has a spatial perception problem, be aware that he or she may have neglect, a spatial perception problem in which the patient doesn't see the affected side as part of his or her body.

AREA/PA SKILL	NORMAL FINDINGS	ABNORMAL FINDINGS
Cerebral Function (Consider the age and the educational and cultural background of your client.) ***Behavior***		
Note facial expression, posture, affect, and grooming.	Well-groomed, erect posture, pleasant facial expression, affect appropriate	Lack of facial expression, or inappropriate expression for speech

(continued)

AREA/PA SKILL	NORMAL FINDINGS	ABNORMAL FINDINGS
Cerebral Function *Behavior (Continued)*		
	Normal findings vary depending on situation	content: Psychiatric disorder (e.g., depression or schizophrenia) or neurological impairment affecting cranial nerves Masklike expression: Parkinson's disease Poor grooming or slumped posture: Psychiatric origin, as in depression; or physiological origin, as in cerebrovascular accident (CVA) with hemiparesis ***Safety is an issue for patients with right-side brain injury because they tend to be impulsive and not know their own limits***
Level of Consciousness		
Assess arousal state using minimal stimuli first, then increasing intensity as needed (Table 13–2). Document appropriately (Table 13–3). Test orientation to time, place, and person. **Disorientation to time and place usually occurs before disorientation to person.**	Awake, alert, and oriented (AAO) × 3 (time, place, and person) Older person may be disoriented to time, but note if client reorients easily	Disorientation physical in origin: Exhaustion, anxiety, hypoxia, fluid and electrolyte imbalance, drugs, or neurological problem Disorientation psychiatric in origin: Schizophrenia

(continued)

AREA/PA SKILL	NORMAL FINDINGS	ABNORMAL FINDINGS
Cerebral Function *Memory*		
Test immediate, recent, and remote memory. • Immediate: Ask client to repeat series of numbers. • Recent: Name three objects and ask client to recall later in exam • Remote: Ask client's birth date, major historical event. • **If asking personal data, such as birth date, be able to validate information independently.**	Immediate, recent, and remote memory intact	Memory problems can be benign or signal a more serious neurological problem such as Alzheimer's disease Forgetfulness—especially for immediate and recent events—is frequently seen in older adults. With benign forgetfulness, client can retrace or use memory aids to help with recall Pathological memory loss, as in Alzheimer's disease, is subtle and progressive until ability to function is impaired Temporary loss of memory: Head trauma, concussion, minor head injury Client may experience amnesia for the event causing injury (retrograde amnesia) Postconcussion syndrome can occur anywhere from 2 weeks to 2 months after injury; may cause short-term memory deficits

(continued)

AREA/PA SKILL	NORMAL FINDINGS	ABNORMAL FINDINGS
Cerebral Function *Mathematical and Calculative Ability*		
Have client perform simple mathematical problem, such as 4 + 5, serial 7s or 4s, subtraction from 100.	Calculative skills intact	Inability to calculate at a level appropriate to age, education, and language ability requires evaluation for neurological impairment
General Knowledge and Vocabulary		
Assess vocabulary and general knowledge. Ask how many days in a week? Months in a year? Ask client to define familiar words, such as apple, earthquake, chastise. **Begin with easy words and proceed to more difficult words.**	Vocabulary appropriate and general knowledge intact	Inability to define familiar words requires further evaluation
Thought Process		
Note attention span, logic of speech, ability to stay focused, appropriateness of responses.	Thought process clear; responds appropriately; speech coherent and logical	Incoherent speech, illogical or unrealistic ideas, repetition of words and phrases, markedly and/or repeatedly straying from the topic, and suddenly losing train of thought: Examples of altered thought processes that warrant further evaluation

(continued)

AREA/PA SKILL	NORMAL FINDINGS	ABNORMAL FINDINGS
Cerebral Function *Thought Process (Continued)*		
		Causes of alteration in thought process: Physical disorder (e.g., dementia), psychiatric disorder (e.g., psychosis), or drugs and alcohol
Abstract Reasoning		
Give client a proverb to interpret. Have client identify similarities, such as apples and oranges.	Abstract thinking intact	Impaired ability to think abstractly: Dementia, delirium, mental retardation, psychoses
Judgment		
Assess client's response to hypothetical situations.	Judgment intact	Impaired judgment: Dementia, psychosis, drug and alcohol abuse
Communication		
Note speech and language, enunciation, fluency. Note any dysarthria, dysphasia, dysphonia, neologisms, or circumlocution. *The following, more specific tests assess for a variety of neurological problems. (See Table 13–4.)*	Speech clear, fluent, no dysarthria, dysphasia, dysphonia, neologisms, or circumlocution Communication skills intact: spontaneous speech, motor speech, automatic speech, sound recognition, auditory-verbal comprehension, visual recognition, visual-verbal comprehension, writing, and figure copying	Hesitancy, stuttering, stammering, unclear speech: Lack of familiarity with language, deference or shyness, anxiety, or neurological disorder Dysphasia or aphasia: Neurological problems such as CVA. Drugs and alcohol can also cause slurred speech ***In assessing a possible stroke client, remember that if he or she has dysarthria, he or she probably also has dysphagia.***

(continued)

AREA/PA SKILL	NORMAL FINDINGS	ABNORMAL FINDINGS
Cerebral Function *Communication (Continued)*		
		If you suspect that your client has had a CVA, test gag, swallow, and cough reflexes before allowing him or her to eat, to avoid aspiration.
Test spontaneous speech: Have client describe a picture.		Impaired spontaneous speech: Cognitive impairment
Test motor speech: Have client say "do, re, mi, fa, so, la, ti, do."		Impaired motor speech: Problem with CN XII
Test automatic speech: Have client recite days of the week.Test sound recognition: Have client identify a familiar sound.		Impaired automatic speech: Cognitive impairment or memory problem Impaired sound recognition: Temporal lobe affected
Test auditory-verbal comprehension: Note client's ability to follow directions.		Impaired auditory-verbal comprehension: Temporal lobe affected Expressive aphasia: Frontal lobe affected Auditory-receptive aphasia: Temporal lobe affected
Test visual recognition: Have client identify object by sight.		Impaired visual recognition: Parieto-occipital lobe affected
Test visual-verbal comprehension: Have client read a sentence and explain meaning.		Impaired visual-verbal comprehension: Cognitive impairment
Test writing: Have client write name and address.		Impaired writing ability

(continued)

AREA/PA SKILL	NORMAL FINDINGS	ABNORMAL FINDINGS
Cerebral Function *Communication (Continued)*		
Test figure copying: Have client copy circle, x, square, triangle, star. **Work from simple to complex.** **Cranial Nerves** (Compare side to side. Have client close eyes when testing sensory nerves.) *CN I—Olfactory Nerve*		Impaired figure copying ability
Check patency of nostrils before testing nerve function. Test each nostril separately.	CN I intact	
Have client identify a distinct odor (e.g., coffee, vanilla).	Sense of smell intact	
Note anosmia.		Anosmia: Inherited and nonpathological, or from chronic rhinitis, sinusitis, heavy smoking, zinc deficiency, cocaine use, damage from facial fractures or head injuries, disorders of base of frontal lobe (e.g., tumor), or atherosclerotic changes. **Clients with anosmia usually have a problem with sense of taste also**
CN II—Optic Nerve		
Test visual acuity, visual fields, retinal structures.	CN II intact Visual acuity intact	CN II deficit: CVA or brain tumor *(continued)*

AREA/PA SKILL	NORMAL FINDINGS	ABNORMAL FINDINGS
Cranial Nerves *CN III, IV, VI—Oculomotor, Trochlear, Abducens Nerves*		
Test extraocular movement (EOM) with 6 cardinal fields; check pupillary reaction to light and accommodation. If indicated, test oculocephalic ("doll's eyes") reflex. ***Never perform oculocephalic reflex test on a client with suspected neck injury.*** *CN V—Trigeminal Nerve*	CN III, IV, VI intact EOM intact in both eyes; pupils equal, round, react to light and accommodation—direct and consensual	CN III deficits are seen in changes in pupillary reactions. Increased intracranial pressure (ICP) causes changes in pupillary reaction Abnormal doll's eyes (eyes fixed): Damage to oculomotor nerves (CN III, IV, VI) or brainstem
Test muscle of mastication strength by having client bite down on tongue blade. Test sensations on face (forehead, cheeks and chin). Test corneal reflex.	CN V intact Jaw muscle strength + 5 Facial sensations intact + corneal reflex	Weak or absent contraction unilaterally: Lesion of the nerve, cervical spine, or brainstem ***Patient may pocket food on affected side, increasing the risk for aspiration*** Inability to perceive light touch and superficial pain: Peripheral nerve damage
CN VII—Facial Nerve		
Test motor function of facial muscles: Have client make faces, smile, frown, whistle. Test taste (sweet, sour, salty) on anterior portion of tongue.	CN VII intact Facial movements symmetrical Taste on anterior tongue intact	Asymmetrical or impaired movement: Nerve damage such as Bell's palsy or a CVA Impaired taste or loss of taste: Damage to the nerve, chemotherapy, or radiation therapy to head and neck

(continued)

AREA/PA SKILL	NORMAL FINDINGS	ABNORMAL FINDINGS
Cranial Nerves *CN VIII—Acoustic Nerve*		
Test hearing, balance. If indicated, do cold caloric test for oculovestibular reflex; look for nystagmus.	CN VIII intact Hearing and balance intact	Hearing loss, nystagmus, balance disturbance, dizziness/vertigo: Acoustic nerve damage Nystagmus: CN VIII, brainstem, or cerebellum problem; or phenytoin (Dilantin) toxicity. Abnormal cold caloric test (no movement): Damage to CN III, VI, and VIII
CN IX, X—Glossopharyngeal and Vagus Nerves		
Note quality of voice, ability to swallow and cough. Look for symmetrical rise of the uvula. Test gag reflex.	CN IX and X intact Strong, clear voice, symmetrical rise of uvula, able to swallow and cough + gag reflex	Unilateral movement: Contralateral nerve damage Impaired swallowing: Damage to CN IX, X Diminished or absent gag reflex: Nerve damage. **Evaluate further; these clients are at increased risk for aspiration** Changes in voice quality (e.g., hoarseness): Damage to CN X. CN X damage may also affect vital functions, causing arrhythmias because the vagus innervates most of the viscera through the parasympathetic system

(continued)

AREA/PA SKILL	NORMAL FINDINGS	ABNORMAL FINDINGS
Cranial Nerves *CN IX, X—Glossopharyngeal and Vagus Nerves (Continued)*		
Assess taste on posterior ⅓ of tongue.	Taste intact	Impaired taste on posterior portion of tongue: Problem with CN IX
CN XI—Spinoaccessory Nerve		
Test muscle strength of neck and shoulders.	CN XI intact +5 muscle strength of neck and shoulders	Asymmetrical, diminished, or absent movement; pain; or unilateral or bilateral weakness: Peripheral nerve damage
CN XII —Hypoglossal Nerve		
Test mobility and strength of tongue. Note ability to say d, l, n, t. Note tongue position, atrophy, or fasciculation.	CN XII intact Full ROM of tongue, midline, no atrophy or fasciculation	Asymmetrical, diminished, or absent movement; or tongue deviated from midline or protruded: Peripheral nerve damage Paralysis of the tongue results in dysarthria
Sensory Function (When testing sensory function, have client close eyes. Compare side to side.)		
Light Touch, Pain, and Temperature		
Test light touch, pain, and temperature on various areas of the body. **If touch sensation is intact distally, do not assume it is intact proximally. If pain sensation is intact, no need to test temperature.**	Light touch, pain, and temperature intact in upper and lower extremities	Diminished or absent cutaneous perception: Peripheral nerve damage, or damage to posterior column of spinal cord. Peripheral neuropathies can also cause sensory deficits Increased sensitivity: Hyperesthesia

(continued)

AREA/PA SKILL	NORMAL FINDINGS	ABNORMAL FINDINGS
Sensory Function *Light Touch, Pain, and Temperature (Continued)*		
Avoid using pins, which could break skin. Use toothpicks, sharp and dull sides, to test pain.		Numbness and tingling: Paresthesia Loss of sensation: Aesthesia Diminished or absent temperature perception: Peripheral nerve damage or damage to lateral spinothalamic tract
Deep Sensations		
VIBRATORY: Place vibrating tuning fork on bony joint, great toe, and distal interphalangeal. KINESTHETICS (POSITION SENSE): Move finger and toe up and down, and have client identify direction of movement. **If intact distally, intact proximally.**	Vibratory sensation and kinesthetic sensation intact in upper and lower extremities	Diminished or absent vibration sense: Peripheral nerve damage from alcoholism or diabetes, or damage to posterior column of spinal cord. Diminished or absent position sense: Peripheral nerve damage, or damage to posterior column of spinal cord

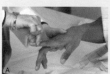
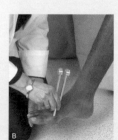

A. Vibrating upper extremity, B. Vibrating lower extremity

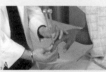
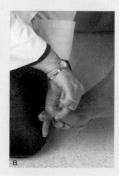

A. Testing position sense in finger, B. Testing position sense in toe

(continued)

AREA/PA SKILL	NORMAL FINDINGS	ABNORMAL FINDINGS
Sensory Function *Discriminatory Sensations*		

STEREOGNOSIS:
Have client identify familiar object (key, paper clip) by touch.

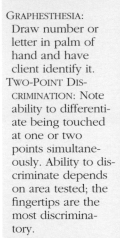

Testing stereognosis

GRAPHESTHESIA:
Draw number or letter in palm of hand and have client identify it.

TWO-POINT DISCRIMINATION: Note ability to differentiate being touched at one or two points simultaneously. Ability to discriminate depends on area tested; the fingertips are the most discriminatory.

POINT LOCALIZATION: Note ability to identify a point touched.

EXTINCTION: Note ability to identify two corresponding areas touched simultaneously.

Stereognosis, graphesthesia, point localization, and extinction intact; 2-point discrimination <5 mm on fingertips

Abnormal findings: Lesion or other disorder involving sensory cortex, or disorder affecting posterior column

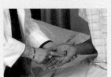

Testing graphesthesia

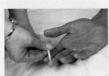

Testing 2-point discrimination

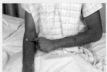

Testing point localization

Extinction: Identification of stimulus on only one side suggests lesion or other disorder involving sensory cortical region in opposite hemisphere

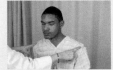

Testing extinction

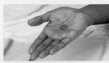

(continued)

AREA/PA SKILL	NORMAL FINDINGS	ABNORMAL FINDINGS
Sensory Function *Deep Tendon Reflexes (DTRs)*		
Grade DTR on 0–4 scale. If difficult to elicit reflex, use reinforcement techniques (e.g., clenching teeth, interlocking hands). Use percussion hammer.		Absent or diminished reflexes: Degenerative disease, damage to peripheral nerve (e.g., peripheral neuropathy), or lower motor neuron disorder (e.g., amyotrophic lateral sclerosis and Guillain-Barré syndrome) Hyperactive reflexes with clonus: Spinal cord injuries and upper motor neuron disease such as multiple sclerosis

Documenting reflex findings

Use these grading scales to rate the strength of each reflex in a deep tendon and superficial reflex assessment.

Deep tendon reflex grades
0 absent
+ present but diminished
+ + normal
+ + + increased but not necessarily pathologic
+ + + + hyperactive or clonic (involuntary contraction and relaxation of skeletal muscle)

Superficial reflex grades
0 absent
+ present

Record the client's reflex ratings on a drawing of a stick figure. The figures here show documentation of normal and abnormal reflex responses.

Normal

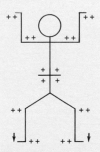

Abnormal

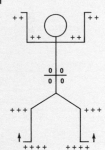

Documenting reflex findings

(continued)

AREA/PA SKILL	NORMAL FINDINGS	ABNORMAL FINDINGS

Sensory Function
Deep Tendon Reflexes (DTRs) (Continued)

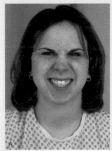

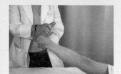

Testing for clonus

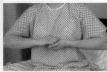

Isometric maneuvers:
(A) Clenching teeth,
(B) Interlocking hands

Biceps Reflex

Place your thumb on biceps tendon and strike. Response: Flexion at elbow.	+2/4	C5, 6 problem

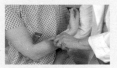

Testing biceps reflex

Triceps Reflex

Strike triceps tendon 1–2′ above elbow. Response: Extension at elbow.	+2/4	C7, 8 problem

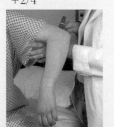

Testing triceps reflex *(continued)*

AREA/PA SKILL	NORMAL FINDINGS	ABNORMAL FINDINGS
Sensory Function *Brachioradialis Reflex*		
Strike brachioradialis tendon 3–5 cm above wrist. Response: Flexion at elbow and supination of hand.	+2/4 *Testing brachioradialis reflex*	C5, 6 problem
Patellar Reflex		
Strike patellar tendon below patella. Response: Extension of knee.	+2/4 *Testing patellar reflex*	L2, 3, 4 problem
Achilles Reflex		
Strike Achilles tendon about 2" above the heel. Response: Plantarflexion of foot	+2/4 *Testing Achilles reflex*	S1, 2 problem
Superficial Reflexes *Grade as positive or negative.*		Absence of superficial reflexes: Pyramidal tract lesions

(continued)

AREA/PA SKILL	NORMAL FINDINGS	ABNORMAL FINDINGS
Superficial Reflexes *Plantar Reflex*		
Stroke sole of foot from heel laterally across ball of foot to great toe. Response: Flexion of toes.	+ plantar reflex Babinski normal in infants *Testing plantar reflex*	Babinski's response, dorsiflexion of great toe, with or without fanning of other toes: In absence of drug or alcohol intoxication, suggests pathology involving upper motor neurons L4 to S2 problem
Abdominal Reflex		
Stroke each quadrant of abdomen toward umbilicus. Response: Umbilicus moves toward stimulus. *Testing abdominal reflex*	+ abdominal reflex May be absent in obese or pregnant clients	T8, 9, 10 problem
Anal Reflex		
Scratch side of anus. Response: Anus puckers.	+ anal reflex	S3, 4, 5 problem
Cremasteric Reflex		
Stroke inner aspect of man's thigh. Response: Elevation of testes.	+ cremasteric reflex	L1, 2 problem

(continued)

AREA/PA SKILL	NORMAL FINDINGS	ABNORMAL FINDINGS
Superficial Reflexes **_Bulbocavernosus Reflex_**		
Gently apply pressure over bulbocavernosus muscle and gently pinch foreskin or glans. Response: Contraction of bulbocavernosus muscle.	+ bulbocavernosus reflex	S3, 4 problem
Primitive or Pathological Reflexes		
		Usually indicate severe underlying neurological problem reflecting cerebral degeneration or late-stage dementia
Grasp: Place your fingers in palm of client's hand; client will close fingers and grasp your fingers.		
Sucking: Gently stimulate client's lips with a mouth swab; client will start sucking.		
Snout: Gently tap oral area with finger; client's lips will pucker.		
Rooting: Gently stroke side of client's face; client will turn toward stimulated side.		
Glabellar: Gently tap on forehead; client will blink.		
Babinski's sign: Stroke lateral aspect of sole of foot; client will dorsiflex great toe and fan toes.		

(continued)

AREA/PA SKILL	NORMAL FINDINGS	ABNORMAL FINDINGS
Meningeal Signs		
		Classic signs of meningitis include nuchal rigidity (extension of neck with resistance to flexion), fever, photosensitivity, headache, and nausea and vomiting
If meningitis is suspected, assess for Kernig's and Brudzinski's signs. To assess for Kernig's sign: With client supine, flex leg and have client attempt to extend while you apply pressure to knee. To assess for Brudzinski's sign: With patient supine, flex head to chest.	*Kernig's sign* *Brudzinski's sign*	Kernig's sign: Contraction and pain of hamstring muscles and resistance to extension are positive signs of meningitis Brudzinski's sign: Flexion of hips is a positive sign of meningitis

PA = physical assessment

Table 13-2. *Painful Stimuli for Assessing Arousal State*

STIMULUS	TECHNIQUE
Trapezius squeeze	Pinch 1 to 2 inches of trapezius muscle and twist. You should get movement if client is going to respond.
Supraorbital pressure	Apply firm pressure with thumbs at notch at center of orbital rim below eyebrows. Because a nerve runs in notch, pressure to this area will cause sinus pain. If you use this stimulus, use it carefully to avoid damage to eyes.

(continued)

Table 13-2. *Painful Stimuli for Assessing Arousal State (Continued)*

STIMULUS	TECHNIQUE
Mandibular pressure	With index and middle finger apply inward and upward pressure at angle of jaw. If responsive, client will experience pain where pressure is being applied.
Sternal rub	Use knuckles of dominant hand and apply pressure in a grinding motion to sternum. You will see movement if the client responds. Repeated use of this site will likely cause bruising, so rotate sites and types of stimulus.
Nail pressure	Apply pressure over moon of fingernail with a pen or pencil. Movement will occur if client responds.
Achilles pinch	Squeeze Achilles tendon between thumb and index finger. Movement will occur if client responds.

Table 13-3. *Terms Used to Describe Client's Level of Consciousness*

TERM	DESCRIPTION OF CLIENT'S RESPONSE
Alert	Follows commands in a timely fashion
Lethargic	Appears drowsy, may drift off to sleep during the examination
Stuporous	Requires vigorous stimulation (shaking, shouting) for a response
Comatose	Doesn't respond appropriately to either verbal or painful stimuli

Table 13–4. *Neurological Problems*

PROBLEM	DEFINITION
Agnosia	Inability to recognize object by sight (visual agnosia), touch (tactile agnosia), or hearing (auditory agnosia)
Akinesia	Complete or partial loss of voluntary muscle movement
Aphasia	Absence or impairment of ability to communicate through speech, writing, or signs
Expressive aphasia	Inability to express language even though person knows what he or she wants to say (also called Broca's, or motor, aphasia)
Fluent aphasia	Words can be spoken but are used incorrectly
Nonfluent aphasia	Slow, deliberate speech, few words
Receptive aphasia	Inability to comprehend spoken or written words (also called Wernicke's, or sensory, aphasia)
Apraxia	Inability to carry out learned sequential movements or commands
Circumlocution	Inability to name object verbally, so patient talks around object or uses gestures to define it
Dysarthria	Defective speech; inability to articulate words; impairment of tongue and other muscles needed for speech
Dysphasia	Impaired or difficult speech
Dysphonia	Difficulty with quality of voice; hoarseness
Neologisms	Made-up, nonsense, meaningless words
Paraphrasia	Loss of ability to use words correctly and coherently; words are jumbled or misused
Tremors	Involuntary movement of part of body
Intention tremor	Involuntary movement when attempting coordinated movements
Fasciculation	Involuntary contraction or twitching of muscle fibers

CHAPTER 14

ASSESSING THE MOTHER-TO-BE

Assessment of the mother-to-be entails assessing both the mother and fetus throughout the perinatal period.

Developmental Considerations

Adolescents

- Careful attention to baseline blood pressure is necessary because teenagers have lower systolic and diastolic pressures than older women.
- Look for signs of physical and sexual abuse in the young adolescent, who may be ashamed or afraid to share this important information.
- The diets of adolescents are often lacking in essential nutrients, such as calcium and iron, needed during pregnancy.
- Mother and fetus are both growing, so they compete for nutrients.
- Cephalopelvic disproportion is a common problem for teen pregnancy because growth of the pelvis lags behind growth in stature.
- For all of these reasons, teen pregnancies are at increased risk for complications.

Older Women

- Risk for maternal or fetal complications increases with the client's age (Table 14–1).

Table 14–1. *Complications of Pregnancy*

SIGNS/SYMPTOMS	POSSIBLE CAUSES
First Trimester	
Severe vomiting	Hyperemesis gravidarum
Chills, fever	Infection
Burning on urination	Infection
Abdominal cramping, bloating, vaginal bleeding	Spontaneous abortion, miscarriage
Second and Third Trimesters	
Severe vomiting	Hyperemesis gravidarum
Leakage of amniotic fluid from vagina before labor begins	Premature rupture of membranes
Vaginal bleeding, severe abdominal pain	Miscarriage, placental separation
Chills, fever, diarrhea, burning on urination	Infection
Change in fetal activity	Fetal distress, intrauterine fetal demise
Uterine contractions before due date (expected date of delivery [EDD])	Preterm labor
Visual disturbances: Blurring, double vision, spots	Hypertensive disorders: PIH
Swelling of face, fingers, eye orbits, sacral area	PIH
Severe, frequent, or continuous headaches	PIH
Muscular irritability or convulsions (seizures)	PIH
Severe stomachache (epigastric pain)	PIH
Glucosuria, positive glucose tolerance test result	Gestational diabetes mellitus

- Pregnant women older than age 35 have an increased risk of developing gestational diabetes, pregnancy-induced hypertension (PIH), gestational bleeding, abruptio placentae, and intrapartal fetal distress.
- Older women also have an increased risk for conceiving a child with chromosomal abnormalities.
- Older women are more likely to have pre-existing medical conditions, such as diabetes and hypertension. In fact, pre-existing conditions appear to pose a greater risk for

maternal well-being and pregnancy outcome than the mother's age.

Cultural Considerations

- Blacks and Southeast Asians are at risk for sickle cell disease.
- Jewish women are at risk for Tay-Sachs disease.
- Mediterranean, Italian, and Greek women are at risk for beta-thalassemia.
- Asians are at risk for alpha-thalassemia.

Pregnancy and Childbearing Practices and Beliefs of Various Ethnic Groups *

AFRICAN-AMERICAN
- Oral contraceptives most popular type of birth control.
- High rate of teen pregnancy.
- Primary advisors are grandmother and maternal relatives.
- Geophagia, eating of earth or clay, is a common practice.
- Taboos/beliefs:
  - If food cravings are not met, baby is marked.
  - Labor is induced by a bumpy ride, a big meal, castor oil, or sniffing pepper.
  - Photographing pregnant woman causes stillbirth or captures baby's soul.
  - Lifting hands over head causes cord to wrap around baby's neck.
  - Amniotic sac over baby's face denotes baby has special powers.
  - Child born after set of twins, the seventh child, or a child born with a physical condition has special powers from God.

AMISH
- Children are a gift from God.
- Average number of children per family is seven.
- Women have high status owing to their role as child producers.
- Birth control seen as interfering with God's will.

---

*Adapted from Purnell, L.D., and Paulanka, B.J.: *Transcultural Healthcare: A Culturally Competent Approach*, ed 2. Philadelphia, F.A. Davis Company, 2003.

- Prenatal care by Amish lay-midwives.
- Fathers expected to be involved and present during delivery and to participate in prenatal classes.
- No major taboos, but showing emotions is considered inappropriate, so woman labors quietly without expressing discomfort.
- Childbirth is not viewed as medical condition, so few have health insurance, keeping hospitalizations very short.
- Family and community are expected to care for mother and baby.

APPALACHIAN
- Contraceptive practices similar to those of the general public, but a common belief is that laxatives facilitate abortion.
- Believe that healthy living during pregnancy leads to a healthy baby.
- Taboos/beliefs:
  - Boys are carried high, girls low.
  - Photo taking causes stillbirth.
  - Reaching over the head causes cord strangulation.
  - Wearing an opal ring may harm baby.
  - Birthmarks are caused by eating strawberries or citrus fruit.
  - Experiencing a tragedy during pregnancy leads to congenital anomalies.
- Birthing is considered a natural process to be endured.
- Family members are expected to care for mother and child during postpartum period.
- A band may be placed around the baby's abdomen to prevent umbilical hernias, and an asafetida bag around the neck to prevent contagious diseases.

ARAB-AMERICAN
- Believe that God decides family size and God provides.
- Procreation is the purpose of marriage, resulting in high fertility rates.
- Irreversible means of contraception and abortions are considered unlawful. Sterility may lead to rejection or divorce. With emphasis on fertility and bearing a son, pregnancy occurs early in marriages.
- Pregnant women are pampered. Unmet cravings are

thought to result in birthmarks. Pregnant women are excused from fasting during sacred days.
- Men are excluded from labor and delivery. Deliveries are often performed at home by midwives because of limited access to hospitals. Breathing and relaxation techniques are not practiced, and labor pain is openly expressed.
- Baby's stomach wrapped after birth to prevent exposure to cold. Male circumcision is a Muslim requirement.
- Postpartum bathing is avoided for fear of mother being exposed to cold.
- Breast-feeding delayed until second or third day to allow mother to rest.
- Postpartum foods include lentil soup to increase milk production and teas to cleanse the body.

CHINESE-AMERICAN
- To control population, Chinese government has one-child law. Contraception is free; abortion is common.
- Pregnancy is seen as a positive experience. Men are not very involved in process. Female midwives are often preferred because of modesty of Chinese women.
- Dietary beliefs:
  - Adding meat to diet makes blood "strong" for fetus.
  - Shellfish cause allergies.
  - Iron makes delivery more difficult.
  - Avoid fruits and vegetables during postpartum period because they are "cold" foods.
  - Mother drinks rice wine to increase strength and has 5 to 6 meals a day with rice, soups, and 7 to 8 eggs. ***Wine may increase bleeding time.***
  - Five- to seven-day hospital stay after delivery, 1 month for recovery. Chinese government allows 6 months maternity leave with full pay. If mother is breast-feeding, time is allowed from work for feedings.
  - Mothers avoid "cold"—don't go outside or bathe, and wear many layers of clothes even in warm weather.

CUBAN-AMERICAN
- Cuba has lowest birth rate in Latin America because of high labor force participation for women and high divorce rate.
- Childbirth is a celebration.

- Beliefs:
  - Must eat for two during pregnancy (leads to excessive weight gain).
  - Eating coffee grounds cures morning sickness.
  - Eating fruit ensures that the baby will have smooth complexion.
  - Wearing necklaces causes umbilical cord to wrap around neck.
- During the postpartum period, family members care for mother for 4 weeks. Mother avoids ambulation and exposure to cold because this is seen as risk for infection.
- Prefer breast-feeding but wean at 3 months and start solid foods. Believe that a fat child is a healthy child.

EGYPTIAN-AMERICAN

- Must have children to make family complete. Three children is the ideal number. Woman are expected to conceive within first year of marriage, and there is much stress until pregnancy occurs. Inability to conceive is grounds for divorce. Pregnancy brings security and respect. Birthing, especially of a son, has status and power.
- Beliefs:
  - Curtail activities during pregnancy to prevent miscarriage.
  - Eat for two.
  - Cravings must be met or baby marked with the shape of the craved food.
  - Maternal mother is expectant mother's source of support during labor and delivery.
  - Men are excluded from the birthing process.
  - Postpartum, avoid cold, such as bathing. Postpartum period is 40 days, and family members tend to mother and baby.

FILIPINO-AMERICAN

- Fertility practices influenced by Catholic faith; rhythm is only acceptable method of contraception; abortion is a sin.
- Child-centered culture. Pregnancy is normal; expectant mothers are pampered. Maternal mother is great source of support and often serves as labor coach.
- Beliefs:
  - Use healthcare providers but also a massage therapist.
  - Cravings should be met to avoid harm to baby.

- Baby takes on characteristics of craved foods, (e.g. dark-colored foods, dark skin).
- If mother has a sudden scare or stress it can harm fetus.
- Postpartum beliefs:
  - Chicken soup stimulates milk production.
  - Showers may cause arthritis, but sponge baths are allowed.
  - Family cares for new mother and baby during post-partum period.

FRENCH-CANADIAN

- Fertility practices influenced by Catholic faith. Abortion considered morally wrong by many.
- Fear of labor and delivery. Fathers are encouraged to be present during delivery. Use of analgesia is high.
- Breast-feeding has regained popularity.
- Both maternity and paternity leaves are available.
- Beliefs:
  - Washing floors can trigger labor; so can full moon.
  - Hyperglycemia during pregnancy means you are likely to give birth to a boy. Hyponatremia during pregnancy means you are likely to give birth to a girl.

GREEK-AMERICAN

- Limited family size because of desire to provide for family and ensure education for children.
- Greek-Orthodox faith condemns birth control and abortion.
- Infertility causes great stress.
- Pregnant mother is greatly respected and protected.
- Birthing usually by midwife or female relatives; fathers remain uninvolved.
- Mother considered impure and susceptible to illness for 40 days postpartum. Remains at home. Breast-feeding is common.
- Beliefs:
  - Eat foods high in iron and protein.
  - Child will be marked if food cravings are unmet.
  - Breast-feeding mothers who shower may cause diarrhea or milk allergy in baby.
  - Silver objects or coins placed in crib bring good luck.

IRANIAN-AMERICAN

- Hot and cold influence pregnancy practices.
- Women are expected to have children early in marriage.
- Infertility blamed on woman.
- Breast-feeding used as method of contraception.
- Birthing a child, especially a boy, is prestigious.
- Beliefs:
    - Cravings must be met with balance for hot and cold foods.
    - Heavy work causes miscarriages.
    - Much support from female relatives. Father usually not present during delivery. The postpartum period is 30 to 40 days.
- Postpartum beliefs:
    - Baby boys are "hotter" than baby girls.
    - Baby may be kept at home for first 40 days until he or she is strong enough to defend against environmental pathogens.
    - Ritual baby bath given between 10th and 40th day.

IRISH-AMERICAN

- Fertility practices influenced by Catholicism. Sexual relationships are often seen as a duty. Abstinence and rhythm are the only acceptable methods of birth control, and abortion is considered morally wrong.
- Beliefs:
    - Eating a well-balanced diet during pregnancy is important.
    - Not eating right leads to deformities.
    - Lifting hands above the head wraps cord around baby's neck.
    - Experiencing a tragedy during pregnancy results in congenital anomalies.
    - Going to bed with wet hair or wet feet causes illness in pregnant woman.

JEWISH-AMERICAN

- Children are a gift and duty; boys are more important. Sterility is a curse.
- Birth control pill is acceptable form of contraception.
- Orthodox Jews condone abortion if mother's health is at risk. Reform Jews believe women have control over their own bodies; therefore it is their decision.

- Hasidic husbands are not allowed to touch the mother during delivery or view her genitals; therefore, they may give only verbal support or choose not to be present during delivery.
- Male circumcision performed the eighth day by a mohel—a person trained in circumcision, asepsis, and the religious ritual.

MEXICAN-AMERICAN

- Fertility practices influenced by Catholicism. Abstinence and rhythm are acceptable methods of birth control. Breast-feeding is also seen as method of birth control. Abortion is considered morally wrong.
- Multiple births are common; childbearing age between 19 and 24 years is seen as best time; woman older than 24 years may be considered too old.
- A large family is a sign of a man's virility. Pregnancy is a natural and desirable condition, so many do not seek prenatal care; extended family provides advice and support.
- Beliefs:
  - Hot food provides fetus with warmth.
  - Cold foods should be eaten during postpartum period.
  - Pregnant women sleep on back to prevent harm to baby.
  - Frequent intercourse during pregnancy keeps vaginal canal lubricated and eases delivery.
  - Walking in moonlight and viewing lunar eclipses lead to deformities.
  - Pregnant women should avoid becoming cold.
  - Lifting hands over head causes cord to wrap around baby's neck.
  - The pregnant woman may wear a safety pin or metal object to prevent deformities.
- The father is not included in delivery. Mothers are very verbal during labor and do not practice breathing techniques. Mother puts legs together after delivery and wears cotton binder or girdle to prevent air from entering the womb.
- The postpartum period is 40 days, warmth preferred, showers avoided.
- Lactating mothers exposed to pesticides have decreased milk production and increased risk of breast cancer.

- Postpartum belief: Cutting baby's nails causes blindness and deafness.

NAVAJO NATIVE AMERICAN
- Large families are favorable; many do not practice birth control. Having twins is not favorable and traditionally one must die; now, however, one may be placed for adoption.
- Beliefs:
  - Mothers are reluctant to deliver in hospital because hospitals are associated with sickness and death.
  - Birthing necklaces worn during labor to ensure a safe birth. Mother holds onto woven sash when ready to push.
  - Chanting may occur during delivery.
  - Baby clothes not bought before baby's birth.
- Postpartum beliefs:
  - Placenta is buried after birth to protect the baby from evil spirits.
  - The baby is given special mixtures after birth to rid mouth of mucus.

VIETNAMESE-AMERICAN
- High fertility rate as a result of long period of childbearing (up to age 44).
- Taboos/beliefs:
  - Dietary practices influenced by hot/cold, wind/tonic. Wind foods are cold, tonic foods are hot and sweet. Maintaining balance between hot and cold restores bodily balance. First trimester, woman considered weak and cold, so she eats hot foods. Second trimester is neutral state. Third trimester, woman considered hot, so she eats cold foods.
  - Woman remains physically active but avoids heavy lifting and raising hands above the head (thought to pull on placenta).
  - Sexual intercourse late in pregnancy is believed to cause respiratory distress.
  - It is taboo to attend weddings and funerals while pregnant.
- Early prenatal care is not the norm. Labor is usually short, may prefer squatting or walking while in labor.
- Postpartum beliefs:

- Head of mother and baby considered sacred, so cannot be touched.
- Placenta buried to protect baby's health.
- Ritual cleansing of mother without water. Showers avoided for a month after delivery because of cold influence.
- Family helps care for mother and child.
- Breast-feeding is a common practice, but the mother may discard colostrum. May alternate breast with bottle because of hot and cold influence (hot foods benefit mother's health, whereas cold foods promote healthy breast milk).

Assessment

History

Key points to remember when obtaining a prenatal history:

- Focus on the current pregnancy and the presenting presumptive symptoms. Take a detailed obstetric and gynecological history.
- Use the past medical history to identify anything that would affect or be affected by pregnancy.
- Pay special attention to the nutritional history.
- Pay special attention to prescribed, over-the-counter, and illegal drug use because it may have a major impact on the developing fetus.
- Determine the client's reaction to pregnancy—was this a planned pregnancy?
- Identify major supports—family, spouse, significant other?
- Assess for history or risk of physical abuse.
- After you have completed your questions, ask the client if she has any problems or concerns that have not been covered, and give her an opportunity to discuss them.

Diagnosis of Pregnancy

The diagnosis of pregnancy (Table 14–2) is based on the following indicators:

- Presumptive signs (experienced by the client)
- Probable signs (observed by the examiner)
- Positive signs (attributed only to the presence of the fetus)

Table 14–2. *Signs and Symptoms of Pregnancy*

SIGNS AND SYMPTOMS	DESCRIPTION/TIME FRAME
Presumptive Signs	
Cessation of menses (amenorrhea)	Uterine lining does not slough off; women may experience spotting during implantation
Nausea, vomiting	From weeks 2 to 12; usually subsides after 12 weeks
Frequent urination	Bladder irritability caused by enlarging uterus
Breast tenderness	Starts at 2–3 weeks; soreness; tingling
Perception of fetal movement (quickening)	Occurs at 16–18 weeks; sensation of "fluttering" in abdomen perceived by mother-to-be
Skin changes	Increased pigmentation; striae gravidarum
Fatigue	Starts at 12 weeks
Probable Signs	
Abdominal enlargement	Palpated at 12 weeks
Piskacek's sign	Palpated at 4–6 weeks; uterus asymmetrical with soft prominence on implantation side
Hegar's sign	6 weeks; palpable softening of the lower uterine segment
Goodell's sign	Palpated at 8 weeks; softening of the cervix
Chadwick's sign	Seen at 6–8 weeks; bluish hue on vulva, vagina, cervix from increased venous congestion
Braxton Hicks contractions	Painless, irregular, intermittent uterine contractions that typically start after the fourth month and last through remainder of pregnancy
Pregnancy test	Positive 7–10 days after conception
Ballottement	Occurs at 16–18 weeks; passive movement of the unengaged fetus
Positive Signs	
Fetal heartbeat	By ultrasound, fetal heart motion is noted by 4–8 weeks after conception; by Doppler, auscultated by 10–12 weeks; by fetal stethoscope, auscultated by 17–19 weeks

(continued)

Table 14–2. *Signs and Symptoms of Pregnancy (Continued)*	
SIGNS AND SYMPTOMS	**DESCRIPTION/TIME FRAME**
Visualization of the fetus	By ultrasound, at 5–6 weeks; by radiograph, by 16 weeks (rarely used to diagnose pregnancy because of teratogenic effects)

Calculation of Estimated Date of Conception

To calculate the estimated date of conception (EDC), apply Naegele's rule: Add 7 days to the first day of the last menstrual period (LMP), then subtract 3 months from that date. Considerations in calculating the EDC include the following:

- Find out the first day of the LMP. Make sure the client is sure of the date because the EDC is based on the LMP. Conception usually occurs around 2 weeks after the LMP in a 28-day cycle.
- Review the client's menstrual history, including frequency of menses, length of flow, normalcy of the LMP, and contraceptive use.
- Ultrasound studies may also be used to estimate the gestational age.

Prenatal Laboratory Tests

URINE TESTS
- Clean-catch midstream urine specimen, for glucose (to assess for diabetes), protein (to assess for PIH), and nitrites and leukocytes (to assess for infection).

BLOOD TESTS
- CBC, blood type and screen, Rh status, rubella titer, serological test for syphilis, and hepatitis B surface antigen.
- Clients of African ancestry are also referred for a sickle cell anemia screen.
- Clients who are at high risk for HIV infection should be screened for this infection.
- Between 16 and 18 weeks' gestation, a multiple marker or "triple screen" for maternal serum level of alpha-fetoprotein (MSAFP), human chorionic gonadotropin (hCG), and

unconjugated estriol (uE3) is usually obtained. High levels of alpha-fetoprotein are associated with neural tube defects; low triple screen values with Down syndrome and other chromosomal abnormalities.

Head-to-Toe Physical Assessment

APPROACH: Inspection, palpation, percussion, auscultation

POSITION: Sitting, supine, lithotomy

TOOLBOX: Stethoscope, light for pelvic examination, tape measure, fetoscope or fetal Doppler, and equipment for pelvic exam (speculum, gloves, lubricant, glass slides, KOH, normal saline, and cytology fixative).

SYSTEM/AREA, APPROACH, AND NORMAL FINDINGS	ABNORMAL FINDINGS
Integumentary: Inspection Linea nigra, striae gravidarum, chloasma, spider nevi, palmar erythema. Increased growth, softening, thinning of hair and nails.	Pale skin: Anemia *Client is anemic if hemoglobin drops below 10 g/dL*

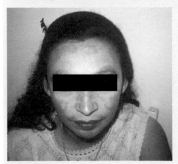

Chloasma

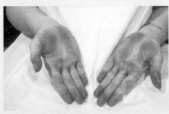

Palmar erythema

(continued)

SYSTEM/AREA, APPROACH, AND NORMAL FINDINGS	ABNORMAL FINDINGS
HEENT *Head and Neck: Palpation*	
Palpable smooth, nontender, small cervical chain lymph nodes. Slight thyroid gland enlargement. *Ears: Inspection*	Hard, tender, fixed or prominent cervical nodes: Cancer Marked thyroid enlargement: Hyperthyroidism
Tympanic membranes clear, landmarks visible. *Nose: Inspection*	Tympanic membranes red and bulging with pus: Infection
Mucosal swelling and redness, epistaxis (nosebleeds) common because of increased estrogen. *Mouth/Throat: Inspection*	Purulent discharge: Upper respiratory infection
Gums: Gingival hypertrophy and epulis usually regress spontaneously after delivery. Throat: Pink, no redness or exudates.	Bleeding gums: Gingivitis Redness in throat: Exudate present Enlarged tonsils: Infection

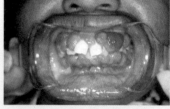

Gingival hypertrophy

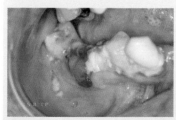

Epulis

(continued)

SYSTEM/AREA, APPROACH, AND NORMAL FINDINGS	ABNORMAL FINDINGS

Respiratory: Inspection, Palpation, Percussion, Auscultation

Increased anteroposterior chest diameter, thoracic breathing, slight hyperventilation, shortness of breath in late pregnancy, lung sounds clear bilaterally.	Dyspnea, crackles, rhonchi, wheezes, rubs, absence of breath sounds, unequal breath sounds, respiratory distress: Pulmonary complications, such as pulmonary edema or acute respiratory distress syndrome

Cardiovascular: Palpation, Auscultation

Point of maximal impulse (PMI) may be displaced upward and laterally in the latter stages of pregnancy.	Enlarged PMI: Hypertension (HTN)
Normal sinus rhythm.	Irregular rhythm: Cardiac disease
Soft systolic murmur caused by increased blood volume.	Dyspnea, palpitations, markedly decreased activity tolerance: Cardiovascular disease
	Midsystolic click and late systolic murmur: Mitral valve prolapse

Breasts: Inspection, Palpation

Venous congestion with prominence of Montgomery's tubercles.	Nipple inversion may be problematic for breast-feeding women
Increased size and nodularity; increased sensitivity; colostrum secretion in the third trimester.	Localized redness, pain, and warmth: Mastitis
Hyperpigmentation of nipples and areolar tissue.	Bloody nipple discharge and skin retraction: Cancer

Abdomen: Inspection, Palpation, Auscultation

Note cesarean scars and location; obtain previous pregnancy records to confirm type and location of uterine incision. Note striae, linea nigra.	Note any scars that may indicate previous abdominal surgery and influence type of delivery

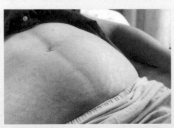

Linea nigra

(continued)

SYSTEM/AREA, APPROACH, AND NORMAL FINDINGS	ABNORMAL FINDINGS

Abdomen: Inspection, Palpation, Auscultation (*Continued*)

Enlargement caused by fetus; in later pregnancy, uterine shape may suggest fetal presentation and position. Palpable uterus at 10 to 12 weeks.	Abnormal palpable masses: Uterine fibroids or hepatosplenomegaly
Fetal movement noticed by mother at 18 to 20 weeks (earlier for multipara).	No fetal movement felt: Wrong EDC or fetal demise
Uterine contractions may be present; intensity is described as mild, moderate, or firm to palpation.	Regular contractions before 37 completed weeks of gestation: Preterm labor
What is the duration of the client's contractions? Time them from beginning to end of same contraction. How frequent are they? Time them from beginning of one contraction to beginning of next.	
Fundal height measurement: Place zero point of tape measure on symphysis pubis and measure to top of fundus. Fundal measurement should approximately equal number of weeks of gestation; measurements may vary by 2 cm; measurements by different examiners should be approximately the same.	Measurements greater than 4 cm from the estimated gestational age warrant further evaluation Measurements greater than expected: Multiple gestation, polyhydramnios, fetal anomalies, macrosomia Smaller than expected: Fetal growth restriction

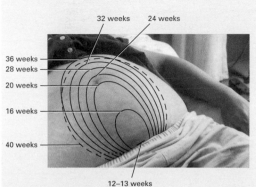

Fundal height assessment

(continued)

SYSTEM/AREA, APPROACH, AND NORMAL FINDINGS	ABNORMAL FINDINGS

Abdomen: Inspection, Palpation, Auscultation (*Continued*)

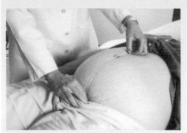

Fundal height measurement

Fetal heart tones (FHTs) are best auscultated through the back of the fetus. A fetal Doppler can be used after 10 to 12 weeks' gestation; a fetoscope may be used after 18 weeks' gestation.

Inability to auscultate FHT with a fetal Doppler at 12 weeks: Retroverted uterus, uncertain dates, fetal demise, false pregnancy

Fetal heart rate (FHR) range: 120 to 160 beats per minute. In the third trimester, FHR accelerates with fetal movement.

FHR decelerations: Poor placental perfusion

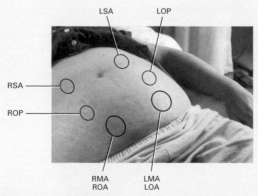

Fetal heart tones
Intensity varies according to fetal position. RSA = right sacrum anterior, LSA = left sacrum anterior, ROP = right occipitoposterior, LOP = left occipitoposterior, RMA = right mentum anterior, LMA = left mentum anterior, ROA = right occipitoanterior, LOA = left occipitoanterior

(continued)

SYSTEM/AREA, APPROACH, AND NORMAL FINDINGS	ABNORMAL FINDINGS

Abdomen: Inspection, Palpation, Auscultation (*Continued*)

Fetal position: Use Leopold's maneuvers to palpate the fundus, lateral aspects of the abdomen, and lower pelvic area. Leopold's maneuvers assist in determining fetal lie, presentation, size, and position. A longitudinal lie is expected. Fetal presentation may be cephalic, breech, or shoulder. Fetal size is estimated by measuring fundal height and by palpation.

First maneuver: Face the client's head and place your hands on the fundal area. You should palpate a soft, irregular mass in the upper quadrant of the mother's abdomen. The soft mass is the fetal buttocks; the round, hard part is the fetal head.

Second maneuver: Next, move your hands down to the lateral sides of the mother's abdomen. On one side you will palpate round, irregular nodules—the fists and feet of the fetus. Expect to feel kicking and movement. The other side of the mother's abdomen feels smooth—this is the fetus's back.

Third maneuver: Now move your hands down to the mother's lower pelvic area and palpate just above the symphysis pubis to determine the presenting part of the fetus. Grasp the presenting part with your thumb and third finger. If it is the fetus's head, it will be round, firm, and ballottable. If it is the fetus's buttocks, it will be soft and irregular.

Oblique or transverse lie: Breech presentation

If you hear fetal heart sounds above the umbilicus, it is a breech presentation; below the umbilicus, a vertex presentation

(continued)

SYSTEM/AREA, APPROACH, AND NORMAL FINDINGS	ABNORMAL FINDINGS

Abdomen: Inspection, Palpation, Auscultation (*Continued*)

Fourth maneuver: Next, face your client's feet, and place your hands on her abdomen, pointing your fingers toward her feet. Try to move your hands toward each other while applying downward pressure. If they move together easily, the fetus's head is not descended into the pelvic inlet. If they do not move together and stop because of resistance, the fetus's head is engaged into the pelvic inlet.

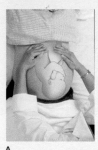
A

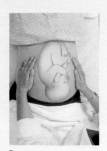
B

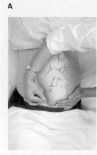
C

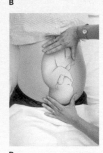
D

Fetal presentation/position

Extremities: Inspection, Palpation

In the third trimester, dependent edema is normal; varicose veins may also appear.

Calf pain, presence of Homans' sign, generalized edema, diminished pedal pulses: Deep venous thrombophlebitis (DVT)

(continued)

SYSTEM/AREA, APPROACH, AND NORMAL FINDINGS	ABNORMAL FINDINGS
Genitourinary: Inspection, Palpation *External Genitalia*	
Labial and clitoral enlargement, parous relaxation of introitus, scars from episiotomy or perineal lacerations (multiparous women).	Labial varicosities: Venous congestion
Bartholin's and Skene's Glands	
No discomfort or discharge.	Discharge and tenderness: Infection
Vaginal Orifice	
Small amount of whitish discharge (leukorrhea).	Thick, purulent vaginal discharge: Gonorrheal infection Thick, white, cheesy discharge: Yeast infection Gray-white discharge, sweet smell, positive clue cells: Bacterial vaginosis infection
Cervix	
Smooth, pink or bluish, long, thick, closed; 2.3 to 3 cm long. Softening of lower uterine segment (Hegar's sign) should be present. Bluish color (Chadwick's sign) indicates increased blood flow to pelvic area and is probable sign of pregnancy.	Effaced, opened cervix: Preterm labor or incompetent cervix if not a term gestation

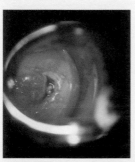

Chadwick's sign

(continued)

SYSTEM/AREA, APPROACH, AND NORMAL FINDINGS	ABNORMAL FINDINGS

Genitourinary: Inspection, Palpation
Cervix (Continued)

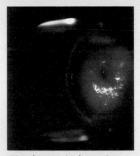

Circular cervical opening: nulliparous

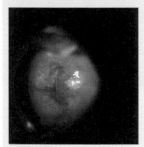

Slitlike cervical opening: multiparous

Uterus

Uterus is size of orange at 10 weeks; grapefruit at 12 weeks.	Uterine size not consistent with dates: Wrong dates, fibroids, multiple gestation
No masses in left and right adnexa; some discomfort because of stretching of round ligaments.	Palpable masses: Ectopic pregnancy

Musculoskeletal

Accentuated lumbar curve (lordosis), wider base of support.	Diastasis recti abdominis: Separation of abdominal muscles from pregnancy

(continued)

SYSTEM/AREA, APPROACH, AND NORMAL FINDINGS	ABNORMAL FINDINGS
Neurological	
+ 1–2 deep tendon reflex.	Hyperreflexia, clonus: Pre-eclampsia, eclampsia
Phalen's or Tinel's sign is absent.	Presence of Phalen's or Tinel's sign: Carpal tunnel syndrome

HEENT = head, eyes, ears, nose, and throat

Postpartal Physical Assessment

SYSTEM/AREA AND NORMAL FINDINGS	ABNORMAL FINDINGS
HEENT: Neck	
Thyroid nonpalpable	Thyromegaly
	Palpable nodules: Thyroiditis; hypothyroidism
Respiratory	
Equal bilateral breath sounds	Unequal bilateral breath sounds: Infection
Cardiovascular	
Normal sinus rhythm	Murmurs
Extremities	
Nontender, no swelling, no increased warmth to any area	Phlebitis; varicosities
Breasts	
Lactating: Full, milk expressible	Erythema, masses
Nonlactating: Soft, without lymphadenopathy; bilateral galactorrhea (up to 3 months)	Lymphadenopathy: Mastitis
	Hard, masses, lymphadenopathy: Mastitis
Gastrointestinal/Musculoskeletal	
No tenderness, masses, hernias, enlarged lymph nodes; diastasis recti; uterus nonpalpable	Costovertebral angle tenderness: Kidney infection, subinvolution

(continued)

SYSTEM/AREA AND NORMAL FINDINGS	ABNORMAL FINDINGS

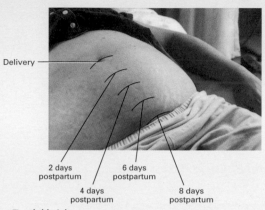

Delivery

2 days postpartum
4 days postpartum
6 days postpartum
8 days postpartum

Fundal heights postpartum

Genitourinary: External/Internal Genitalia

No edema, lesions, tenderness; episiotomy site intact; internal cervical os closed; uterine corpus nonpregnant size

Infection

HEENT = head, eyes, ears, nose, and throat

CHAPTER 15

ASSESSING THE NEWBORN AND INFANT

During the first year of life, the infant experiences rapid growth and developmental changes. Many physical, gross motor, fine motor, primitive reflex, sensory, communication, and socialization changes are seen.

Developmental Considerations

- Psychosocial development focuses on establishing trust; infant establishes trust when his or her needs are met.
- Cognitive development during first year, also called the sensorimotor phase of development, involves three tasks:
  - Separation—realizing that self is separate from other objects
  - Object permanence—realizing that objects are permanent even when not in sight
  - Mental representation—recognizing symbols of objects without actually experiencing the object
- Infant develops body image by exploring and playing with different parts of his or her body.
- Social development includes developing attachment to parents or caregivers and experiencing separation anxiety and fear of strangers.
- Communication and language development also occur.
- Denver Developmental Screening Test-II (DDST-II) and growth charts are frequently used to assess and track growth and development during well-baby check-ups.

- As you assess the infant, be sure to note if his or her physical development is appropriate for his or her age and whether he or she is performing appropriate developmental tasks for the age. Because growth and development are so rapid during the first year of life, even the slightest developmental delay may signal an underlying problem and warrant further investigation.
- Key physical changes:
  - Birth weight doubles by 6 months, triples by 12 months.
  - Height increases by 1 inch per month for first 6 months.
  - Fontanels are closing.
  - Lumbar curve develops with a lordosis once infant begins to walk.
  - Drooling and teething occur.
  - Primitive reflexes disappear as neurological system matures.
- Gross motor changes:
  - Rolls, crawls
  - Pulls to sit
  - Begins to walk
  - Achieves head control
- Fine motor changes:
  - Grasps objects
  - Puts objects in mouth
  - Holds bottle
  - Plays with toes
  - Develops pincer grasp
- Sensory changes:
  - Develops better vision
  - Follows objects
  - Responds to sounds
- Communication changes:
  - Initially cries to convey needs
  - Babbles
  - Laughs
  - Says three to five words by 12 months
  - Begins to comprehend simple directions
  - Imitates sounds
- Socialization changes:
  - Identifies parents

- Develops social smile
- Is aware of strange situations
- Has increasing difficulty separating from parents
- Becomes more fearful of strangers
- Begins to develop memory
- Shows emotions

Cultural Considerations

Cultural or ethnic influences may affect your assessment findings. You need to be aware of these normal variations so that you do not mistake them for abnormal findings. Cultural or ethnic influences may also affect the relationship between child and parent and define the roles of both parent and child within the family. They may also affect the infant's health and wellness.

Cultural and Ethnic Variations in Infants *

AFRICAN-AMERICAN
- Mongolian spots and other birthmarks more prevalent than in other ethnic groups.

AMISH
- Babies seen as gifts from God. Have high birth rates, large families.

APPALACHIAN
- Newborns wear bands around abdomen to prevent umbilical hernias and asafetida bags around neck to prevent contagious diseases.

ARAB-AMERICAN
- Children "dearly loved."
- Male circumcision is a religious requirement.

CHINESE-AMERICAN
- Children highly valued because of one-child rule in China.
- Mongolian spots occur in about 80% of infants.

---

*Adapted from Purnell, L.D., and Paulanka, B.J.: *Transcultural Healthcare: A Culturally Competent Approach, ed 2*. Philadelphia, F.A. Davis Company, 2003.)

- Bilirubin levels higher in Chinese newborns than in others, with highest levels seen on day 5 or 6.

CUBAN-AMERICAN
- Childbirth is a celebration. Family takes care of both mother and infant for the first 4 weeks.
- Tend to bottle-feed rather than breast-feed. If breast-fed, child is weaned early, around 3 months. If bottle-fed, weaned late, around 4 years.

EGYPTIAN-AMERICAN
- Children very important.
- Mother and infant cared for by family for the first 50 days.

FILIPINO-AMERICAN
- Eyes almond shaped, low to flat nose bridge with mildly flared nostrils. Mongolian spots common.

FRENCH-CANADIAN
- Five mutations account for 90% of phenylketonuria (PKU) in French-Canadians. High incidence of cystic fibrosis and muscular dystrophy.

GREEK-AMERICAN
- High incidence of two genetic conditions: thalassemia and glucose-6-phosphate dehydrogenase (G-6-PD).

IRANIAN-AMERICAN
- Believe in hot and cold influences, with baby boys "hotter" than baby girls. Infant may be confined to home for first 40 days. Ritual bath between 10th and 40th day.

JEWISH-AMERICAN
- Children seen as valued treasure.
- High incidence of Tay-Sachs disease.
- Male circumcision is a religious ritual.

MEXICAN-AMERICAN
- Wears stomach belt (ombliguero) to prevent umbilicus from popping out when infant cries.
- Believe that cutting nails in the first 3 months after birth causes blindness and deafness.

NAVAJO NATIVE AMERICAN
• Infants kept on cradle boards until they can walk.
• Mongolian spots common.

VIETNAMESE-AMERICAN
• Mongolian spots common.

Assessment of Newborns

Apgar Scoring of Newborns

HEART RATE	0 = absent	1 = <100 beats/ minute	2 = >100 beats/ minute
RESPIRATIONS	0 = absent	1 = <30, irregular	2 = strong cry, regular
MUSCLE TONE	0 = flaccid	1 = some flexion in arms and legs	2 = full flexion, active movement
REFLEX IRRITABILITY	0 = no response	1 = grimace, weak cry	2 = vigorous cry
COLOR	0 = pale, blue	1 = body pink, extremities blue	2 = totally pink

Newborn Health History

MATERNAL HEALTH HISTORY	SIGNIFICANCE
General health, prenatal diseases or conditions, prenatal care, number of pregnancies	Maternal health problems (e.g., gestational diabetes, cardiac, or kidney disease) may cause potential risk factors in newborn.
Use of prescribed or over-the-counter (OTC) medications, tobacco, alcohol, illegal drugs	Medications and other agents may affect physiological systems (e.g., smoking during pregnancy related to low birth weights, alcohol use related to fetal alcohol syndrome).
Duration of pregnancy and labor, type of anesthesia, type of delivery, complications	Details of labor and delivery alert nurse to observe for potential newborn problems.

Physical Assessment of Newborns

APPROACH: Inspection, palpation, percussion, auscultation. Perform techniques that may evoke crying (e.g., otoscopic examination) at the end of the assessment. Be sure to keep the room and the baby warm.

TOOLBOX: Tape measure, stethoscope, thermometer, blood pressure cuff, penlight, otoscope, ophthalmoscope, and baby scale.

AREA/SYSTEM AND NORMAL VARIATIONS	ABNORMAL FINDINGS
General Survey/Anthropometric Measurements/Vital Signs: Inspection, Auscultation, Measurement	
Posture	
Head and extremities flexed.	Limp posture with extension of extremities: Birth injuries, anesthesia, acidosis, hypoglycemia, hypothermia, or congenital problems
Head Circumference	
Measure head circumference from occiput to forehead. 33–35 cm. Molding can affect measurement. 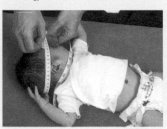 *Measuring head circumference*	Head circumference <10% of normal: Microcephaly related to congenital malformation or infection Head circumference >90% of normal: Macrocephaly related to hydrocephalus
Chest Circumference	
Measure chest at nipple line. 30.5–33 cm (2–3 cm less than head). Breast engorgement can affect measurement.	

(continued)

AREA/SYSTEM AND NORMAL VARIATIONS	ABNORMAL FINDINGS

General Survey/Anthropometric Measurements/Vital Signs: Inspection, Auscultation, Measurement
Chest Circumference (Continued)

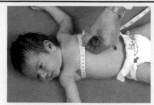

Measuring chest circumference

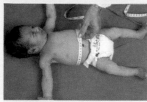

Measuring abdominal circumference

Abdominal Circumference

Measure abdomen above the umbilicus.
Similar to chest measurement. Should not be distended.

Length

Crown to rump: 31–35 cm (about equal to head circumference).
Head to heel: 45–55 cm (18–22 inches) at birth.
Molding can affect measurement.

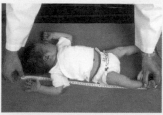

Measuring length

(continued)

AREA/SYSTEM AND NORMAL VARIATIONS	ABNORMAL FINDINGS
General Survey/Anthropometric Measurements/Vital Signs: Inspection, Auscultation, Measurement *Weight*	
Newborn weight is usually between 2500 and 4000 g (5 lb, 8 oz and 8 lb, 13 oz).	Birth weights <10% or >90% are abnormal Low birth weight (small for gestational age): Associated with prematurity Macrosomic infant (large for gestational age): Associated with gestational diabetes in mother
Temperature	
Axillary: 36.5–37.2°C.	Hypothermia leads to cold stress. Sepsis, environmental extremes, and neurological problems can cause hypothermia or hyperthermia
Pulse	
Apical rate 120–160 BPM. Rate increases with crying and decreases with sleep.	Irregular rhythms, such as bradycardia (<100 BPM) and tachycardia (>160 BPM) Most murmurs are not pathological and disappear by age 6 months
Respirations	
30–60 breaths/minute; irregular. Anesthesia during labor and delivery can affect respirations.	Respirations <30 or >60 breaths/minute Periods of apnea >15 seconds
Blood Pressure	
Systolic: 50–75 mm Hg Diastolic: 30–45 mm Hg Crying and moving increase systolic pressure.	Low blood pressure: Hypovolemia Late clamping of umbilical cord can increase blood pressure because of expanded blood volume from the "placental transfusion"
Integumentary: Inspection *Skin*	
Skin may be red, smooth, edematous, mottled (cutis marmorata). Hands and feet may be cyanotic (acrocyanosis).	Persistent acrocyanosis: Thermoregulation problem or hypoglycemia Extensive desquamation: Post-term baby.

(continued)

AREA/SYSTEM AND NORMAL VARIATIONS	ABNORMAL FINDINGS

Integumentary: Inspection
Skin (Continued)

Physiologic jaundice occurs after 24 hours.	Pathological jaundice occurs within first 24 hours.
Color may change with position (Harlequin sign).	Plethora: Polycythemia
Cheesy substance (vernix caseosa) decreases as baby's gestational age increases to term.	Pallor: Anemia, hypothermia, shock, or sepsis
Desquamation, ecchymosis, and petechiae may occur from trauma during delivery.	Persistent ecchymosis or petechiae: Thrombocytopenia, sepsis, or congenital infection
Milia (white papules) may occur on face.	Poor turgor: Intrauterine growth retardation or hypoglycemia
Miliaria or audamina (papules or vesicles on face) are caused by blocked sweat ducts.	Café-au-lait spots: >6 or larger than 4 × 6 cm may indicate neurofibromatosis; can become precancerous with age
Mongolian spots (bluish discoloration in sacral area) are commonly seen in African, Asian, Latin, and Native American newborns.	Nevus flammeus (port-wine stain): Disfigures face; may be associated with cerebral vascular malformation
Telangiectatic nevi.	Giant hemangiomas and nevus vasculosus ("strawberry marks") tend to trap platelets and lower circulating platelet counts. They usually disappear by age 5
Flat hemangiomas ("stork bites") may be present at nape of neck.	Reddish-blue round mass of blood vessels (cavernous hemangioma) must be monitored. If size increases, surgery may be necessary.

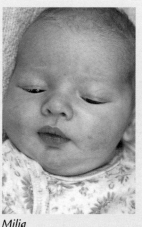

Milia

Erythema toxicum, a common newborn rash of red macules and papules, usually disappears in 1 week

Bullae or pustules: Infections such as syphilis or staphylococcus

Thin, translucent skin and vernix caseosa are signs of prematurity

Genetic disorders may cause extra skin folds

(continued)

AREA/SYSTEM AND NORMAL VARIATIONS	ABNORMAL FINDINGS
Integumentary: Inspection *Skin (Continued)*	

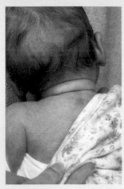

Stork bite

Hair

Some fine hair (lanugo) is normal.	Abundant lanugo: Prematurity Genetic disorders may cause abnormal hair distribution unrelated to gestational age

Nails

	Long nails seen in post-term babies

HEENT
Head/Face: Inspection, Palpation

Molding in birth canal may cause asymmetry of face and skull and should resolve within 1 week.	Fused sutures
Anterior fontanel: Diamond shaped, 2.5–4 cm. Posterior fontanel: Triangle shaped, 0.5–1 cm. Soft and flat.	Large fontanels: Hydrocephaly, osteogenesis imperfecta, congenital hypothyroidism Small fontanels: Microcephaly Bulging fontanels: Increased intracranial pressure Depressed fontanels: Dehydration Craniosynostosis (premature closure of sutures)

(continued)

AREA/SYSTEM AND NORMAL VARIATIONS	ABNORMAL FINDINGS

HEENT
Head/Face: Inspection, Palpation (Continued)

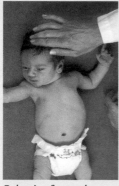

Palpating fontanel

Cephalohematoma (hematoma between periosteum and skull with unilateral swelling): Most uncomplicated cephalohematomas totally resolve within 2 weeks to 3 months

Caput succedaneum (edema of soft scalp tissue from birth trauma) decreases gradually in several days

Symmetrical facial movements.

Asymmetrical facial movements: Damage to facial nerve during forceps delivery

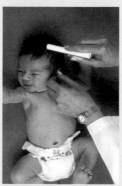

Transilluminating fontanel

Neck: Inspection, Palpation

Positive tonic reflex.
Short neck.

Absent tonic reflex: Erb's palsy if unilateral or dislocation of cervical spine or fractured clavicle

Able to hold head up with "pull-to-sit" test.

Head lag with "pull-to-sit" test: Muscle weakness
Torticollis (wry neck)

(continued)

AREA/SYSTEM AND NORMAL VARIATIONS	ABNORMAL FINDINGS

HEENT
Eyes: Inspection

Avoid bright light because it will cause the newborn to avoid opening his or her eyes and make assessment difficult. Eyes may be edematous after vaginal delivery.

Eyes equal and symmetrical.

Blue/gray or brown iris; white or bluish-white sclera.
Antimongolian slant; Mongolian slant seen in Asian infants.
Positive red light reflex.
Positive blink reflex.
Positive corneal reflex.
No tears (tear production begins by 2 months).
Positive fixation on close objects.
Positive pupillary reaction to light.
Strabismus and searching nystagmus caused by immature muscular control.

Subconjunctival hemorrhage: Trauma during delivery
Brushfield spots, epicanthal fold, and Mongolian slant: Down syndrome
Absent red light reflex: Congenital cataract
Ptosis: Neuromuscular weakness
Sun-setting (crescent of sclera over iris from retraction of upper lid): Hydrocephalus
Yellow sclera: Jaundice
Blue sclera: Osteogenesis imperfecta
Persistent nystagmus, absent blink reflex, inability to follow objects: Vision problem, such as blindness
Dilated or fixed pupil: Anoxia or neurological damage
Chemical conjunctivitis from eye prophylaxis may occur during first 24 hours

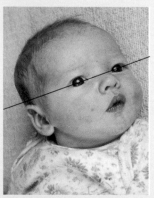

Normal eye line

(continued)

AREA/SYSTEM AND NORMAL VARIATIONS	ABNORMAL FINDINGS
HEENT	
Ears: Inspection, Palpation, Hearing Testing	
Pinna flexible, without deformity, aligns with external canthus of eyes.	Low-set ears: Down syndrome. **The ears and kidneys develop at the same time in utero, so malformed ears may be accompanied by renal problems**
Presence of the startle reflex. American Academy of Pediatrics recommends hearing screening by auditory brainstem response or evoked otoacoustic emissions on newborns before discharge.	Absent startle reflex: Possible hearing problem
Nose: Inspection	
Nares patent. Small amount of thin white mucus. May be flattened and bruised from birth.	Because infants are obligatory nose breathers, large amounts of mucus drainage may obstruct nostrils and result in respiratory difficulty Nasal flaring: Sign of distress
Mouth/Throat: Inspection	
Mucous membranes pink and moist. Frenulum of tongue and lip intact. Palate intact, uvula midline. Strong sucking reflex; positive rooting, gag, extrusion, and swallowing reflexes. Minimal saliva. Strong cry. Natal teeth may be benign or associated with congenital defects. ***Natal teeth must be removed by a specialist because they usually fall out and can cause choking.*** Small white, pearl-like epithelial cysts on the palate (Epstein's pearls) disappear within a few weeks.	Cyanotic mucous membranes: Hypoxia *Candida albicans* (thrush): Contracted during vaginal delivery Weak sucking, swallowing reflex: Maternal anesthesia or perinatal asphyxia Opening in palate or lips: Cleft palate or lip. Any opening is abnormal. A series of surgical interventions will be necessary ***Cleft lip or palate will cause newborn to have difficulty with feeding.*** Weak cry: Neuromuscular problem, hypotonia, and prematurity

(continued)

AREA/SYSTEM AND NORMAL VARIATIONS	ABNORMAL FINDINGS

HEENT
Mouth/Throat: Inspection (Continued)

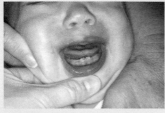

Natal teeth

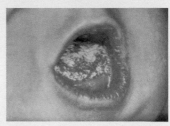

Thrush

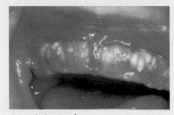

Epstein's pearls

Chest: Inspection, Auscultation

Anteroposterior:lateral (1:1).
Equal chest excursion.
Breast engorgement.
Clear or milky liquid from nipples ("witch's milk") develops from maternal hormones in utero.
Supernumerary nipples.

Funnel chest (pectus excavatum): Congenital anomaly
Pigeon chest (pectus carinatum): Obstructed respiration in infancy
Asymmetrical excursion, retraction: Respiratory distress
Red, firm nipples

Respiratory: Auscultation

Lungs clear, bronchial breath sounds audible.

Persistent crackles, wheezes, stridor, grunting, paradoxical

(continued)

AREA/SYSTEM AND NORMAL VARIATIONS	ABNORMAL FINDINGS

Respiratory: Auscultation (*Continued*)

Cough reflex absent at birth, but present 1–2 days later.

Scattered crackles a few hours after birth.

breathing, decreased breath sounds, prolonged periods of apnea (>15–20 seconds) are signs of respiratory problems

Cardiovascular: Auscultation

S1, S2, normal rhythm with respiratory variations.

Point of maximal impulse (PMI): 4th left intercostal space mid-costal line.

Quiet but clearly audible murmurs occur in 30% of newborns but should disappear in 2 days.

Dextrocardia (heart on right side)

Cardiomegaly: Displaced PMI

Murmurs often heard at base or along left sternal border and are usually benign, but need to be evaluated to rule out cardiac disorder.

Thrills

Abdomen: Inspection, Palpation

Abdomen round.

Positive bowel sounds.

Liver edge palpable 2 to 3 cm.

Tip of spleen, kidneys palpable.

Cord bluish white with two arteries and one vein.

Positive femoral pulses.

Umbilical hernias and diastasis recti more common in African-Americans; often resolves within a year.

Abdominal distention, ascites, distended veins: Portal hypertension

Green umbilical cord: Infection

Absence of umbilical vessels: Associated with heart and kidney malformations

Rectum: Inspection

Anus patent.

Passage of meconium stool within 48 hours.

Positive anal reflex ("anal wink").

Anal fissures or fistulas

No stools: Malformation in gastrointestinal (GI) tract

Imperforate anus (absent anus) requires immediate surgical repair

Female Genitourinary: Inspection, Palpation

Urination within 24 hours.

Urinary meatus midline and uninterrupted stream noted on voiding.

Labia majora and minora may be edematous. Place thumbs on either side of labia and gently separate tissues to visualize perineum.

Inability to urinate within 24 hours

Fused labia or absent vaginal opening

Ambiguous genitalia

Meconium from vaginal opening

(continued)

AREA/SYSTEM AND NORMAL VARIATIONS	ABNORMAL FINDINGS

Female Genitourinary: Inspection, Palpation (*Continued*)

Blood-tinged vaginal fluid may be noted (pseudomenstruation).	
Note presence of clitoris, vagina, and hymen.	A newborn clitoris larger than 0.5 cm is abnormal

Male Genitourinary: Inspection, Palpation

Urination within 24 hours.	Inability to urinate within 24 hours
Foreskin retracts.	Inability to retract foreskin
Urethral opening at tip of penis.	Hypospadias
Scrotum edematous.	Epispadias
Smegma.	Chordee
Palpable testes.	Hydrocele
	Undescended testicles
	Inguinal hernia
	Ambiguous genitalia
	Meconium from scrotum

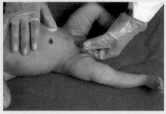

Palpating scrotum

Musculoskeletal: Inspection, Palpation

10 fingers and 10 toes.	Polydactyly: Extra digits
Full range of movement.	Syndactyly: Webbed digits
No clicks in joints.	Phocomelia: Hands and feet attached close to chest
Equal gluteal folds.	Hemimelia: Absence of distal part of extremity
C curve of spine, no dimpling.	
When arms and legs are extended, muscles symmetrical with equal muscle tone, and arms and legs symmetrical in size and movement.	Talipes (club foot): Foot is permanently twisted out of shape
	Severe bowing of legs is abnormal
Hands held as fists until after 1 month, when grasp becomes strong and equal.	Unequal gluteal folds and positive Barlow-Ortolani: Associated with congenial hip dislocation. Requires immediate referral
Position in utero may affect appearance.	Decreased range of motion (ROM) and muscle tone
	Swelling, crepitus, neck tenderness: Possible broken clavicle
	Simian (transverse palmar) creases: Down syndrome

(continued)

AREA/SYSTEM AND NORMAL VARIATIONS	ABNORMAL FINDINGS

Musculoskeletal: Inspection, Palpation (*Continued*)

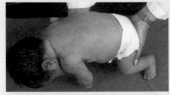

Checking for C curve

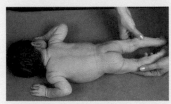

Checking gluteal folds

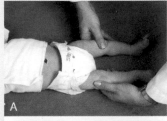

A. Barlow-Ortolani maneuver #1

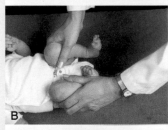

B. Barlow-Ortolani maneuver #2

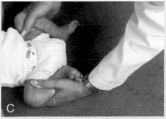

C. Barlow-Ortolani maneuver #3

(continued)

AREA/SYSTEM AND NORMAL VARIATIONS	ABNORMAL FINDINGS
Neurological: Inspection, Palpation, Percussion	
Positive newborn reflexes (Table 15–1). Positive knee reflex.	Hypotonia: Floppy, limp extremities Paralysis Marked head lag Tremors Asymmetrical posture Hypertonia: Tightly flexed arms and stiffly extended legs with quivering Opisthotonic posture: Arched back Dimpling of spine, tuft of hair: Spina bifida or pilonidal cyst

HEENT = head, eyes, ears, nose, and throat

Table 15-1. *Newborn/Infant Reflexes*

REFLEX AND TECHNIQUE	NORMAL RESPONSE	ABNORMAL RESPONSE
Moro Present at birth and lasts 1–4 months *Technique:* Startle infant by suddenly jarring bassinet, or with infant in semi-sitting position, let head drop back slightly.	Quickly abducts and extends arms and legs symmetrically. Makes "C" with index finger and thumbs. Legs flex up against trunk.	Premature or ill infants may have sluggish response. Positive response beyond 6 months indicates neurological problem. Asymmetrical response may be caused by injury to clavicle, humerus, or brachial plexus during delivery.

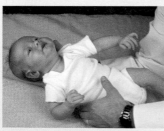

Moro reflex

(continued)

Table 15-1. *Newborn/Infant Reflexes (Continued)*		
REFLEX AND TECHNIQUE	**NORMAL RESPONSE**	**ABNORMAL RESPONSE**
Startle Present at birth and lasts 4 months *Technique:* Startle infant by making loud noise.	Hands clenched, arms abducted, flexion at elbow.	Same as Moro.

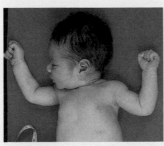

Startle reflex

Tonic Neck Present between birth and 6 weeks; disappears at 4–6 months. *Technique:* With infant supine, rotate head to one side so that chin is over shoulder.	Infant assumes "fencing position," with arm and leg extended in direction where head was turned.	Response after 6 months may indicate cerebral palsy.

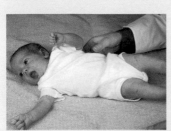

Tonic neck reflex

(continued)

Table 15-1. *Newborn/Infant Reflexes (Continued)*

REFLEX AND TECHNIQUE	NORMAL RESPONSE	ABNORMAL RESPONSE
Palmar Grasp Present at birth; disappears at 3–4 months. *Technique:* Place object or finger in palm of infant's hand.	Infant grasps object tightly. If he or she grasps your fingers with both hands, he or she can be pulled to a sitting position.	Negative grasp seen with hypotonia or perinatal asphyxia.

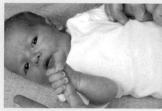

Palmar grasp reflex

| **Plantar Grasp** Present at birth; disappears at 3–4 months. *Technique:* Place thumb firmly against ball of infant's foot. | Toes flex tightly downward in a grasping motion. | Negative grasp seen with hypotonia or spinal cord injury. |

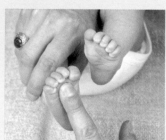

Plantar grasp reflex

| **Babinski** Present at birth; disappears at 1 year. *Technique:* Stroke lateral surface of sole of infant's foot. | Toes should fan. | Diminished response associated with neurological problem. |

(continued)

Table 15-1. *Newborn/Infant Reflexes (Continued)*

REFLEX AND TECHNIQUE	NORMAL RESPONSE	ABNORMAL RESPONSE

Babinski (*Continued*)

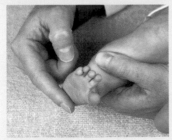

Babinski reflex

Stepping or Dancing

Present at birth; disappears at 3–4 weeks. *Technique:* Hold infant upright with feet touching a flat surface.	Infant steps up and down in place.	Poor response caused by hypotonia.

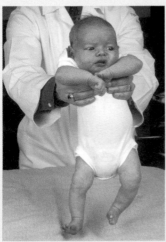

Stepping or dancing reflex

(continued)

Table 15-1. *Newborn/Infant Reflexes (Continued)*

REFLEX AND TECHNIQUE	NORMAL RESPONSE	ABNORMAL RESPONSE
Rooting Present at birth; disappears at 3–6 months. *Technique:* Brush cheek near corner of mouth.	Infant turns head in direction of stimulus and opens mouth.	Prematurity or neurological problem may cause weak or absent response.

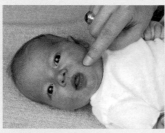

Rooting reflex

REFLEX AND TECHNIQUE	NORMAL RESPONSE	ABNORMAL RESPONSE
Sucking Present at birth; disappears at 10–12 months. *Technique:* Touch lips. **Don't check for rooting or sucking responses immediately after a feeding—they will be difficult to elicit.**	Sucking motion occurs.	Weak or absent response associated with prematurity or neurological defect.

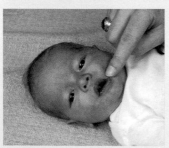

Sucking reflex

(continued)

Table 15-1. *Newborn/Infant Reflexes (Continued)*

REFLEX AND TECHNIQUE	NORMAL RESPONSE	ABNORMAL RESPONSE
Swallowing Present at birth and lasts throughout life. *Technique:* Automatically follows sucking response during feeding.	Sucking and swallowing should occur without coughing, gagging, or vomiting.	Weak or absent response associated with prematurity or neurological problem.
Extrusion Present at birth to 4 months. *Technique:* Touch tip of tongue.	Tongue protrudes outward.	Absence may indicate neurological problem. Continued extrusion of large tongue associated with Down syndrome.

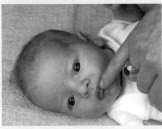

Extrusion reflex

Glabellar Present at birth *Technique:* Tap on forehead.	Newborn blinks for first few taps.	Persistent blinking with repeated taps indicates extrapyramidal problem.

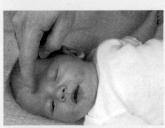

Glabellar reflex

Crawling Present at birth; disappears at 6 weeks. *Technique:* Place infant on abdomen.	Newborn attempts to crawl.

(continued)

Table 15-1. *Newborn/Infant Reflexes (Continued)*

REFLEX AND TECHNIQUE	NORMAL RESPONSE	ABNORMAL RESPONSE

Crawling (*Continued*)

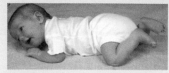

Crawling reflex

Crossed Extension

Present at birth; disappears at 2 months. *Technique:* Infant supine with leg extended. Stimulate foot.	Flexion, adduction, then extension of opposite leg.	Peripheral nerve damage causes weak response. Spinal cord lesion causes absent response.

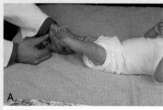

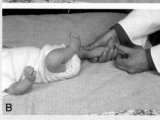

A. Crossed extension, B. Stimulate foot

Pull-to-Sit

Present at birth *Technique:* Pull infant to sitting position.	Head lags as infant is pulled to sitting position, but then infant is able to hold up head temporarily.	Inability to hold up head suggests prematurity or hypotonia.

(continued)

Table 15-1. *Newborn/Infant Reflexes (Continued)*

REFLEX AND TECHNIQUE	NORMAL RESPONSE	ABNORMAL RESPONSE

Pull-to-Sit (*Continued*)

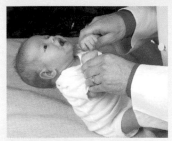

Pull-to-sit reflex

Trunk Incurvation Present at birth; disappears in a few days to 4 weeks. *Technique:* With infant prone, run finger down either side of spine.	Flexion of trunk with hip moving toward stimulated side.	Absent response indicates neurological or spinal cord problem.

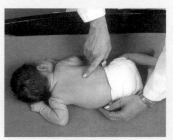

Trunk incurvation reflex

Magnet Present at birth *Technique:* With infant supine, flex leg and apply pressure to soles of feet.	Extends legs against pressure.	Breech birth may diminish reflex. Absent response caused by spinal cord problem.

(continued)

Table 15-1. *Newborn/Infant Reflexes (Continued)*		
REFLEX AND TECHNIQUE	**NORMAL RESPONSE**	**ABNORMAL RESPONSE**
Magnet (*Continued*)		

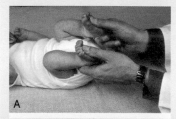

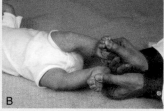

A. Flex legs, B. Apply pressure to soles of feet

Diagnostic/Screening Tests for Newborns

TEST	SIGNIFICANCE
Phenylketonuria: Measures amount of phenylalanine amino acids in blood	Test is collected after several days of feedings. High phenylalanine levels can cause brain damage.
Galactosemia: Transferase deficiency	Elevated galactose and low fluorescence may result in mental retardation, blindness, or death from dehydration and sepsis.
Maple syrup urine disease	Elevated leucine can result in acidosis, seizures, mental retardation, and death.
Homocystinuria	Elevated methionine can lead to mental retardation, seizures, and behavioral disorders.

(continued)

TEST	SIGNIFICANCE
Congenital adrenal hyperplasia	Elevated 17-hydroxyprogesterone can lead to hyponatremia, hypokalemia, hypoglycemia, and ambiguous female genitalia.
Biotinidase deficiency	Decreased activity of biotinidase on colorimetric assay causes mental retardation, skin changes, hearing and vision problems, even death.
Thyroxine	Thyroxine is a thyroid hormone necessary for growth, development, and metabolism. Low values are associated with brain defects.
Blood type	RH and ABO incompatibility can cause hemolysis and subsequent jaundice. If mother is RH− and newborn is RH +, mother must be treated promptly to avoid sensitization to future RH+ fetuses.
Sickle cell anemia	Detects presence of hemoglobin S. Electrophoresis identifies whether infant has the trait or disease.
Audiometric testing	Identifies hearing disorders early.
HIV: Newborns of mothers with HIV are tested for virus.	Early virus detection can permit start of early treatment that may enhance survival.
Gestational age: Normal gestational age is 38–42 weeks. Newborn less than 38 weeks is premature. A screening test, such as Ballard test, estimates fetal gestation.	Accurate estimate of gestational age influences care management and special monitoring needs. Full-term infant should have creases over entire sole of foot, full breast areolas, firm ear cartilage. Boys should have pendulous testes and deep scrotal rugae. In girls, the labia majora should cover clitoris and labia minora.

Assessment of Infants

Infant Health History

A complete health history can be obtained from the newborn's chart and from a parent or guardian. Review the chart, paying special attention to prenatal care, gestational or family health problems, and supports. The infant health history also addresses developmental milestones, home safety, and immunizations, which are critical for primary prevention of childhood diseases. Table 15–2 reviews the immunizations recommended for infants. For the most recent information about vaccines, visit the National Immunization Program Home Page at *http://www.cdc.gov/nip/,* or call the National Immunization Hotline at 800-232-2522 (English) or 800-232-0233 (Spanish).

Table 15-2. *Recommended Immunizations for Infants*

IMMUNIZATION	SCHEDULE
Hepatitis B	First dose within 2 months of age, second dose 1 month after first dose, and third dose 6 months after second dose.
Diphtheria, pertussis, tetanus toxoid (DPT)	Doses at 2 months, 4 months, and between 6 and 18 months.
Haemophilus influenzae Type B (hib)	Doses at 2 months, 4 months, and 6 months (check with manufacturer if third dose at 6 months is required).
Inactivated polio vaccine	Doses at 2 months, 4 months, and between 6 and 18 months.
Pneumococcal conjugate (PCV)	Doses at 2 months, 4 months, and between 6 and 18 months.

AREAS AND QUESTIONS TO ASK	SIGNIFICANCE
General Health Status How is your infant doing now?	Determining the parents' view of their infant's general well-being provides a baseline for you to begin your assessment.

(continued)

AREAS AND QUESTIONS TO ASK	SIGNIFICANCE
Body Weight	
Has infant been gaining weight?	Weight gain within normal parameters is an indicator of nutritional status.
Integumentary	
Does the infant have good skin turgor?	Skin tenting denotes dehydration.
Does skin appear healthy?	Scaly skin may be caused by an underlying medical condition or dryness from soaps or lotions.
Do hair and nails appear healthy or brittle?	Brittle hair and nails may be caused by poor protein intake.
Head and Neck	
Is head shape symmetrical?	Symmetry is normal.
Can infant hold head upright while sitting and move head from side to side?	Head control is a necessary motor development milestone.
Eyes, Ears, Nose, and Throat	
Can infant recognize toys you give him or her? Do eyes focus symmetrically?	Refer infants with signs of visual difficulties to specialist.
Is there eye exudate?	Infants are highly susceptible to eye infections and may require medications.
Does infant turn head when his or her name is called? Can he or she vocalize?	Ability to hear and speak is critical for development. If you notice signs of hearing or speaking problems, refer infant to specialist.
Is there exudate from the nose?	Nose exudate may signal infection or allergies or may be normal mucus production.
Respiratory	
Is breathing labored?	Monitor abnormal breathing patterns carefully.
Cardiovascular	
Is infant active? Is skin ever blue-tinged?	Infants should be active and lively when awake. Lethargy may be related to cardiac difficulties, of which cyanosis is a warning sign.
Gastrointestinal	
How is the infant's appetite?	Appetite denotes good health.
What does he or she usually eat and drink each day?	Adequate daily nutrient intake is necessary for growth.

(continued)

AREAS AND QUESTIONS TO ASK	SIGNIFICANCE
Gastrointestinal (*Continued*)	
How many bowel movements a day does he or she have?	Regular bowel movements suggest normal gastrointestinal activity.
Genitourinary	
Is urination pattern consistent with fluid intake?	Adequate urination pattern denotes normal kidney function.
How many diaper changes a day?	Usually about eight diapers a day is normal, depending on fluid intake.
Musculoskeletal	
Does infant roll over, sit unsupported, transfer toy from one hand to the other? Can he or she creep forward or backward on tummy?	Body movements should be within developmental norms.
Neurological	
Have you noticed any unusual movements such as tremors? Problems with sucking, swallowing?	Tremors or other unusual movements may indicate seizures. Diminished sucking or swallowing reflexes may indicate an underlying neurological problem.
Infections	
Has infant had any colds, fevers, infections?	Usual infant infections may not be preventable. However, teach parents infection-control methods.
Development	
Does infant prefer to play with people rather than toys? Does he or she search for an object that is out of sight? Is he or she afraid of strangers?	Deviations from these developmental milestones may impair social activities.
Relationships	
How do you feel about the new baby and about being a mother or father?	Mother may cry, feel irritable, and have loss of appetite and sleeplessness for first 10 days or so after delivery. If these problems persist for more than 2 weeks, it may signal postpartum depression and warrants referral.

Physical Assessment of Infants

AREA/PA SKILL	NORMAL FINDINGS	ABNORMAL FINDINGS
Anthropometric Measurements *Head and Chest*		
Apply tape measure around widest part of head, just above eyebrows.	Head circumference increases by 1.5 cm each month for first 6 months and by 0.5 cm per month until age 12 months	Greater than normal head circumference: Hydrocephalus Smaller than normal head circumference: Microcephaly
Measure chest at nipple line.	Chest circumference equals head circumference by 12 months	
Height and Weight		
Measure length from head to heels. Weigh without clothing or diaper.	Height should increase 50% by age 12 months. Birth weight should double by 6 months and triple by 12 months	Anthropometric measurements deviating from normal: Underlying disease or inadequate eating or nutritional pattern
Integumentary *Skin*		
Inspect skin appearance, folds, turgor.	Skin pigmentation varies. Newborns of dark-skinned parents may appear light skinned at birth. True skin color develops by 3 months of age Good skin turgor in newborns and infants is a sign of adequate hydration	Persistent cyanosis in the warm infant is never normal and requires immediate referral Red, excoriated skin: Diaper rash (diaper dermatitis). Secondary yeast infection (*Candida*) causes bright, round scaling patches Dry, itchy patches on face and skin folds in infants with allergies: Eczema (atopic dermatitis)

(continued)

AREA/PA SKILL	NORMAL FINDINGS	ABNORMAL FINDINGS
Integumentary *Skin (Continued)*		
		Flat, greasy scales on scalp: "Cradle cap" (seborrheic dermatitis); may be caused by infrequent shampooing
		Depressed fontanels and skin tenting: Signs of severe dehydration
Note axillary temperature. *Never use a mercury thermometer on a newborn or infant. Mercury is highly toxic.*	Axillary temperature range for newborns and infants is 35.9°C to 36.7°C (96.6°F to 98.0°F)	Low temperature: Hypothermia High temperatures can cause seizures in newborns and infants
Hair and Nails		
Inspect amount and characteristics of hair. Check for presence of nails.	As baby grows, amount of hair varies Nails present	Dry, brittle hair: Malnutrition or malabsorption
HEENT *Head, Face, and Neck*		
Inspect and palpate infant's head, face, and neck. Some cultures fear touching fontanel area.	Face and skull symmetrical Fontanels flat and soft. At birth, anterior fontanel is 2.5–4 cm across; it closes between 12 and 18 months of age. Posterior fontanel is initially 2 cm and closes by 3 months Neck is short and should rotate left to right	Sunken fontanel: Dehydration Bulging fontanel: Increased intracranial pressure

(continued)

AREA/PA SKILL	NORMAL FINDINGS	ABNORMAL FINDINGS
HEENT		
Eyes		
Inspect and palpate external eye, eyelids, lacrimal ducts, conjunctiva, and sclera.	Bilateral blinking Corneal reflex positive Transient strabismus common	Continued strabismus after 6 months is abnormal
Test visual acuity using the DDST II. *CHECK VISUAL ACUITY.*	No tearing in first month Sclera may be blue. tinged	Lack of tears after 2 months: Clogged lacrimal ducts; requires medical attention
	Pupils constrict with light and are round and equal in size Infants have full binocular vision	Fixed or dilated pupils: Neurological problem
Ears		
Inspect and palpate external and internal ear.		
Check hearing.	Infant should respond to noise	Lack of response to noise: Hearing problem
To perform otoscopic examination, place infant flat and restrain arms above head. Pull auricle down and back to observe tympanic membrane.	Pinna flexible	
Nose		
Inspect nose. Check patency by closing one nostril, then the other.	Infants are nose breathers Thin white mucus discharge and sneezing are normal	Flaring of nares: Sign of respiratory distress Bloody discharge or large amount of nasal secretions may obstruct nares
Mouth/Throat		
Inspect oral cavity: Palate, tongue, gums, tonsils. Use light and tongue blade.	White nodules (Epstein's pearls) may be found on hard palate and usually disappear by 3 months	Protruding tongue: Associated with congenital disorders, such as Down syndrome or hypothyroidism

(continued)

AREA/PA SKILL	NORMAL FINDINGS	ABNORMAL FINDINGS
HEENT *Mouth/Throat (Continued)*		
	Tongue should not protrude from mouth No coating in mouth Suck should be strong First primary teeth usually appear at 6 to 8 months	
Chest/Back/Shoulders		
Inspect spinal curvature.	Convex spinal curvature (C-curve) By 12–18 months, lumbar curve develops and lordosis is present as walking begins	Limited ROM may result from injury Dimpling in spine may be associated with neural tube defects
Note blemishes or skin openings.	No blemishes or skin openings	
Respiratory Inspect chest. Percuss chest lightly. Use direct percussion. Palpate back with two fingers while newborn is crying. Auscultate lungs.	Respiratory rate 25–50 breaths per minute Apnea less common than in newborns Normal breath sounds more bronchial Infants are abdominal breathers Anteroposterior:lateral diameter is equal	***Apnea >15 seconds accompanied by decreased heart rate is abnormal Stressful breathing with flaring nares and sighing with each breath are signs of respiratory distress and require immediate attention*** Inspiratory stridor, expiratory grunts, retractions, paradoxical (seesaw) breathing, asymmetrical or decreased breath sounds, wheezing, and crackles are abnormal Depressed sternum may affect normal respiration

(continued)

AREA/PA SKILL	NORMAL FINDINGS	ABNORMAL FINDINGS
Cardiovascular		
Auscultate heart and peripheral pulses. Use a stethoscope with a small diaphragm and perform exam when infant is quiet.	Apical pulse felt in fourth or fifth intercostal space just medial to midclavicular line	
	Heart rate range 80–160 beats per minute	Abnormal heart rate range requires attention
	Capillary refill <1 second	Murmurs accompanied by cyanosis: Congenital heart defects
	Peripheral pulses present	Capillary refill times >2 seconds: Dehydration or hypovolemic shock
		Evaluate newly discovered murmurs
		Infant who eats poorly may have cardiovascular problem
Gastrointestinal		
Inspect, palpate, percuss, and auscultate abdomen.	Bowel sounds present Bowel soft Tympany may be heard because of air swallowing	
	Umbilicus flat	Umbilical hernias >2 cm wide may require further evaluation
		Abdominal pain may indicate childhood illnesses
	Liver edge 1–2 cm below right rib cage (costal margin)	Enlarged liver or palpable spleen may indicate disease
Extremities		
Inspect hands, arms, feet, legs, and hips. Test ROM.	Feet flat Legs equal in length	Inadequate ROM may indicate congenital malformation or birth injury or may result from pulling or lifting infant

(continued)

AREA/PA SKILL	NORMAL FINDINGS	ABNORMAL FINDINGS
Extremities (*Continued*)		
	Transfers objects from one hand to other by 7 months	Inability to meet developmental milestones may indicate neurological or environmental deficits
	Crawls and sits unsupported by 7 months	
	Pulls to standing position and holds on to furniture by 11 months	
Genitourinary		
	Note infant's sex	Ambiguous genitalia abnormal
Boys		
Inspect and palpate penis and urethra.	In uncircumcised infant, foreskin may not be fully retractable until 1 year of age	Phimosis (tight foreskin) can constrict penis. Instruct parents on gentle retraction of foreskin to prevent phimosis
	Urethra midline	
	Urine flow straight and strong	Weak urine stream or dribbling: Stricture at urinary meatus
	No palpable masses in testes	Solid scrotal masses are abnormal
	Two testes should be palpated in scrotum or brought down from inguinal ring	Hernias present as scrotal masses
		Testes not palpable: Undescended testicles
		If scrotum swollen, transilluminate to determine if fluid (hydrocele) present
Girls		
Inspect external genitalia.	External genitalia pink and moist	Blood-tinged fluid from vagina abnormal after 1 week
		Vaginal discharge or labial redness or itching may be caused by diaper or soap irritation or sexual abuse

(continued)

AREA/PA SKILL	NORMAL FINDINGS	ABNORMAL FINDINGS
Anus and Rectum Inspect anus and rectum.	Bowel movements may occur with each feeding. By 1 year, they occur once or twice a day Breast-fed babies have stools that are mustard colored and soft Formula-fed babies have stools that are yellow-green and more formed	Watery stools and explosive diarrhea: Infection Constipation or hard stools: Inadequate hydration or nutrition
Neurological Inspect and test muscle strength, sensory function, and reflex movements. (See Table 15–1 for newborn/infant reflexes.)	Infant's body stays erect when you support him or her with both hands under axilla. Motor control develops from head to toe Infant opens eyes to noise and responds to touch Presence of infantile reflexes denotes healthy neurological system	Delays in motor or sensory activity: Brain damage, mental retardation, illness, malnutrition, or neglect Asymmetrical posture or spastic movements need further evaluation Maintenance of infant reflexes past usual age is abnormal

PA = physical assessment

Diagnostic/Screening Tests for Infants

TEST	SIGNIFICANCE
Developmental testing: Should occur regularly throughout childhood. Denver Developmental Screening Tool 2 assesses skills in areas of personal/social, fine motor, language, and gross motor.	If delays are noted, refer child to specialist for further testing. Medications, malnutrition, neurological, and emotional conditions affect test results.
Urine screening: Dipstick screening test is usually sufficient.	Any abnormalities require full urinalysis.
Hemoglobin or hematocrit.	Hemoglobin below 10 g/dL is low and infant is considered anemic. Hematocrit below 29% is low.
Lead screening: Only if environmental exposure is suspected.	Elevated blood lead levels can cause neurological damage.

CHAPTER 16

ASSESSING THE TODDLER AND PRESCHOOLER

The toddler years extend from 12 to 36 months and the pre-school years from 3 to 5 years. The toddler years are often referred to as the "terrible 2s" as the child struggles to gain control; in the preschool years, the child is preparing for school.

Psychosocial and Emotional Changes

- Toddlers are struggling to develop a sense of autonomy.
- Toddlers work to gain control over bodily functions, tolerate separation from parents, differentiate self from others, develop socially acceptable behavior, develop verbal communication skills, become less egocentric, and tolerate delay in gratifying needs.
- Failure in developing autonomy results in doubt and shame.
- The negativism associated with this period often explains the term "the terrible 2s," when "No" seems to be the only word in the child's vocabulary.
- The child also looks for consistency in "ritualism," or sameness within his or her environment. This sameness provides a sense of safety and comfort.
- Sex role imitation, such as dressing-up, is common during toddler and preschooler years.
- The next developmental stage, initiative versus guilt, is a

time of playing and learning. If the child goes beyond set limits, guilt results.

- Ability to tolerate a delay in satisfying needs reflects ego development in the child.
- Superego development is in its early stages.
- Behavior is seen as good or bad based on the outcome, either reward or punishment.
- Rapid cognitive development occurs during this time.
- The child begins to see causal and spatial relationships, and develops object permanence.
- Language skills continue to develop during the preschool years.
- Play is an important means of expression and of learning.
- Preschoolers' perceptions of God are concrete and based on parental influence.

Health Promotion and Risk Factors for the Toddler and Preschooler

Common health issues seen with the toddler and pre-schooler include toilet training, sibling rivalry, temper tantrums, negativism and regression, fears, stress, and aggression. Health problems seen with toddlers and preschoolers include communicable diseases, accidents (such as poisonings), and injuries. Abuse or neglect can occur at any age, but younger children are more dependent on the parents for all needs, physical and psychological, and therefore they are more vulnerable to neglect or abuse.

Assessment of the Toddler and Preschooler

Health History

CURRENT HEALTH STATUS
Ask about the health status of the child. Has the child been healthy, or is there an acute problem?

CURRENT MEDICATIONS
Ask about all prescription and over-the-counter medications.

PAST HEALTH HISTORY
Include questions that relate to the pregnancy and the delivery of the child.

IMMUNIZATIONS

Additional immunizations recommended by or during the preschool years include:

- Polio dose 3 by 18 months
- Diphtheria, tetanus, and pertussis (DTP) between 15 and 18 months
- Measles, mumps, and rubella (MMR) between 12 and 15 months
- Chickenpox (VZV) between 1 and 12 years
- *Haemophilus influenzae* between 12 and 15 months
- Hepatitis B (HBV) dose 3 between 6 and 18 months

SIGNIFICANT FAMILY MEDICAL HISTORY

Ask about heart disease, strokes, cancer, and other serious health conditions within the family that present later in life.

SYSTEM AND QUESTIONS TO ASK	SIGNIFICANCE
General Health Status How has child been feeling? How much does child weigh? Changes in behavior are good indicators of how a child is feeling.	Screen for any obvious problems. Changes in weight are closely monitored to evaluate normal growth and development.
Integumentary Any skin rashes, lesions, excessive itching?	Tinea capitis, ringworm, or contagious disorders can occur in toddlers and preschoolers, especially if the child is in day care. Eczema is often associated with allergies and has a familial tendency. Diaper rashes occur from prolonged exposure to an irritant, such as urine or feces. Head lice can occur in preschoolers in day care or preschool. Playing dress-up or sharing hats can increase transmission.

(continued)

SYSTEM AND QUESTIONS TO ASK	SIGNIFICANCE
Integumentary *(Continued)*	
Sun exposure? Use of sunblock?	Excessive exposure to sun (UV rays) without sunblock increases the risk for skin cancer later in life.
HEENT	
Eyes	
Does child have vision problems? Crossed eyes? When was child's last eye exam?	Normal visual acuity is 20/40 for toddler. Depth perception is developing. Vision should be tested routinely during physical examinations.
Ears	
Does child have any hearing problems? Does child respond to sounds? Is child talking, making sounds? When was child's last hearing examination? Does child have frequent ear infections? Does he or she exhibit irritability, poor appetite, poor sleeping?	Hearing should be tested routinely during physical examinations. Toddlers and preschoolers have a high incidence of otitis media, with the highest incidence between 6 months and 2 years.
Teeth	
How many teeth does child have? Has child had first dental examination?	All 20 primary teeth should be complete by 2½ years. The first dental examination should occur shortly after onset of eruption of primary teeth. The child should have at least annual dental examination.
Does child brush teeth?	Review tooth-brushing technique with child and parent.
Is your water fluoridated?	Fluoride decreases tooth decay. ***Fluoride is toxic if ingested. Advise parents not to allow child to eat toothpaste.***
Does child go to bed with a bottle?	Bedtime bottles, nocturnal breast-feeding, or coating pacifiers with sweet substance can cause baby-bottle caries; occurs most frequently between 18 months and 3 years.

(continued)

SYSTEM AND QUESTIONS TO ASK	SIGNIFICANCE
Respiratory	
Does child have a cough, sneezing, runny nose, or fever?	Upper respiratory infections (URIs) are common in toddlers and preschoolers. Respiratory syncytial virus (RSV) causes $\frac{1}{2}$ of all bronchiolitis, usually occurring in children younger than age 2 years.
Does child ever wheeze or have trouble breathing?	Asthma is the most common disease among children. Onset usually occurs between ages 3 and 8.
Is child exposed to air pollutants (e.g., smoke or second-hand smoke)?	Exposure to second-hand smoke increases risk for respiratory and ear infections and asthma attacks.
Cardiovascular	
Were you ever told that child had a heart murmur?	Although cardiovascular disease is not common in children, murmurs are a common finding. Most murmurs are innocent, functional murmurs, but follow-up is indicated to rule out pathology.
Has child ever turned blue?	Change in skin color may indicate a cardiopulmonary problem.
Gastrointestinal	
Is child potty trained? What is child's bowel pattern?	Bowel control usually achieved before age 3 years. Bowel control usually precedes bladder control.
Genitourinary	
Does child have bladder control?	Bladder control usually achieved by age 3 years.
Musculoskeletal	
Is the child walking?	The child should be able to walk without difficulty. *Even though the child is able to walk, the child still does not have refined coordination and full depth perception and therefore is still at risk for falls.*

(continued)

SYSTEM AND QUESTIONS TO ASK	SIGNIFICANCE
Neurological	
Is child speaking? Using complete sentences?	Cognitive skills continue to develop. The child should be speaking. Speech development usually occurs between ages 2 and 4 years.
Does child have any fears?	Fears, real and imaginary, are common (e.g., fear of dark).
Does child have temper tantrums or aggressive behavior?	Acting-out, aggressive behavior, temper tantrums: May need to provide education to parents regarding effective ways to deal with child's behavior.
Lymphatic/Hematological	
Have you noticed any lumps in child's neck, groin, or underarms?	Enlarged nodes may indicate an infection.

Psychosocial History

HEALTH PRACTICES

When was the child's last health examination? Recommend health examinations every year.

TYPICAL DAY

Can you tell me what your child's day is like? Does the child go to day care or preschool?

NUTRITION

Screen diet by asking for a 24-hour recall. Is the child still nursing or bottle feeding? If yes, how often? Because breast milk contains immunoglobulin A (IgA) and breast-feeding minimizes reflux of milk into the eustachian tube, breast-feeding decreases the risk of otitis media and respiratory viruses and allergies. Ask about eating patterns: "How often do you eat breakfast?"; "What is a usual lunch for you?"; "What are your favorite snacks?" For the toddler, protein and caloric requirements are still high for growth, and calcium, iron, and phosphorus are needed for bone growth. After 18 months, the toddler's appetite decreases (physiological anorexia) in response to decreased nutritional needs. For the preschooler, an average of 1800 calories, with reduced fat, is needed per day. Calcium and minerals are still needed for bone growth. During the toddler and preschool years, the child develops taste preferences and may become a picky eater.

ACTIVITY/EXERCISE
Toddlers and preschoolers are usually very active. With this increased activity, close supervision is needed.

SLEEP/REST
Ask about sleep patterns and naps, bedtime rituals, sleep problems (nightmares, night or sleep terrors, somnambulism, enuresis). The toddler and preschooler usually sleep about 12 hours per day. The toddler usually requires a nap; the preschooler does not.

PERSONAL HABITS/BEHAVIORS
Investigate personal habits of parents or caregivers, such as smoking or alcohol or drug use. Exposure to these substances (such as through second-hand smoke) places the child at risk for health problems. If drug or alcohol abuse is an issue, both the caregiver's ability and the home environment need to be assessed to ensure the child's safety. Referrals may be warranted.

RECREATION/HOBBIES
Safety is a major concern for the toddler and preschooler. If recreational activities or hobbies increase the risk for injury, ask if protective measures, such as bike helmets, are used. Also question the parent's hobbies; for example, ask about the presence of weapons in the home, and gun and hunting safety.

Play for the toddler is parallel; play for the preschooler is associative, group play. There is more social interaction in the play of preschoolers. With both age groups, safety is paramount, supervision is needed, and toys must be age appropriate.

ROLES AND RELATIONSHIPS
If there are siblings, ask the parent about the relationship. Sibling rivalry is not uncommon.

SEXUALITY/REPRODUCTIVE

Toddlers and preschool children are curious by nature and exhibit sex-role imitation. They are also curious about their own bodies, and it is not uncommon for them to masturbate. How this behavior is addressed is important because it can have lasting effects.

COPING AND STRESS TOLERANCE

Does the child have aggressive behavior or temper tantrums? If the child's behavior is destructive to self or others, he or she needs to learn effective coping strategies.

VALUE/BELIEF PATTERN

The toddler's and preschooler's perception of God is rather concrete and based on the beliefs and practices of the parents or caregivers. Prayer can be a source of comfort for a child; for example, prayers are often part of bedtime rituals.

PHYSICAL ASSESSMENT

SYSTEM/ASSESSMENT	NORMAL VARIATIONS/ ABNORMAL FINDINGS
Anthropometric Measurements and Vital Signs	
Weigh child and take measurements of height and head and chest circumference.	Toddler usually gains 4–6 lb a year and 3 inches a year in height. Head and chest circumferences are usually equal by age 2. The preschooler gains 5 lb a year and 2½–3 inches a year in height.
Check child's vital signs	Changes in vital signs include a gradual and slight increase in blood pressure and a slight decrease in temperature, pulse, and respirations.
General Health Survey	
Inspect overall appearance, noting appropriate growth and development for child's age.	Toddler's general appearance: "Pot belly" and wide base of support are normal. Preschooler loses pot belly and becomes taller and leaner. Detect any delays or premature maturation. Note any obvious weight problems.

(continued)

SYSTEM/ASSESSMENT	NORMAL VARIATIONS/ ABNORMAL FINDINGS
Integumentary	
Inspect skin for lesions.	Lesions, such as tinea capitis or ringworm, need treatment.
Inspect hair and scalp for lice.	Pediculosis common among preschoolers. ***Suspect abuse if you find unexplained bruising or injury.***
HEENT *Head and Face*	
Inspect head and face. Palpate anterior fontanel.	Head size growth slows to 1 inch a year by end of age 2, then ½ inch a year until age 5. Anterior fontanel closes by 18 months.
Eyes	
Test visual acuity. Test for "lazy eye"(strabismus) with corneal light reflex or cover-uncover test.	Visual acuity is 20/40 during toddler years. Vision screening should begin between 3 and 4 years. Visual deficits warrant follow-up Referral needed for strabismus to prevent amblyopia (reduction or dimness in vision).
Ears	
Test hearing with pure tone audiometer. Inspect external ear canal and tympanic membrane. You may want to leave the otoscopic examination until the end of the physical assessment.	Hearing deficits warrant follow-up. Hearing should be tested by age 3–4 years. Toddlers and preschoolers have a high incidence of otitis media.
Nose	
Inspect the nasal septum and mucosa.	Chronic rhinorrhea can result from allergic rhinitis. Boggy, bluish purple or gray turbinates are consistent with allergic rhinitis. **When inspecting the nares or the external ear canal, always be alert for the presence of foreign objects.**

(continued)

SYSTEM/ASSESSMENT	NORMAL VARIATIONS/ ABNORMAL FINDINGS
HEENT *Mouth*	
Inspect oral mucosa and pharynx.	Generally, the tonsils are large.
Inspect number and condition of teeth.	Primary teeth eruption usually complete by 2½ years.
	Note any nursing/baby-bottle caries.
	Review dental hygiene with parent and child.
Neck	
Palpate the neck for lymph nodes.	Enlarged lymph nodes may be associated with an infection or lymphoma.
Respiratory	
Inspect and measure size and shape of chest.	Anteroposterior to lateral diameter 1:2 by end of second year.
Auscultate lungs.	Toddlers and preschoolers have a high incidence of respiratory infections.
Cardiovascular	
Auscultate heart; note rate and rhythm.	Children often have a sinus arrhythmia and a split second heart sound. Both the arrhythmia and split second sound change with respiration. This is a normal variation.
	Systolic innocent murmurs and venous hum are common findings.
	If murmur is detected, refer for follow-up to rule out pathology.
Gastrointestinal	
Inspect, auscultate, and palpate abdomen.	A pot belly is normal for a toddler; the condition disappears as the abdominal muscles strengthen.
Genitourinary	
Inspect external genitalia.	If child is still in diapers, inspect for diaper dermatitis.

(continued)

SYSTEM/ASSESSMENT	NORMAL VARIATIONS/ ABNORMAL FINDINGS
Musculoskeletal	
Inspect gait.	Toddlers usually can walk alone by 12–13 months. Balance is unsteady with wide base of support. Genu valgus or varus may be present. Preschooler's gait more balanced, smaller base of support; walks, jumps, climbs by 3 years.
Test muscle strength.	Strength increases during preschool years.
Neurological	
Test balance, coordination, and accuracy of movements.	During toddler and preschool years, the child's balance and coordination improve, with refinement of fine motor skills.

HEENT = head, eyes, ears, nose, and throat

CHAPTER 17

ASSESSING THE SCHOOL-AGE CHILD AND ADOLESCENT

THE SCHOOL-AGE CHILD

The school-age child is the child between the ages of 6 and 12 years. This period is known as the "latency period." During this time, growth and development occur at a slower, steadier pace.

Growth and Developmental Changes

The changes that take place during the school-age years are subtle as the toddler and preschooler transforms into a child approaching preadolescence.

Physical Growth

- Measurements become more proportional as baby fat disappears.
- Child becomes more agile and coordinated.

Psychosocial and Emotional Changes

- Task of this stage is industry versus inferiority.
- Child becomes more independent, developing skills and competencies.
- Social skills also develop during this time as child becomes more involved in school and community activities.
- Peer acceptance is very important: The child needs a sense of belonging, of fitting in.

- Peer pressure often has a greater influence on child than parents do.
- Sex roles are established through peer relationships.
- Child chooses same-sex best friends.
- School provides the child with the opportunity to see different perspectives, argue, negotiate, resolve conflicts, work together, and develop friendships.
- Belonging to clubs, teams, and peer groups is important.
- Parents still have a major role in child's development. Child will test parents, and limits and restrictions are needed to give child a sense of security.
- Play involves team play, either active (such as sports) or quiet games.
- Sports, art, reading, collections, cooking, sewing, and the like are also important activities and often carry through adolescence and into adulthood.
- The child needs to feel special for a positive self-concept to develop.
- The child moves from preconceptual thinking to conceptual thinking, mastering the tasks of conservation and classifications.
- Reading is the most important skill that child develops during this stage.
- The child becomes less egocentric and begins to develop a conscience. Initially, child's views are black and white, right or wrong, based upon parents' moral values.
- God is seen in concrete terms. Child may see illness or injury as a punishment.

Health Promotion and Risk Factors

Common health problems seen with the school-age child include injuries related to accidents; drug, alcohol, and nicotine abuse; eating disorders; learning disorders; and emotional problems.

Cultural Considerations

The following information on various cultures and their perspectives on children is adapted from Purnell, L.D. and Paulanka, B.J. (2003): *Transcultural Healthcare: A Culturally Competent Approach* (2nd ed.). Philadelphia, F. A. Davis Company.

CULTURE	PERSPECTIVE ON CHILDREN
African-American	Good behavior, respectfulness, obedience, and conformity to rules are stressed. In violent communities, mothers try to protect children and keep them off the streets.
Amish	Children are seen as gift from God. Parents very directive of child throughout school.
Appalachian	Subscribe to physical punishment, which may be perceived as abuse. Having children associated with sense of importance.
Arab-American	Child's character and success dependent on parental influence. Taught conformity and cooperation. A "good" child is an obedient child; behavior that would bring dishonor is avoided. Subscribe to physical punishment.
Chinese-American	Boys and girls play together when young but separate when older. Pressure on children to succeed. Boys are more valued than girls. Help parents at home.
Cuban-American	Children are expected to study and respect parents.
Egyptian-American	Children are expected to be studious and goal oriented; respectful and loyal to family.
Filipino-American	Children are expected to honor and respect parents.
French-Canadian	Children are well educated and a source of pride for family.
Greek-American	Children are center of family. Children are disciplined through "teasing."
Iranian-American	Culture is child oriented. Children expected to be respectful.
Irish-American	Boys are expected to be more aggressive than girls. Children are expected to show self-restraint, discipline, respect, and obedience.
Jewish-American	Children are seen as a valued treasure. Children are expected to respect and honor parents.
Mexican-American	Children are highly valued. Children must respect parents.
Navajo Native American	Children are allowed to make decisions that might seem irresponsible, such as taking medicine.
Vietnamese-American	Children are prized and valued. Children are expected to be obedient and devoted.

Assessment

Health History

CURRENT HEALTH STATUS

This is addressed in essentially the same way as with an adult.

CURRENT MEDICATIONS

Ask about all prescription and over-the-counter medications.

PAST HEALTH HISTORY

Check with the parents or guardians for specifics of past health history questions.

IMMUNIZATIONS

Additional immunizations recommended by or during the school-age years include:

• Polio dose 4 by 6 years of age
• Tetanus-diphtheria (TD) between 11 and 16 years
• Measles, mumps, and rubella (MMR) between 11and 12 years, if second MMR shot not given between 4 and 6 years
• Chickenpox (VZV) between 1 and 12 years

SIGNIFICANT FAMILY MEDICAL HISTORY

Ask about heart disease, strokes, cancer, and other serious health conditions within the family. It is also important to ask if anyone died at an early age (younger than age 35 years) from a sudden heart attack. This may be a risk factor for sports participation and may require additional investigation if present.

REVIEW OF SYSTEMS

SYSTEM AND QUESTIONS TO ASK	SIGNIFICANCE
General Health Status	
How have you been feeling?	Screen for any obvious problems.
Any recent weight changes?	Changes in weight, especially gains, may indicate poor eating habits.

(continued)

SYSTEM AND QUESTIONS TO ASK	SIGNIFICANCE
Integumentary	
Any skin rashes, lesions, excessive itching?	Tinea capitis, ringworm, verruca (warts); contact dermatitis; and poison ivy, oak, and sumac frequently seen in school-age children.
	Pediculosis capitis (head lice) common in school-age children.
Sun exposure? Use of sunblock?	Excessive exposure to sun (UV rays) without sunblock increases the risk for skin cancer later in life.
HEENT	
Eyes	
Any visual problems? Do you wear glasses or contact lenses?	Visual acuity reaches 20/20 by school age.
If yes, ask if child wears glasses consistently, especially while at school.	Many times children may not consistently wear glasses for fear of being teased by other children.
	May identify teaching need about care of contact lenses.
When was last eye examination?	Eyes should be tested routinely during physical examinations.
Ears	
Do you have any hearing problems? Do you listen to loud music?	Cochlear damage can result from excessive exposure to loud noise, such as CD players and rock concerts.
	May identify teaching need about noise pollution's effect on hearing.
When was last hearing examination?	Hearing should be tested routinely during physical examinations.
Teeth	
When was your last visit to the dentist? Orthodontist?	Should have at least annual dental examination.
How many second teeth do you have?	Primary teeth are lost during school-age years and replaced by secondary teeth.
	This stage is called "age of loose tooth" or "ugly duckling stage"

(continued)

SYSTEM AND QUESTIONS TO ASK	SIGNIFICANCE
HEENT *Teeth (Continued)*	
	because secondary teeth initially are too big for face. Common dental problems during school-age years include dental caries, periodontal disease, malocclusion, and dental injury. *In secondary tooth evulsion, tooth should be replanted as soon as possible. If replanted within 30 minutes, 70% successful.*
Respiratory Do you have asthma? Do you ever have trouble breathing or wheeze when exercising or running? Are you exposed to air pollutants, smoke, or second-hand smoke?	Allergies and asthma are likely to become apparent during school-age years. Asthma is the most common disease among children. Exercise-induced bronchospasm is acute, reversible, self-terminating airway obstruction that occurs after vigorous exercise, peaks 5–10 minutes once activity stops, and then ceases within 30 minutes.
Cardiovascular Do you have any chest pain? Does your heart ever skip a beat?	Although cardiovascular disease is not common in children and adolescents, it can occur. Prolonged QT syndrome can cause sudden cardiac death in a seemingly healthy child.
Gastrointestinal Any stomach problems?	Recurrent abdominal pain is common during childhood and is often psychosomatic. Child usually has poor self-image. School can precipitate attacks. *If child presents with recurrent abdominal pain, first rule out physiological causes.*

(continued)

SYSTEM AND QUESTIONS TO ASK	SIGNIFICANCE
What is your bowel pattern?	Encopresis (fecal incontinence and voluntary or involuntary loss of bowel control) is more common in boys, usually secondary to constipation.
Genitourinary Do you have bladder control? Bedwetting?	Nocturnal bedwetting, often self-limiting, ends by age 6–8 years. More common in boys.
Musculoskeletal Do you have any back problems? Have you ever been told you had a spinal problem?	Heavy backpacks have been associated with low back problems in children. Scoliosis occurs more frequently in girls than in boys. Screening usually occurs in middle and high school. If present, determine if scoliosis is structural or postural (see Chapter 12). Physical maturity varies and does not always correlate with emotional or social maturity.
Neurological How would you describe your mood?	Stress, anxiety, and fears can be seen in children. Depression, conversion reactions, and even schizophrenia can occur during childhood and be difficult to detect.
Lymphatic and Hematological Have you been tired? Any lumps in neck, underarms, or groin?	Non-Hodgkin's lymphomas occur most frequently in children before age 15 years.

Psychosocial History

HEALTH PRACTICES

When did you have your last health examination? (Recommend health examinations every 2 years.)

TYPICAL DAY

Can you tell me what your day is like? How are you doing in school? This allows you to see the child through his or her eyes. You may be able to identify stresses confronting the child in everyday life. A change in academic perform-ance or a sudden disinterest in school may reflect a more serious problem. Ask children what subjects they like, which ones they dislike. If they are having problems with a partic-ular subject, have they sought help for this? How many days of school do they miss in a term? Attention deficit hyperac-tivity disorder (ADHD) and LD may become more apparent once the child starts school, and appropriate referrals should be made as indicated. School phobias are common at age 10 years, with child trying to avoid school with somatic com-plaints such as nausea, headache, or abdominal pain. Char-acteristically, these complaints quickly subside once the child is assured that he or she does not have to go to school. If the child is a "latchkey child," one who is left without adult supervision after school, identify what the child does with his or her time until the parent or guardian returns home. Safety is an issue for children who are left home alone, which places them at higher risk for injury or delinquent behavior.

NUTRITION
Screen diet by asking for a 24-hour recall. Ask about eating patterns: "How often do you eat breakfast?" "What is a usual lunch for you?" "What are your favorite snacks?" Junk and fast food amount to empty calories and contribute to the high incidence of obesity among children.

ACTIVITY AND EXERCISE (SUCH AS SPORTS, IF APPLICABLE)
Ask about what children enjoy doing outside of the home. What sports do they play, if any? What do they like to do with their friends? How often do they watch TV during the week? How much time do they spend on the computer? You may identify a need for health education regarding the importance of routine exercise. If a child does participate in sports, does he or she use protective equipment? Is it a con-tact sport? Contact sports may increase the risk for injury. **If a child plays sports, he or she should engage in sports appropriate for his or her age.**

SLEEP AND REST
Ask about when the child usually goes to bed and when he or she awakens. The school-age child, age 8 to 11, may

resist going to bed. Does he or she have a bedtime routine? Remember that enuresis can continue into adolescence.

PERSONAL HABITS AND BEHAVIORS
Substance abuse is occurring at younger and younger ages, so it is not uncommon for the school-age child to have tried smoking or alcohol. Experimentation is common for this age group, and peer pressure can be great. So you need to ask about substance use (drugs, alcohol, and nicotine). Ask, "If you smoke cigarettes, how many do you smoke in an average day?" "If you use alcohol, how much do you usually drink during the week?" "If you use drugs, what type and what method (smoking, snorting, huffing, ingesting, injecting)?" Asking questions in this way is less threatening to the child, and he or she is more likely to give an honest response.

RECREATION AND HOBBIES
Ask, "What do you do for fun? Do you have any hobbies?" If recreational activities or hobbies increase the risk for injury, ask if protective measures (e.g., bike helmets) are used. Ask about presence of weapons in the home and gun and hunting safety courses, if appropriate.

SELF-PERCEPTION AND SELF-CONCEPT
Ask the child to describe himself or herself—"Tell me about yourself." A child's self-image and body image are often influenced by his or her perception of how he or she is seen by others, peers, and family. Anything out of the norm may become an easy target for teasing, and such teasing can have lasting effects on a child.

ROLE AND RELATIONSHIP
Ask the child to tell you about the family—"Who lives at home with you?" If there are siblings, ask about the relationship. Ask, "Is there an adult in your life whom you feel comfortable talking with?" Teachers can have a major influence on a child's development, either positive or negative. Ask about peer relationships. Ask if the child has a special friend and what things he or she enjoys doing with that friend. It is during the school-age years that a child develops close friendships with same-sex peers.

SEXUALITY AND REPRODUCTIVE ISSUES

The school-age child is curious by nature, and it is not unusual for school-age children to include some form of sexuality into play. This is the best time to begin sex education, and as a nurse you are in an ideal position to educate both children and parents.

COPING AND STRESS TOLERANCE

Ask questions such as "What do you do when you get angry?" and "What makes you angry?" Also ask questions such as "What do you do when you want to relax or have fun?" You need to identify whether the child has healthy coping strategies to deal with feelings and stresses in life. Violence is ever present in our society: in the home, at school, and within the community. If your client uses violence as a coping mechanism, you may need to make referrals to help him or her develop more effective coping strategies.

VALUE AND BELIEF PATTERN

The school-age child's values and beliefs are often guided by those of the parents. God has to be depicted in concrete terms. Illness may be perceived as a punishment. Prayer can be a source of comfort for a child; for example, prayers are often part of bedtime rituals.

Physical Assessment

SYSTEM/ASSESSMENT	NORMAL VARIATIONS/ ABNORMAL FINDINGS
Anthropometric Measurements and Vital Signs	
Obtain height and weight and vital signs. Plot height and weight on growth charts to note growth and development of child.	During school-age years, child will grow about 5 cm a year and gain about 4½ to 6½ lb a year. Boys and girls are relatively equal in size until they reach preadolescence, when girls tend to pass boys in both height and weight. Boys catch up during adolescence, but until then, this situation can be distressing for both boys and girls.

(continued)

SYSTEM/ASSESSMENT	NORMAL VARIATIONS/ ABNORMAL FINDINGS
General Health Survey Inspect overall appearance, noting appropriate growth and development for child's age.	General appearance more slender, loss of baby fat. Detect any delays or premature maturation. Note any obvious weight problems.
Integumentary Inspect skin for lesions. Inspect hair and scalp for lice.	Lesions, such as tinea capitis or ringworm, need treatment. Pediculosis common among school-age children.
HEENT *Head and Face*	
Inspect head and face.	Head size becomes more proportionate to body.
Eyes	
Test visual acuity.	Visual acuity 20/20 by age 6. Visual deficits warrant follow-up.
Ears	
Test hearing with pure tone audiometer.	Hearing deficits warrant follow-up. Use opportunity to teach hazards of listening to loud music.
Nose	
Inspect nasal septum and mucosa.	Chronic rhinorrhea can result from allergic rhinitis. Boggy, bluish purple, or gray turbinates are consistent with allergic rhinitis.
Mouth and Throat	
Inspect oral mucosa and pharynx. Inspect occlusion. Inspect number of teeth.	Generally, the tonsils are large. If malocclusion is present, refer to orthodontist. Child loses first teeth during school age. Secondary teeth begin to erupt around age 6 years (with the 6-year molars): Most secondary teeth have grown in by the time 12-year molars erupt.

(continued)

SYSTEM/ASSESSMENT	NORMAL VARIATIONS/ ABNORMAL FINDINGS
HEENT *Mouth and Throat (Continued)*	
	Also assess for orthodontic devices and brushing technique around them.
Neck	
Palpate the neck for lymph nodes.	Enlarged lymph nodes may be associated with an infection or lymphoma.
Respiratory Auscultate lungs.	Children with exercise-induced asthma require bronchodilators before activity. Usually, albuterol administered through a metered-dose inhaler is given 20–30 minutes before exercise.
Cardiovascular Auscultate heart; note rate and rhythm.	Children often have a sinus arrhythmia and a split second heart sound. Both the arrhythmia and split second sound change with respiration. This is a normal variation.
Gastrointestinal Inspect, auscultate, and palpate abdomen.	Appendicitis is the most common illness during childhood that requires surgery.
Genitourinary Inspect external genitalia.	Precocious puberty—sexual development before age 8 in girls and age 9 in boys— warrants follow-up evaluation.
Musculoskeletal Inspect and palpate spinal curves. Test for spinal deformities. (See Chapter 12.)	Scoliosis is the major variation within the musculoskeletal system. Screening for scoliosis should be done in the preadolescent period, generally during the fifth and sixth grade. Any significant curvature should be referred for evaluation and follow-up.
Test muscle strength.	Strength doubles during school-age years.

(continued)

SYSTEM/ASSESSMENT	NORMAL VARIATIONS/ ABNORMAL FINDINGS
Neurological Test balance, coordination, and accuracy of movements.	During school-age years, the child's balance and coordination greatly improve with refinement of fine motor skills.

Abuse

Abuse can occur at any age and comes in many different forms: neglect, physical injury, sexual abuse, or psychological abuse. You must be constantly alert for the following signs or symptoms of abuse or neglect in all children:

- Obvious physical signs of abuse or neglect
- Repeated emergency room visits
- Siblings blamed for injury
- Inconsistent accounts of how injury occurred
- Report of abuse by child
- Inappropriate response by child or parent to injury
- Inconsistency between physical findings and cause of accident
- Inconsistency between injury and child's developmental level
- Previous history of abuse

A sudden change in a child's behavior may reflect an underlying problem that warrants further investigation.

THE ADOLESCENT

Stages of Adolescence

- Early adolescence begins at puberty (as early as 8 or 9 years but more typically 11–14 years for girls and 12–16 years for boys). This is a period of rapid physical growth and corresponds with the onset of menstruation in girls and sperm production in boys.
- Middle adolescence typically ranges from ages 14 to 16 in girls and 16 to 18 in boys. Girls have generally achieved adult height, but boys may continue their linear growth.

- Late adolescence typically starts around age 17 and can continue into the early 20s.
- Prepubescence is the 2-year period before puberty in which preliminary physical changes are occurring.
- Puberty is the time when sexual maturity occurs, reproductive organs begin to function, and secondary sexual characteristics develop.
- Postpubescence occurs 1 to 2 years after puberty, when skeletal growth is completed and reproductive function is regular.

Growth and Developmental Changes

Physical Growth

- There is a rapid period of growth in height, weight, and muscle mass.
- Sexual maturation occurs during this period and can be tracked by using the Tanner scale.
- For girls, the first sign of sexual maturation is breast development, and menstruation generally begins within 2 years of the onset of breast development.
- For boys, sperm production (spermatogenesis) corresponds with increased testicular size and penile enlargement. Nocturnal emissions ("wet dreams") typically start about 1 year after the penis begins to enlarge in size.
- The achievement of Tanner Stage 5 for both girls and boys corresponds with adult sexual maturity.
- The rapid physical growth is responsible for much of the clumsiness and awkwardness associated with the adolescent period.

Psychosocial and Emotional Changes

- Adolescence is also a period of tremendous psychosocial and emotional changes.
- The developmental task of adolescence is "identity versus identity diffusion."
- Adolescents become preoccupied with "what others think about them" in an attempt to be accepted. The focus of influence shifts from the family to the peer group, and it is with this group that the adolescent begins to form a sense of identity.

- Ideally, the adolescent moves through this stage developing an internal set of personal values and a sense of self-competency while beginning to plan for a future career.
- Cognitive development is termed the "formal operational stage." The adolescent now begins a process of more logical thought.
- Conflicts begin to occur between adolescents and their parents. Traditional values of the adolescent's family may be challenged by the exposure to new ideas and values from peers.
- The adolescent struggles to develop his or her own set of moral principles, questioning established moral codes.
- Peers often have more influence on the adolescent than do his or her parents, but often pre-established values and morals persist.
- The adolescent questions his or her spiritual beliefs, often turning away from formal religion, and eventually resolving the questions and identifying his or her own sense of spirituality.
- Adolescence is also a time of increased risk-taking behavior. This is a result of several factors, including the desire to separate from parental influence, peer pressure and the need to "belong," and a thought process in which the adolescent does not see himself or herself as vulnerable ("It can't happen to me").
- A number of undesirable behaviors—such as unprotected sexual activity, substance use, and unsafe driving—are examples of risky behavior that is often exhibited by teens.

Health Promotion and Risk Factors

Common health problems seen with this age group include eating disorders, obesity, pregnancy, sexually transmitted diseases (STDs), emotional disorders, substance abuse, and violence.

Cultural Considerations

Cultural influences may affect adolescent behaviors by establishing expectations. The following information on various cultures and their perspectives on adolescents is adapted from Purnell and Paulanka: *Transcultural Healthcare: A Culturally Competent Approach* (2nd ed.). Philadelphia: F. A. Davis Company, 2003.

CULTURE	PERSPECTIVES ON ADOLESCENTS
African-American	Adolescents are often expected to assume some responsibility for household chores and are encouraged to get jobs. Premarital teen pregnancy is not condoned, but it is accepted once child is born.
Amish	Adolescent may want to break away from cultural norms (e.g., dress), but it is expected that this is experimental and teen will return and assume adult role adhering to prescribed norms.
Appalachian	Formal education is not stressed; adolescent expected to get job and support family. Adolescents marry young, 15 years and even as young as 13 years. Having children associated with sense of importance. Underage alcohol abuse common.
Arab-American	Chastity and decency expected.
Chinese-American	Expected to score well in national tests by age 18 years. Must make career choice during adolescent years. Teenage pregnancy not common. Expected to respect elders.
Cuban-American	At age 15, girls have "rite of passage" (quince party) and are ready for courting. Unmarried couples may have chaperones.
Egyptian-American	Loss of virginity affects marriageability, so parents very restrictive.
Filipino-American	Short courtships.
Greek-American	Girls have less freedom in dating than boys. Dating is often prohibited until upper grades of high school.
Iranian-American	Girls are expected to maintain virginity.
Irish-American	Expected to remain loyal to family.
Jewish-American	Rite of passage at age 13 for boys and age 12 for girls.
Navajo Native American	Menarche for a teenage girl seen as passage to adulthood. Older children taught to be stoic and not complain.
Vietnamese-American	Teens are expected to respect elders.

Assessment

Health History

CURRENT HEALTH STATUS
This is addressed in essentially the same way as with an adult.

CURRENT MEDICATIONS
Ask about all prescription and over-the-counter medications. Many teens (especially those involved in athletics) take vitamin or protein supplements, and it is important to assess for these. Ask girls if they take oral contraceptives, get monthly "shots" (Depo-Provera), or have a contraceptive implant (Norplant). Also, ask all female clients about Accutane (an acne medication) because the risk of serious birth defects with this medication necessitates counseling about pregnancy prevention.

PAST HEALTH HISTORY
The questions are the same as for the adult, although the adolescent may not be aware of all his or her past health history.

IMMUNIZATIONS
Additional immunizations recommended by or during adolescence include:

- Tetanus-diphtheria (TD) between 11 and 16 years
- Measles, mumps, and rubella (MMR) between 11 and 12 years, if second MMR shot not given between 4 and 6 years
- Chickenpox (varicella zoster virus {VZV}) between 11 and 12 years
- Meningitis vaccine (Menomonee) administered before start of college.

SIGNIFICANT FAMILY MEDICAL HISTORY
If the teen is being interviewed alone, he or she may have limited knowledge in this area. Most, however, will be aware of heart disease, strokes, cancer, and other serious health conditions within the family. It is also important to ask if anyone died at an early age (younger than age 35

years) from a sudden heart attack. This may be a risk factor for sports participation and may require additional investigation, if present.

REVIEW OF SYSTEMS

SYSTEM AND QUESTIONS TO ASK	SIGNIFICANCE
General Health Status	
How have you been feeling?	Screen for any obvious problems.
Any recent weight changes?	Changes in weight, either loss or gain, may indicate an eating disorder.
Integumentary	
Any skin problems, such as acne?	Adolescents are very self-conscious about appearance and acne may affect self-image.
Changes in body hair growth?	Secondary sexual changes include increased growth of body hair (i.e., pubic hair, axillae, legs, and facial hair for boys).
Piercing or tattoos?	Body piercing and tattooing can increase risk for HIV or hepatitis B.
Sun tanning? Use of sunblock? Tanning salons?	Excessive exposure to sun (UV rays) without sunblock increases the risk for skin cancer later in life.
HEENT	
Eyes	
Any visual problems?	Visual refractive problems peak during adolescence.
Do you wear glasses or contact lenses?	May identify teaching need about care of contact lenses.
When was your last eye examination?	Eyes should be tested routinely during physical examinations.
Ears	
Do you have any hearing problems? Do you listen to loud music?	Cochlear damage can result from excessive exposure to loud noise, such as CD players and rock concerts. May identify teaching need about noise pollution's effect on hearing.

(continued)

SYSTEM AND QUESTIONS TO ASK	SIGNIFICANCE
HEENT *Ears (Continued)*	
When was your last hearing exam?	Hearing should be tested routinely during physical examinations.
Teeth	
When was your last visit to the dentist? Orthodontist?	Should have at least an annual dental examination. The need for orthodontic work usually becomes apparent during adolescence and can make the teenager even more self-conscious about appearance.
Respiratory Do you have asthma? Do you ever have trouble breathing or wheeze when exercising or running?	Asthma is the most common disease among children and adolescents. Exercise-induced bronchospasm is acute, reversible, self-terminating airway obstruction that occurs after vigorous exercise, peaks in 5–10 minutes once activity stops, and then ceases within 30 minutes.
Are you exposed to air pollutants, smoke, or second-hand smoke?	
Cardiovascular Do you have any chest pain? Does your heart ever skip a beat?	Although cardiovascular disease is not common in children and adolescents, it can occur. Prolonged QT syndrome can cause sudden cardiac death in a seemingly healthy child.
Breasts *Girls*	
Do you have any tenderness of the breasts? Have they increased in size? Are they growing equally?	Need to determine if normal breast development is occurring. May identify areas for health teaching. Initially, breast development may be asymmetrical, but it will even out.

(continued)

SYSTEM AND QUESTIONS TO ASK	SIGNIFICANCE
Breasts *Boys*	
Have your breasts enlarged?	During early puberty, boys may experience temporary gynecomastia, which usually disappears within 2 years. Because appearance is of great concern, gynecomastia can be very alarming for boys and make them very self-conscious.
Gastrointestinal	
Any stomach problems? What is your bowel pattern?	Identify underlying eating disorder.
Do you use laxatives?	Excessive use of laxatives associated with eating disorders.
Genitourinary *Girls*	
Did your periods start? When? Frequency? Description of flow?	Need to identify menarche and determine if cycle is normal.
Do you use pads or tampons?	Use of tampons has been associated with risk for toxic shock syndrome.
Do you have burning when you go to the bathroom? Urinary tract infections (UTIs)?	A history of frequent UTIs in girls can be the result of sexual activity and a clue to follow up more thoroughly in this area.
Are you sexually active? Have you had sex? Are you practicing safe sex?	May identify teaching need about sexually transmitted diseases (STDs) and safe sex practices.
	Pubertal delay for girls: No breast development by age 13 or no menarche within 4 years of initial breast changes.
Boys	
Are you sexually active? Have you had sex? Are you practicing safe sex?	May identify teaching need about STDs and safe sex practices.
	Pubertal delay for boys: No changes in testes or scrotum by age $13\frac{1}{2}$ to 14, incomplete genital growth within 4 years of initial change.

(continued)

SYSTEM AND QUESTIONS TO ASK	SIGNIFICANCE
Musculoskeletal	
Do you have any back problems? Have you ever been told you had a spinal problem?	Heavy backpacks have been associated with low back problems in children and adolescents.
	Scoliosis occurs more frequently in girls than in boys. Screening usually occurs in middle and high school. If scoliosis is present, determine if it is structural or postural (see Chapter 12).
Neurological	
How would you describe your mood? Do you feel sad a lot?	Adolescence is a time of change, and emotional response to these changes varies. Depression and suicidal ideations need to be identified and treated.
Endocrine	
Any swelling in neck? Difficulty swallowing? Hoarseness?	Thyroid is more active during puberty.
	Enlarged thyroid may indicate hypothyroid or hyperthyroid disease. Lymphocytic thyroiditis (Hashimoto's disease or juvenile autoimmune thyroiditis) peaks in adolescence.
	Graves' disease occurs between ages 12 and 14.
	If sexual maturation is not progressing, endocrine problems should be considered.
Lymphatic and Hematological	
Have you been tired? Have you any lumps in neck, underarms, or groin?	Rapid growth and poor dietary habits increase the risk of iron deficiency anemia during adolescence.
	Hodgkin's lymphoma is prevalent between ages 15 and 19. Non-Hodgkin's lymphomas occur more frequently before age 15.

HEENT = head, eyes, ears, nose, and throat

Psychosocial History

HEALTH PRACTICES

When did you have your last health examination? (Recommend health examinations every 2 years.)

TYPICAL DAY

Can you tell me what your day is like? How are you doing in school? This allows you to see the teen through his or her eyes. You may be able to identify stresses confronting the teen in everyday life. A change in academic performance or a sudden disinterest in school may reflect a more serious problem. Ask teens what subjects they like, which ones they dislike. If they are having problems with a particular subject, have they sought help for this? How many days of school do they miss in a term? High absenteeism (except for serious illness) correlates with other risky behaviors.

NUTRITION

Screen diet by asking for a 24-hour recall. Ask questions about realistic body image, such as, "How much do you think you should weigh?" Further explore this issue if the response is unrealistic. Ask about eating patterns: "How often do you eat breakfast?" "What is a usual lunch for you?" "What are your favorite snacks?" These open-ended questions will provide a much clearer picture of the adolescent's nutritional status and potential risks. Dietary needs are greater for calcium, iron, and zinc. Calcium is needed for bone growth and the bone mass that develops during adolescence: It also influences the development of osteoporosis later in life. You need to assess for both overeating and undereating problems. Ask about dieting. Girls tend to be more concerned about losing weight, whereas boys may want to "bulk-up" and improve strength.

ACTIVITY AND EXERCISE (SUCH AS SPORTS, IF APPLICABLE)

Ask about what teens enjoy doing outside of the home. What sports do they play, if any? What do they like to do with their friends? How often do they watch TV during the week? How much time do they spend on the computer? You may identify a need for health education regarding the importance of routine exercise. If a teen does participate in sports, does he or she use protective equipment? Is it a contact sport? Contact sports may increase the risk for injury.

SLEEP AND REST

Ask about when they usually go to bed and when they awaken. Do they feel refreshed in the morning or are they still tired? How does this pattern change on weekends? Even though sleep needs increase during growth spurts, teens often get less than ideal amounts of sleep during the week and sleep late into the day on weekends. Also ask about bedwetting, which is not entirely uncommon in teens, especially boys. Asking, "Many young people find they sometimes wet themselves during their sleep—does this ever happen to you?" is a less threatening and less embarrassing way to assess for this.

PERSONAL HABITS AND BEHAVIORS

Ask about substance use (drugs, alcohol, and nicotine). Ask, "If you smoke cigarettes, how many do you smoke in an average day?" "If you use alcohol, how much do you usually drink during the week?" "If you use drugs, what type and what method (smoking, snorting, huffing, ingesting, injecting)?" Asking questions in this way is less threatening to the teen, and he or she is much more likely to give an honest response.

If the teen drives, did he or she attend a driver's education program? Does he or she wear seat belts? Is he or she aware of the hazards of driving under the influence of drugs or alcohol? If drug or alcohol use is identified, make appropriate referrals as indicated.

RECREATION AND HOBBIES

Ask, "What do you do for fun? Do you have any hobbies?" If recreational activities or hobbies increase the risk for injury, ask if protective measures (e.g., bike helmets) are used. Ask about presence of weapons in the home and gun/hunting safety courses if appropriate.

SELF-PERCEPTION AND SELF-CONCEPT

Ask the teen to describe himself or herself—"Tell me about yourself: What do you like best about yourself, and what would you like to change?"

ROLE AND RELATIONSHIP

Ask the teen to tell you about his or her family—"Who lives at home with you?" If there are siblings, ask about the relationship. Ask, "Is there an adult in your life whom you feel comfortable talking with?" Ask about peer relationships. Ask if the teen has a special friend and what things he or she enjoys doing with that friend. Ask about dating or other significant relationships.

SEXUALITY AND REPRODUCTIVE ISSUES

For girls, ask about menarche, and if they have any questions or concerns about menstrual issues. For boys, ask about physical changes and if they have questions about this. For example, one could ask a young man, "Many young men have questions about some of the changes in their bodies; do you have any questions I could answer for you?" Ask about sexual activity: "If you are sexually active, how do you protect yourself against sexually transmitted diseases and unwanted pregnancy?" Sex role identity becomes established during adolescence. Sexual preferences—heterosexual, homosexual, or bisexual—become apparent during adolescence.

COPING AND STRESS TOLERANCE

Ask questions such as "What do you do when you get angry?" and "What makes you angry?" Also ask questions such as "What do you do when you want to relax?" You need to identify whether the teen has healthy coping strategies to deal with feelings and stresses in life.

VALUE AND BELIEF PATTERN

Ask about what is important to them—do they have specific beliefs about God or a "higher power?"

Physical Assessment

The physical assessment of the adolescent does not differ greatly from the adult assessment, but there are specific variations that are unique to this developmental period. **It is important that weight measurements be done in private. Often, particularly in school settings, this is not done, and it is the source of much anxiety for adolescents, especially those who are overweight or who think they are.**

SYSTEM/ASSESSMENT	NORMAL VARIATIONS/ ABNORMAL FINDINGS
General Health Survey	
Inspect overall appearance, noting appropriate growth and development for client's age.	Detect any delays or premature sexual maturation. Note any obvious weight problems.
Integumentary	
Inspect skin for lesions. Note piercings and tattoos.	Acne is a common problem and a major concern for adolescents. This condition should be treated and not dismissed as insignificant. Severe acne can result in permanent scarring. Many effective treatments are now available for all types of acne.
Note body hair distribution.	Absence of or excessive body hair may relate to a problem with sexual maturation.
HEENT	
Eyes	
Test visual acuity.	Many adolescents are reluctant to wear prescribed eyeglasses, yet many have some degree of myopia.
Ears	
Test hearing with pure tone audiometer.	Adolescents often listen to very loud music (often in very close ear contact using earphones); this can result in early hearing loss. Use opportunity to teach hazards of listening to loud music.
Nose	
Inspect nasal septum and mucosa.	Chronic rhinorrhea can result from allergic rhinitis. Boggy, bluish purple turbinates are consistent with allergic rhinitis. Also assess for cocaine-induced rhinorrhea or mucosal damage.
Mouth	
Inspect oral mucosa and pharynx.	Hypertrophied tonsils of early childhood have usually shrunk to more normal proportions.

(continued)

SYSTEM/ASSESSMENT	NORMAL VARIATIONS/ ABNORMAL FINDINGS
HEENT *Mouth (Continued)*	
Inspect occlusion.	If malocclusion is present, refer to orthodontist.
Inspect number of teeth and presence of wisdom teeth.	Adolescents should have 28 permanent teeth, and third molars ("wisdom teeth") may erupt during this period. Referral may be needed if wisdom teeth are impacted. Also assess for orthodontic devices and brushing technique around them.
Neck	
Palpate the thyroid.	A tender, enlarged thyroid gland can signal acute thyroiditis.
Respiratory Auscultate lungs.	Adolescents with exercise-induced asthma will require bronchodilators before activity. Usually, albuterol administered through a metered-dose inhaler is given 20–30 minutes before exercise.
Cardiovascular Auscultate heart and note rate and rhythm.	Adolescents often have a sinus arrhythmia and a split second heart sound. Both the arrhythmia and split second sound change with respiration. This is a normal variation.
Breasts Inspect and palpate breasts.	Breast examinations should begin during adolescence, along with instruction in breast self-examination. Gynecomastia occurs in about $1/3$ of boys.
Gastrointestinal Inspect, auscultate, and palpate abdomen.	No specific variations occur with the abdomen during adolescence, except for pregnancy. It

(continued)

SYSTEM/ASSESSMENT	NORMAL VARIATIONS/ ABNORMAL FINDINGS
Gastrointestinal	is not unusual to detect pregnancy during a routine examination of the abdomen in an adolescent who is denying this possibility. By 20 weeks' gestation, the fundus is at the level of the umbilicus.
Genitourinary Inspect external genitalia. For girls: Perform pelvic examination at age 18 or earlier if sexually active. For boys: Perform testicular examination.	Sexually active teens should be examined for STDs. Sexually active girls should have annual gynecological examinations. Instruction in testicular self-examination should be provided to all adolescent boys. Tanner staging should be noted for both boys and girls.
Musculoskeletal Inspect and palpate spinal curves. Test for spinal deformities. (See Chapter 12.)	Scoliosis is the major variation within the musculoskeletal system. Screening for scoliosis should be done in the preadolescent period, generally during the fifth and sixth grade. Any significant curvature should be referred for evaluation and follow-up.
Neurological Focus on affect and cognitive functioning.	Depression and suicidal ideations warrant immediate intervention.

18

ASSESSING THE OLDER ADULT

Developmental Considerations

- Erikson identifies the final stage of development as ego integrity versus despair, and this stage of life correlates well with Maslow's Theory of Human Needs self-actualization need, in which self-fulfillment of one's potential is actualized.
- Ideally, adults older than age 65 will be able to do a life review with a sense of satisfaction and accomplishment and will be able to accept their own mortality.

Cultural Considerations

The following information on various cultures and their perspectives on aging is adapted from Purnell and Paulanka (2003): *Transcultural Healthcare: A Culturally Competent Approach* (2nd ed.). Philadelphia: F. A. Davis Company.

CULTURE	PERSPECTIVE ON AGING
African-American	Elders are valued and treated with respect. Grandmother has central role, often offers economic and child care support. Grandchildren often raised by grandmother.
Amish	Elders are respected members of the community. Grandparents turn over farming responsibilities to their children, live close to them, and assist with child care. Elder care usually within the family setting, and Amish prefer to die at home.
Appalachian	Elders respected and honored. Live close to children and participate in child care.
Brazilian-American	Elders live with children and are included in all activities.
Chinese-American	Elders are highly valued, respected, and considered very wise. Children are expected to care for parents.
Cuban-American	Elders live with children. Multigenerational households are common.
Egyptian-American	Elders are respected and are thought to become wiser with age. Family expected to take care of elders. Women gain status with age and childbearing; however, older women are expected to care for older men.
European-American	Value is on youth and beauty, so elders are seen as less important and little attention is paid to their problems.
Filipino-American	Multigenerational households are common. Grandparents act as surrogate parents while parents work.
Greek-American	Elders well respected. Children are expected to care for parents, who actively participate in family activities.
Iranian-American	Believe that with age come experience, worldliness, and knowledge; so elders seen with respect. Caring for them is children's obligation.
Irish-American	Elders are well respected, and their opinions are valued. Elders are cared for in home.
Jewish-American	Elders respected and seen as having wisdom. Honoring and caring for parents is important. Old age is a state of mind.
Korean-American	60 is considered old age, and one is expected to retire then.
Mexican-American	Elders live with children. Large extended family.

(continued)

CULTURE	PERSPECTIVE ON AGING
Navajo Native American	Elders with many children seen with respect. They have important role in teaching and keeping rituals to children and grandchildren.
Vietnamese-American	Elders are honored, have key role in family activities, and are consulted on major family decisions.

Assessment

Health History

Remember that older adults may not present in the same way as younger people when ill.

- Older adults may minimize or ignore symptoms.
- They often have several concurrent medical problems.
- They often present with atypical signs and symptoms of disease.

Key points to remember when obtaining a history from an older adult:

- Realize that age differences between you and your client may influence his or her response.
- Be aware of your own views and values associated with aging.
- Explain what you are doing and why.
- Allow more time than with younger clients.
- Realize that you may need to obtain the history over several visits.
- Ask the client if he or she can hear you.
- Sit at same level in front of client without invading his or her personal space.
- Maintain eye contact.
- Speak slowly and clearly, the lower the pitch the better.
- Set time limits for your interview.
- Redirect the interview as needed, but respect the client's need to reminisce.
- Allow the client to respond to each question before asking another.
- Listen to what your client is saying, being alert for any signs of fatigue or discomfort.

- Use lay terminology that is culturally relevant to elicit more comprehensive information (e.g., "sugar" rather than "glucose" in diabetes).

The history and physical assessment are essentially the same as with other adults, but keep in mind:

- Symptom reporting may differ because the older client may be either a health pessimist or health optimist.
- Cost of health care is a concern.
- The older client may delay treatment.
- The older client may have multiple pathologies.
- Disease presentation may differ in older adults.
- Polypharmacy may account for many of your client's symptoms.
- Common surgeries for older adults include cataracts, joint replacement, and skin lesion removal.
- History should include functional assessment, and family history should include history of Alzheimer's disease and dementia.
- The client needs to be asked about advance directives.
- History taking should begin with questions that focus on orientation and past information, as a way of establishing the client's cognitive status.

REVIEW OF SYSTEMS

SYSTEM AND QUESTIONS TO ASK	SIGNIFICANCE
General Health Status How would you describe your usual state of health? Are you able to do what you usually do? Have you noticed any changes in your height or weight? Do you notice any difference in how your clothes fit?	Helps to identify current heath status and activity tolerance. Loss of height (normally 6–10 cm) occurs with aging. Changes in weight distribution occur with age; a decrease of subcutaneous fat is seen on the face and extremities with an increase on the abdomen and hips. Differences in the way clothes fit may signal subtle changes in weight that warrant further investigation.

(continued)

SYSTEM AND QUESTIONS TO ASK	SIGNIFICANCE
Integumentary *Skin*	
Have you noticed any changes in your skin; for example, dryness, itching, rashes, blisters?	There are many age-related changes in the skin, some of which are also caused by the environment. They result in uncomfortable symptoms such as pruritus and xerosis (dry skin), which occur frequently in older adults during the winter.
How often do you bathe? What type of soap do you use? Do you use lotions, sunscreens? Have you been in the sun a great deal? What type of work did you do?	Skin care practices, sun exposure, and occupational history may influence current skin condition.
Have you noticed any skin changes such as changes in size of growths or open, sore, cracked, itchy, bleeding areas that won't heal?	The incidence of skin cancer increases with age.
Have you noticed any new rough areas of your skin that do not seem to go away?	**Remember that visual changes that occur with aging may make early recognition of skin changes more difficult.**
Hair	
Any hair loss, increased hair growth, graying, dry scalp, or other hair changes? What are your usual patterns of hair care? Have you undergone hair replacement treatments?	Changes in hair growth and distribution are commonly associated with aging. Dry scalp is a normal and common complaint. Hair loss may be distressing for both men and women. Women may also be concerned about increased facial hair. You need to differentiate normal changes from possible disease.
Nails	
How do you care for your nails? Do you cut them yourself? Do you see a podiatrist?	Nails thicken with age and may be more difficult to trim. Fungal nail infections are common. A podiatry consult may be indicated, especially if the client has a history of diabetes or vascular disease.

SYSTEM AND QUESTIONS TO ASK	SIGNIFICANCE
HEENT *Head, Face, and Neck*	
Do you have facial pain?	Increased incidence of temporal arteritis in older adults may explain pain over temporal artery.
Can you move your head easily?	Range of motion (ROM) in the head and neck may be limited because of musculoskeletal (MS) changes or osteoarthritis.
Eyes	
Have you noticed any changes in your vision? Can you read normal-sized print or large-print materials? Do you have problems going from light to dark areas? Do you drive at night?	Common problems (e.g., cataracts, macular degeneration, and glaucoma) can affect vision. Normal age changes include increased sensitivity to glare and decreases in visual acuity, lens elasticity, peripheral vision, color intensity (specifically blue, green, and purple), night vision, accommodation to changes in lighting, tear production and viscosity, depth perception; and presbyopia. Dry eyes are very common. They may be caused by decreased tear production or blocked tear ducts, so further investigation is warranted.
Do your eyes feel dry? Do you have floaters? Do you see flashes of light? Does it look like a shade is being pulled over your eye?	There are several eye complaints that require immediate attention, such as a sudden onset of floaters or flashes of light peripherally, with decreased visual acuity. The client may describe this as like a curtain coming down over the field of vision (amaurosis fugax). These symptoms indicate retinal detachment or transient ischemic attack (TIA) or cerebrovascular accident (CVA). A complaint of a sudden onset of painless unilateral loss of vision also requires immediate attention because this may be caused by retinal vein occlusion.

(continued)

SYSTEM AND QUESTIONS TO ASK	SIGNIFICANCE
HEENT	
Ears	
Do you have any problems with your hearing?	Problems with pitch discrimination are common, especially with high-pitched sounds (s, t, f, and g). Presbycusis is common in older adults.
Do you have balance problems?	Balance problems may be caused by a problem in the inner ear or a more serious neurological problem.
Nose	
Have you noticed any changes in your sense of smell?	Anosmia—a decreased ability to identify and discriminate odors—occurs with aging.
Do you have a runny nose? Do you sneeze frequently? Do you have postnasal drip?	Atrophic changes associated with aging may cause vasomotor rhinitis.
Mouth and Throat	
Do you have difficulty chewing, swallowing, tasting, smelling, or enjoying food?	Age-related changes on the surface of the tongue and atrophy of taste buds affect the ability to eat and enjoy food. In particular, there is a decrease in the ability to taste sweets and salt. Gums become thinner and recede, resulting in loose teeth and exposure of the roots.
Do you wear dentures? Do they fit properly? Do you have any sores in your mouth? When was the last time you saw your dentist?	Poorly fitted dentures may lead to poor nutrition and mouth sores. May identify need for referral.
When you are eating, do you ever cough or choke? Does this occur with liquids and/or solids? Do you have problems swallowing?	Dysphagia may be related to a variety of underlying problems and is not a normal part of aging. It warrants further investigation.
Does your mouth always feel dry with a bad taste? Do you have difficulty swallowing dry food or speaking for long periods?	Dry mouth (xerostomia) is a very common problem in older adults, caused by medication, decreased production of saliva, inadequate fluid intake, atrophy of the oral mucosa, vitamin deficiencies, poor nutrition, and

(continued)

SYSTEM AND QUESTIONS TO ASK	SIGNIFICANCE

HEENT
Mouth and Throat (Continued)

	poor oral hygiene. Burning mouth syndrome is also common in the older adult. It causes dry mouth, altered taste, thirst, difficulty swallowing, swelling in the face and cheeks, and altered sense of smell.

Respiratory

Do you have any difficulty breathing? If yes, when does it occur and with how much exertion? Has it affected your ability to perform usual activities?	Respiratory disorders are common in older adults. Clients may describe themselves as having breathing difficulties or trouble getting a deep breath or sufficient air. With chronic obstructive pulmonary disease (COPD), dyspnea is usually insidious in onset and progressive.
Do you have a cough?	Lung cancer most frequently occurs between ages 55 and 74 years. There has been a recent increase in tuberculosis among older adults. If there is a new-onset cough, determine if the client has been exposed to a change in environment or has taken any new medications, such as angiotensin-converting enzyme (ACE) inhibitors.

Cardiovascular

Do you get short of breath when walking or making the bed? Do you have swelling in the feet, hands, face, or abdomen; weight gain; or shoes or clothing that no longer fit? Does the swelling get worse as the day goes on and disappear in the morning? Do you get dizzy? When? Does the dizziness get worse when going from lying to standing, or is it worse with exertion? Are there any changes in your energy level?	Cardiovascular disease is not a normal change associated with aging, but it is the most common problem. Unfortunately, it often does not exhibit the typical signs and symptoms found in younger people. For example, an older adult may present with atrial fibrillation but have no symptoms at all or complain vaguely of just not feeling right. If the client reports swelling, explore if this is related to his or her activity level or to a change in medication or diet.

(continued)

SYSTEM AND QUESTIONS TO ASK	SIGNIFICANCE
Cardiovascular (*Continued*)	
Do you have a cough? Is it worse at night? Do you get more short of breath when lying flat? Do you need to sleep with several pillows?	Cough may be related to congestive heart failure or a cardiac medication. Vascular disease increases with age.
Do you have headaches?	Headaches may be associated with hypertension (HTN), CVA, or temporal artery disease.
Do you have leg pain when walking? Skin changes, swelling, ulcers, or varicose veins in your legs?	Intermittent claudication (pain in legs when walking) and skin changes (thin, shiny, and hairless) suggest arterial vascular disease. High incidence of venous disease in older adults.
Gastrointestinal	
What is your typical diet for a day? Any change? Any food intolerance?	Food intolerance is a common complaint and may be associated with hiatal hernia and esophageal reflux.
What are your usual bowel patterns? Diet and fluid intake? Medications, prescribed and OTC?	Constipation is one of the most common digestive complaints in the older adult, and accounts for 2.5 million physician visits annually. The prevalence of constipation increases with age, is more common in women than in men, in nonwhites than in whites, and in those with lower family income and education. Constipation may have dangerous complications in older adults, including acute changes in cognition, urinary retention, urinary incontinence, and fecal impaction. Fecal impaction can result in intestinal obstruction, ulceration, and urinary problems. Chronic straining to defecate can have adverse effects on cerebral, coronary, and peripheral vascular circulation. Constipation can be categorized as functional (slow transit of stool) or

(continued)

SYSTEM AND QUESTIONS TO ASK	SIGNIFICANCE
Gastrointestinal (*Continued*)	
	rectosigmoid outlet delay (anorectal dysfunction, 10 minutes or more needed to defecate). Bowel changes associated with bleeding and weight loss suggest a malignancy.
Genitourinary *Urinary*	
Do you have trouble getting to the bathroom on time? Do you need to wear a pad? If so, how many times a day do you have to change it? Does the incontinence occur with coughing or sneezing, on the way to the bathroom, or at night? Does it interfere with your ability (or desire) to do daily activities or engage in social activities? Ask men about frequent urination, hesitancy, weak or intermittent stream, a sensation of incomplete emptying of the bladder, dribbling after voiding, and nocturia.	Urinary incontinence is not a normal aspect of aging, but it is a common problem. Approximately 10 million Americans suffer from urinary incontinence. Report of new-onset incontinence, loss of appetite, vomiting, falls, nocturia, difficulty urinating, or behavioral and cognitive changes should alert you to a possible urinary tract infection. Prostate enlargement can cause incontinence. See Table 18–1 for types of incontinence.
Female Reproductive	
Do you have any vaginal discharge? If so, what is the type, color, odor, and consistency of the discharge?	Changes in vaginal secretions, amount, and pH increase the risk for vaginal infections.
Do you have vaginal pressure, or an uncomfortable, bearing-down sensation, in addition to symptoms of urinary incontinence?	Symptoms may be related to the presence of a uterine prolapse, cystocele, or rectocele.
Do you have any vaginal bleeding? Are you taking hormone replacement therapy? When did you go through menopause? When was your last Pap test?	Bleeding may be related to hormone replacement therapy. If client is not on hormones, bleeding that occurs after one year postmenopause is abnormal and needs follow-up.

(continued)

SYSTEM AND QUESTIONS TO ASK	SIGNIFICANCE

Genitourinary
Female Reproductive (Continued)

Do you do breast-self-examinations? When was your last mammogram? Do you get them yearly?	Incidence of breast cancer increases with age. Yearly mammograms are recommended for women older than age 50. May identify teaching needs.
Are you satisfied with your sexual activity? Do you have pain during intercourse (dyspareunia) or vaginal dryness?	Older adults continue to be sexually active, unless they no longer have a sexual partner, have a disease, or are exposed to a treatment that decreases libido or makes intercourse uncomfortable. None of the age-related changes in either men or women precludes the continuation of a satisfying sexual life. Decreased vaginal secretions may result in dyspareunia. If it is present, an appropriate plan of care should be developed.
Have you ever had a sexually transmitted disease? Do you practice safe sex?	Because older women do not fear pregnancy, they are less likely to ask their partners to use condoms as a form of protection.

Male Reproductive

When was the last time you had your prostate checked? Have you ever had a prostate specific antigen (PSA) test? Do you have any urinary changes or problems?	Increased incidence of prostate cancer in older men. Yearly prostate examinations should begin at age 40. May identify need for health teaching.
Are you satisfied with your sexual activity? Have you been feeling more tired than usual?	Sexuality does not normally decrease with age. However, the physical act and response may require more time and be less intense. Be alert for vague complaints. Give men the opportunity to talk about impotence and associated feelings so that individualized plans can be developed.

(continued)

SYSTEM AND QUESTIONS TO ASK	SIGNIFICANCE
Musculoskeletal	
Do you have pain, stiffness, joint enlargement, decreased ROM, and functional changes? Do you have pain, stiffness, and decreased ROM in the neck, shoulders, or hips that persists for at least one month? Do you have severe headache, visual loss, scalp tenderness, and mouth pain?	Osteoarthritis is the most common joint disease in the older adult and affects over 80% of those age 65 and older. Rheumatoid arthritis also increases with age. Gout is also common, exacerbated by use of diuretics or alcohol. Common problems in older adults include polymyalgia rheumatica, a syndrome that involves the musculoskeletal system; giant cell arteritis, a vasculitic disorder of the cranial arteries associated with polymyalgia rheumatica; and osteoporosis.
Have you had any fractures, bone pain, or loss of height? Do you take calcium and vitamin D? Do you exercise? If so, what type of activity do you do? Are you taking any additional bone building medication?	Identifies participation in measures to prevent further bone loss and possible teaching needs.
Do you have balance problems or a history of falls?	Refer to Box 18.1 for the checklist *Evaluating the Risk Factors for Falls*. This can help determine whether the fall is caused by a gait or balance disorder or another underlying problem for which the client needs to be evaluated and treated.
Do you have any foot problems? How do your shoes fit? Do you see a podiatrist? How do you care for your feet?	Foot problems are common in older adults and may result from poorly fitted shoes or poor foot care. Referrals may be warranted.
Neurological	
Do you have problems with balance, mobility, coordination, sensory interpretations, level of consciousness, intellectual performance, personal-	Changes in the neurological system may be normal or the result of disease. CVA (stroke) is the most common neurological problem in older adults.

(continued)

SYSTEM AND QUESTIONS TO ASK	SIGNIFICANCE
Neurological (*Continued*)	
ity, communication, comprehension, emotional responses, and thoughts?	Parkinson's disease is the most common extrapyramidal problem.
Do you have dizziness? Feel the room is spinning or you're spinning?	Vertigo is a common problem, and diagnosis is based mainly on clinical symptoms.
Do you have a known history of seizures? Do you have repetitive shaking or muscle contractions, brief lapses of consciousness, or any abnormal sensations?	Incidence of seizures significantly increases in people over age 65 because of an increase in strokes, tumors, subdural hematomas, metabolic disorders, dementia, and medications.
Endocrine	
Have you been feeling depressed? Experiencing weight loss/gain?	Thyroid disease presents differently than in younger adults. Signs of hyperthyroidism include apathy, depression, and emaciation rather than hyperactivity. Atrial fibrillation also often occurs. Hypothyroidism is the most frequent thyroid disorder in older adults, but it is easy to miss because signs (dry skin and hair, hypotension, slow pulse, sluggishness, depressed muscular activity, goiter, weight gain) are often attributed to aging.
Does your heart ever flutter, race, or skip beats?	
Do you have increased thirst, urination, and appetite?	The incidence of diabetes mellitus increases with age.
Immune and Hematological	
Have you been feeling more tired than usual?	When an older person becomes sick, symptoms may be vague because of changes in the immune system. Fatigue may be associated with anemia, a common problem in older adults, usually caused by iron deficiency.

HEENT = head, eyes, ears, nose, and throat

Table 18–1. *Types of Incontinence*

TYPE OF INCONTINENCE	DEFINITION	PATHO-PHYSIOLOGY	SIGNS AND SYMPTOMS
Stress	Involuntary loss of urine caused by urethral sphincter failure with increases in intra-abdominal pressure.	Usually caused by weakness and laxity of pelvic floor musculature or bladder outlet weakness. Also may be caused by urethral hypermobility.	Urine is lost during coughing, sneezing, laughing.
Urge	Leakage of urine because of inability to delay voiding after sensation of bladder fullness is perceived.	Associated with detrusor hyperactivity, central nervous system disorders, or local genitourinary conditions.	Urine is lost on the way to the bathroom or as soon as the urge to void is felt.
Overflow	Leakage of urine resulting from mechanical forces on an overdistended bladder.	Results from mechanical obstruction or an acontractile bladder.	Variety of symptoms including frequent or constant dribbling, increased incontinence at night, frequency, and urgency.
Functional	Urine leakage caused by inability to get to toilet because of cognitive or physical impairment.	Cognitive and physical functional impairment.	Client is aware of the need to void, but urine is lost on the way to the bathroom.

Psychosocial History

A psychosocial history of the older adult client should address subjects such as a description of the client's typical day, nutritional history, physical activity and exercise, sleep/rest patterns (see Box 18.2), personal habits (see Box 18.3), support systems, and possible environmental hazards.

BOX 18.1. Evaluating the Risk Factors for Falls

Client's name _____

Age_____ Gender_____ Date_____

1. History of previous falls:
   ☐ Yes   ☐ No
2. Medications:
   ☐ Four or more prescriptions
   ☐ New prescription in the last 2 weeks
   ☐ Use of any of the following medications: tranquil-
     izers, sleeping pills, antidepressants, cardiac med-
     ications, antidiabetic agents
3. Known gait problem or muscular weakness:
   ☐ Yes   ☐ No
4. Dizziness, vertigo, or loss of consciousness at time of
   fall:
   ☐ Yes   ☐ No
5. Visual changes:
   ☐ Yes   ☐ No
6. Environmental problems:
   ☐ Clutter
   ☐ Dim lighting
   ☐ Uneven flooring
   ☐ Inappropriate footwear/lack of footwear
   ☐ Inappropriate assistive device
7. Major illnesses:
   ☐ Neurological: Parkinson's disease, stroke, dementia
   ☐ Musculoskeletal: Arthritis, contracture, fracture
   ☐ Cardiac: Hypotension, arrhythmia, acute infarct
   ☐ New acute illness: Infection
   ☐ Other
8. What was the client doing at the time of the fall?

   _____

   _____

   _____

9. Were there any injuries associated with the fall?
   ☐ Laceration   ☐ Persistent pain
   ☐ Sprain/strain   ☐ Head trauma
   ☐ Fracture   ☐ Other
10. How has course been since the fall?
    ☐ Associated fear of falling
    ☐ Change in function
    ☐ Change in cognition

Is the client able to carry on usual activities? If not, who
is available to help him or her?

_____

_____

BOX 18.2.   How Age Affects Sleep

- Longer time to fall asleep
- Increased time in stages 1 and 2 sleep
- Decreased time in deeper stages of sleep (stages 3 and 4)
- Decreased rapid eye movement (REM) sleep
- Increased and shorter repetition of sleep cycle
- Increased nighttime awakenings
- Altered circadian rhythm with a need to fall asleep earlier and awaken earlier

Functional Assessment

Exploring functional performance is a very important component of the history for older clients. The Katz Index (Box 18.4), the Barthel Index (Table 18–2), and the Instrumental Activities of Daily Living tool (Box 18.5) are examples of instruments that will help you obtain baseline information on your client's ability to perform ADLs and make appropriate referrals for care.

BOX 18.3.   CAGE Questionnaire for Alcohol Abuse

- Have you ever felt you should cut down on your drinking?
- Have people annoyed you by criticizing your drinking?
- Have you ever felt bad or guilty about your drinking?
- Have you ever had a drink first thing in the morning to steady your nerves or get rid of a hangover?

Mayfield, D., et al. (1974). The CAGE questionnaire: Validation of a new alcoholism screening instrument. *American Journal of Psychology, 131,*1121–1123, with permission.

BOX 18.4. The Katz Index of Activities of Daily Living

Abbreviations: I= independent; A= assistance; D= dependent

1. Bathing (sponge, shower, or tub)
   - I: Receives no assistance (gets in and out of the tub)
   - A: Receives assistance in bathing only one part of the body
   - D: Receives assistance in bathing more than one part of the body
2. Dressing
   - I: Gets clothes and gets completely dressed without assistance
   - A: Gets clothes and gets dressed without assistance except in tying shoes
   - D: Receives assistance in getting clothes or in getting dressed or stays partly or completely undressed
3. Toileting
   - I: Goes to bathroom, cleans self, and manages clothes without assistance (may use an assistive device)
   - A: Receives assistance in going to bathroom or in cleaning self, managing clothes, or emptying a bedpan
   - D: Doesn't go to bathroom for elimination
4. Transfer
   - I: Moves in and out of bed or chair without assistance (may use assistive device)
   - A: Moves in and out of bed or chair with assistance
   - D: Doesn't get out of bed
5. Continence
   - I: Controls urination and bowel movements independently
   - A: Has occasional accidents
   - D: Urine or bowel control maintained with supervision; client is incontinent or has catheter
6. Feeding
   - I: Feeds self without assistance
   - A: Feeds self except for cutting meat or buttering bread
   - D: Receives assistance in feeding or is fed partly or completely by tubes or intravenous fluids

Adapted from Katz, S., Ford, A., and Moskowitz, R. (1963). Studies of illness in the aged: The index of ADL. *Journal of the American Medical Association, 185,* 914–919.

Table 18-2. *The Barthel Index*

LEVEL OF CARE	INTACT	LIMITED	HELPER	NULL
Self-Care				
Feed	10	5	3	3
Dress (upper extremities)	5	5	3	0
Dress (lower extremities)	5	5	2	0
Don brace	0	0	−2	0
Grooming	4	4	0	0
Cleanse Perineum	4	4	2	0
Sphincters	Completely voluntary	Urgency/ appliance	Some help needed	Frequent accidents
Bladder	10	10	5	0
Bowel	10	10	5	0
Mobility/Transfer	Easy/No device	With difficulty or uses device	Some help needed	Dependent
1. Chair	15	15	7	0
2. Toilet	6	5	3	0
3. Tub	1	1	0	0
4. Walk 50 yards	15	15	10	0
5. Stairs	10	10	5	0
6. Wheelchair 50 yards	15	5	0	0

Adapted from Mahoney, F., and Barthel, D. (1965). Functional evaluation: The Barthel Index. *Maryland State Medical Journal,* 14(2), 61–65.

Physical Assessment

APPROACH

When examining the older client, make sure the environment is as safe and appropriate as possible. To ensure a senior-friendly environment, do the following:

- Keep examination rooms warm (between 70 and 80 degrees).
- Use bright but nonglaring lights.
- Keep background noise to a minimum.
- Provide higher than standard seating with arm rests on all

BOX 18.5. Instrumental Activities of Daily Living (IADL)

Abbreviations: I= independent; A= assistance, and D= dependent

1. Telephone:
   I: Able to look up numbers, dial, receive, and make calls without help
   A: Able to answer phone or dial operator in an emergency, but needs special phone or help in getting number or dialing
   D: Unable to use the telephone
2. Traveling:
   I: Able to drive own car or travel alone on bus or taxi
   A: Able to travel but not alone
   D: Unable to travel
3. Shopping:
   I: Able to take care of all shopping with transportation provided
   A: Able to shop but not alone
   D: Unable to shop
4. Preparing meals:
   I: Able to plan and cook full meals
   A: Able to prepare light foods, but unable to cook full meals alone
   D: Unable to prepare any meals
5. Housework:
   I: Able to do heavy housework (scrub floors)
   A: Able to do light housework, but needs help with heavy tasks
   D: Unable to do any housework
6. Medication:
   I: Able to take medications in the right dose at the right time
   A: Able to take medications, but needs reminding or someone to prepare it
   D: Unable to take medications
7. Money:
   I: Able to manage buying needs, write checks, pay bills
   A: Able to manage daily buying needs, but needs help managing checkbook and paying bills
   D: Unable to manage money

Duke University Center for the Study of Aging and Human Development. *The Multidimensional Functional Assessment Questionnaire* (2nd ed.), pp 169–170, with permission.

chairs. (Client might have trouble getting up, and if client has degenerative joint disease or has had joint replacement, he or she should not flex joint more than 90 degrees.)

- Use examination tables that mechanically elevate the client from lying to sitting and vice versa and a broad-based step stool to help clients get onto the table.
- Use a private examination room, if possible, or at least pull the privacy curtain if there is a roommate.
- Minimize position changes to keep the client from getting tired.
- Uncover only the area being assessed, making sure that client is warm and covered with blankets or drapes.
- Provide reading materials with large print.
- Allow more time than usual for the examination. The complete examination may need to be scheduled over several meetings.
- Make safety a priority. If your client cannot tolerate or perform what is expected for the examination, adapt the examination to meet his or her needs.
- Take the time to explain to your client everything you are doing.

TOOLBOX

To perform the physical examination, you will need all the tools of assessment.

SYSTEM/AREA, APPROACH, AND NORMAL FINDINGS	ABNORMAL FINDINGS
Integumentary: Inspection, Palpation *Skin*	
Skin color uneven in areas, increased creases, wrinkle lines, and skin lesions. Some common skin lesions include seborrheic keratosis, lentigines (liver spots), and acrochordons. Senile purpura commonly found on hands and forearms is caused by frail capillaries.	Areas of pressure or pressure sores from immobility or splints/appliances. Body folds may develop intertrigo (inflammatory, moist erythema and scaling lesions) or fungal infections. Table 18–3 describes common skin lesions associated with aging.

(continued)

SYSTEM/AREA, APPROACH, AND NORMAL FINDINGS	ABNORMAL FINDINGS

Integumentary: Inspection, Palpation
Skin (Continued)

Temperature: Warm, but hands and feet may be cool.	Cool extremities may signal vascular disease. Unilateral cool temperature may indicate an occlusion and warrants medical attention.
Turgor: Normally decreased. Not a marker of hydration status.	Decreased turgor increases risk for injury and skin breakdown.
Hydration and texture: Dry, flaky, and thin.	Excessive dryness may indicate dehydration.

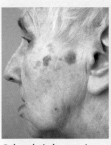 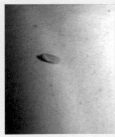 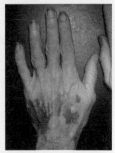

Seborrheic keratosis   *Acrochordon*   *Senile purpura (normal)*

Hair and Scalp

Hair color and distribution: Graying in both sexes; thinning and balding especially in men. Increased facial hair (hirsutism) in women. Coarse, dry hair and dry flaky scalp (senile xerosis).	Changes in hair may also relate to endocrine problems or may occur as a side effect of medications.

Nails

Yellow, dry, brittle nails with longitudinal ridges	Yellow, thick nails may also be caused by vascular disease or a fungal infection.

HEENT: Inspection, Palpation
Head/Neck

May have decreased ROM caused by MS changes.	Decreased ROM of the neck may also be associated with degenerative joint disease (DJD).

(continued)

SYSTEM/AREA, APPROACH, AND NORMAL FINDINGS	ABNORMAL FINDINGS
HEENT: Inspection, Palpation *Lymph Nodes*	
Lymph tissue decreases in size with aging and should be non-palpable.	Palpable nodes warrant referral.
Thyroid	
Nonpalpable.	Palpable thyroid may signal thyroid disease (common in older patients) and warrants referral.
Temporal Artery	
Palpable and nontender.	Pain, nodularity, and presence of a pulse may indicate temporal arteritis.
Eyes	
Presbyopia may cause difficulty reading. Far vision may be intact. Decreased peripheral vision. Dry eyes. Enophthalmos (recession of eyeball into orbit). Arcus senilis (white to yellow deposit at outer edge of the iris), along with xanthelasma (yellowish, raised tumor on upper or lower lids). Senile entropion (inversion of the lashes). Senile ectropion (eversion of the lashes). Xanthelasma (lipid deposits) on lids. Pale or yellow-tinted conjunctiva; pale iris; pingueculae (clear to yellow fleshy lesion on conjunctiva).	Loss of central vision, halos, and eye pain may indicate glaucoma and warrant referral. Visual changes may also occur with cerebrovascular disease. Basal cell carcinoma frequently found on inner third of lower lid. Yellow or opaque lens associated with increased incidence of cataracts. Entropion increases the risk of corneal abrasions. Ectropion increases risk of dryness and conjunctivitis. Macular degeneration. Check for diabetic and hypertensive retinal changes; their incidence increases with age.

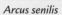

Arcus senilis

(continued)

SYSTEM/AREA, APPROACH, AND NORMAL FINDINGS	ABNORMAL FINDINGS
HEENT: Inspection, Palpation *Eyes (Continued)*	
Pterygium: Similar to pinguecu-lae, but extends over cornea. Increased stimulation needed to elicit corneal reflex. Small pupils; reaction equal but may be less brisk. Fundoscopic—retina and optic disc paler. *Ears*	
Internal	
Gross hearing is intact but di-minished with decreased pitch discrimination. Potential conductive hearing loss (presbycusis). Increased difficulty hearing high-pitched sounds, espe-cially, "s," "t," "f," and "g." Difficulty understanding speech. Equilibrium-balance problems.	Balance problems and tinnitus may indicate a neurological problem. Balance problems increase risk for falls and injury.
External	
Lobes elongate. Increased external ear canal hair in men. *Otoscopic*	Dry ears with scratch marks re-lated to senile pruritus.
Dry cerumen. Diminished cone of light.	Cerumen impaction can de-crease hearing acuity by 40 to 45 dB; removal of cerumen corrects the impairment. Hearing aids can cause contact dermatitis.
Nose	
Elongated nose. Increased nasal hair. Decreased sense of smell (CN I).	Vasomotor rhinitis causes pale nasal mucosa and boggy turbinates.
Mouth and Throat	
"Purse-string" appearance of mouth. Teeth may show staining, chip-ping or erosion.	Gum recession and bleeding (atrophic gingivitis).

(continued)

SYSTEM/AREA, APPROACH, AND NORMAL FINDINGS	ABNORMAL FINDINGS

HEENT: Inspection, Palpation
Mouth and Throat (Continued)

Some teeth may be loose or missing. Buccal mucosa and gums thin and pale. Oral mucosa dry, causing halitosis. Decreased sense of taste (CN VII and CN IX). Decreased gag reflex (CN IX and CN X). Decreased papillae on tongue. Varicose veins under tongue (caviar spots).	Chewing and swallowing difficulty may be caused by poor dentition or poorly fitted dentures, or by more serious problem such as CVA. Leukoplakia (white precancerous lesion) in mouth, particularly under tongue.

Respiratory: Inspection, Palpation, Auscultation

Senile kyphosis (increased anterior to posterior diameter) caused by MS changes, barrel chest appearance. Decreased respiratory excursion. Cheyne-Stokes breathing may occur during sleep. Breath sounds may be decreased with few atelectatic crackles.	Respiratory changes increase risk for pulmonary problems, such as pneumonia.

Cardiovascular: Inspection, Palpation, Auscultation

Increase in premature beats and irregular pulse. Decreased pedal pulses. Stiffer arteries Slight increases in blood pressure and wider pulse pressure. Orthostatic drops in blood pressure more common in older adults.	Increased incidence of vascular disease. If present, carotid bruit and thrills may be detected. Increased varicosities. Abnormal heart sounds: Rate irregular with ectopic beats, S_4 common, systolic murmurs associated with aortic stenosis. Differentiate arterial insufficiency from venous insufficiency.

(continued)

SYSTEM/AREA, APPROACH, AND NORMAL FINDINGS	ABNORMAL FINDINGS
Gastrointestinal: Inspection, Palpation, Percussion, Auscultation	
Bowel sounds may be slightly decreased.	Bruits may be heard over stenotic arteries or aneurysms with palpable enlarged aorta.
Abdomen very soft because of decreased musculature, so organs may be easier to palpate.	Dullness over bladder may signal urinary retention; dullness over bowel may signal stool retention. Do a follow up physical exam to determine that dullness is not caused by tumor.
Rectal examination: Stool negative for occult blood; no fecal impaction; prostate soft and smooth and not enlarged.	Palpable bladder with retention.
	Palpable intestines if filled with stool.
	A pulsatile mass in the abdomen may be an aneurysm. Incidence of abdominal aortic aneurysms increases with age. An aneurysm may have lateral as well as anteroposterior pulsation. Aneurysms are usually wider than 3 cm and often have an associated bruit. Surgical evaluation may be appropriate, particularly if aneurysm is greater than 5 cm.
	Incidence of colorectal cancer peaks between ages 85 and 92 and accounts for 20% of all cancers found in people age 90 and above.
	Benign prostatic hypertrophy and prostatic cancer increase with age. If prostate feels abnormal, refer patient for urological evaluation.
Genitourinary: Inspection, Palpation *Urinary*	
Incontinence is a common problem. Evaluate urinary incontinence with the Pad test: With full bladder, have patient cough forcefully three times while standing. No leakage is normal.	Leakage of urine indicates stress incontinence.
	In urinary retention, bladder may be palpable above the symphysis pubis after voiding. You will also percuss dullness above the symphysis pubis after patient voids.

(continued)

SYSTEM/AREA, APPROACH, AND NORMAL FINDINGS	ABNORMAL FINDINGS
Genitourinary: Inspection, Palpation *Female Reproductive*	
Decreased elasticity, breast sag, cordlike feel to breasts. Decrease in and graying of pubic hair. External genitalia decrease in size, and skin becomes thin, inelastic, and shiny. Pelvic exam reveals pale vaginal walls, narrow, thick, glistening cervix as a result of decreased estrogen. Uterus and ovaries decrease in size. Ovaries should not be palpable.	Palpable ovaries, masses, rectocele, cystocele, or prolapsed uterus require referral.
Male Reproductive	
Gynecomastia may be seen. Decrease and graying of pubic hair Scrotum and penis decrease in size. Testes hang lower and have fewer rugae.	Any mass requires referral.
Musculoskeletal: Inspection, Palpation	
About half of people over 65 have decreased arm swing during gait; a wider base of support; a decline in step length, stride length, and ankle ROM; decreased vertical and increased horizontal head excursions; decrease in spinal rotation and arm swing; increased length of double support phase of walking, and a reduction in propulsive force generalized at the push off phase. Decrease in sensory input, slowing of motor responses, and MS limitations result in an increase in unsteadiness or postural sway under both static and dynamic conditions.	MS changes associated with aging increase the risk for falls and injury. Heberden's nodes, involving the distal interphalangeal joints, are commonly seen with osteoarthritis but are rarely inflamed. Asymmetrical decrease in strength and tone may be associated with TIA or CVA. Diabetes-related ulcerations, fungal infections of the feet or toenails, calluses, bunions, hallux valgus, and other deformities are very common and can affect function.

(continued)

SYSTEM/AREA, APPROACH, AND NORMAL FINDINGS	ABNORMAL FINDINGS

Musculoskeletal: Inspection, Palpation

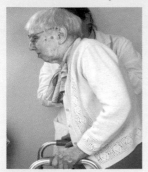

Thoracic curvature (senile kyphosis).

ROM decreased.
Crepitation, stiffness with ROM.
Decreased muscle strength and tone. Muscle strength depends on muscle mass. Strong equal hand grip usually remains intact.
Shoes fit well, wear evenly. No lesions, calluses, or deviations noted. Toenails well groomed.

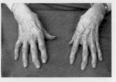

Heberden's nodes

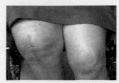

Degenerative joint disease (osteoarthritis)

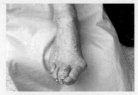

Hallux valgus and bunions

Neurological: Inspection
Mental Status

Cognitive ability intact; benign forgetfulness; short-term memory and long-term memory for new information may decrease with age.

Confusion may be caused by delirium, an underlying dementia, or depression. These conditions may be difficult to differentiate and may occur independently or together. Clients with dementia will work hard to answer questions and confabulate answers. Delirium causes difficulty concentrating on the questions and attending to the task. Clients with depression are often unwilling to try to complete the task or answer the

(continued)

SYSTEM/AREA, APPROACH, AND NORMAL FINDINGS	ABNORMAL FINDINGS
Neurological: Inspection *Mental Status (Continued)*	
	question. Detection of dementia, delirium, or depression warrants referral. Several bedside screening tools are available to differentiate between dementia, delirium, and depression and to evaluate cognitive function. See Tables 18–4 and 18–5 and Boxes 18.6 through 18.8.
Cranial Nerves	
Slower response time bilaterally CN I Olfactory—Decreased CN II Optic—Decreased visual acuity, presbyopia, fundoscopic changes CN III Oculomotor—Pupils smaller and reaction to light not as brisk Extraocular movements should remain intact: • CN III Oculomotor • CN IV Trochlear • CN VI Abducens • CN V Trigeminal—Increased stimulation needed to elicit corneal reflex CN VII Facial—Decreased taste CN VIII Acoustic—Presbycusis, increased loss of high-pitched sounds progresses to loss of all frequencies CN IX Glossopharyngeal—Decreased taste CN X Vagus—Decreased gag reflex CN XI Spinoaccessory—No change, but ROM and strength depend on MS changes CN XII Hypoglossal—No change	Diminished response time on only one side warrants further investigation.

(continued)

SYSTEM/AREA, APPROACH, AND NORMAL FINDINGS	ABNORMAL FINDINGS
Neurological: Inspection *Muscle Function Movements*	
+ drifting with minimal weakness No abnormal movements	Tremors common in older patients. Types include: • Postural or physiological—benign fine tremors • Intention, essential, familial, and senile—visible tremor associated with intentional movements, diminishes with rest • Rest—visible tremor at rest but absent/diminished with movement; "pill-rolling"; associated with Parkinson's disease • Action—large, irregular tremors of limbs, associated with cerebellar dysfunction (e.g., multiple sclerosis)
Cerebellar Function	
Slight increase in swaying—Romberg's sign	Loss of balance may be associated with Parkinson's disease.
Reflexes: Percussion	
Deep tendon reflex may be increased or decreased (+1 or +3). Achilles reflex more difficult to elicit. May need to use reinforcement techniques to elicit response. Superficial abdominal reflexes disappear with age.	Asymmetrical reflexes may indicate an underlying problem.
Older adults may demonstrate the release of some primitive reflexes, including the snout, glabellar, and palmomental.	Positive primitive reflexes may also indicate a severe neurological assault.

HEENT = head, eyes, ears, nose, and throat

Table 18-3. *Common Skin Lesions Associated with Aging*

SKIN LESION	DESCRIPTION
Lentigines	Hyperpigmented macular lesions (liver spots)
Ichthyosis	Dry, scaly, fishlike skin
Acrochordons	Small, benign polyp-growths (skin tags)
Actinic keratosis	Rough precancerous skin macule or papule from sun exposure
Seborrheic keratosis	Benign pigmented lesions with a waxy surface on face and trunk
Senile purpura	Vascular lesion of ecchymoses and petechiae on arms and legs caused by the frail nature of capillaries and decreased collagen support
Venous lakes	Bluish-black papular vascular lesions
Senile ectasias	Red-purple macular or papular lesions (senile or cherry angiomas)
Basal cell carcinoma	Pearly, papular or plaquelike cancerous lesions that may be ulcerated in the center; associated with sun exposure
Squamous cell carcinoma	Erythematous, indurated areas that may be scaly or hyperkeratotic; associated with sun exposure, and tend to grow more rapidly than basal cell

Table 18-4. *Characteristics of Dementia, Delirium, and Depression*

FEATURE	DEMENTIA	DELIRIUM	DEPRESSION
Onset	Gradual (months to years)	Abrupt (hours to a few weeks)	Either
Prognosis	Irreversible	Reversible	Variable
Course	Progressive	Worse in PM	Worse in AM
Attention	Normal	Impaired	Variable
Memory	Impaired recent and remote	Impaired recent and immediate	Selective impairment
Perception	Normal	Impaired	Normal
Psychomotor Behavior	Normal/Apraxia	Hypo/Hyperkinetic	Retardation/Agitation
Cause	Caused by many diseases, including alcoholism, AIDS, cerebral anoxia, and brain infarcts	Caused by acute illness, fever, infection, dehydration, electrolyte imbalance, medications, and alcoholism	Usually coincides with life event, such as death in the family, loss of a friend or a pet, or a move

Table 18-5. *Geriatric Depression Scale*

		YES	NO
*1.	Are you basically satisfied with your life?		
*2.	Have you dropped many of your activities and interests?		
*3.	Do you feel that your life is empty?		
*#4.	Do you often get bored?		
5.	Are you hopeful about the future?		
6.	Are you bothered by thoughts that you just cannot get out of your head?		
*7.	Are you in good spirits most of the time?		
*8.	Are you afraid that something bad is going to happen to you?		
*9.	Do you feel happy most of the time?		
*#10.	Do you often feel helpless?		
11.	Do you often get restless and fidgety?		
*#12.	Do you prefer to stay at home rather than going out and doing new things?		
13.	Do you frequently worry about the future?		
*14.	Do you feel you have more problems with memory than most?		
*15.	Do you think it is wonderful to be alive now?		
16.	Do you often feel downhearted and blue?		
*#17.	Do you feel pretty worthless the way you are now?		
18.	Do you worry a lot about the past?		
19.	Do you find life very exciting?		
20.	Is it hard for you to get started on new projects?		
*21.	Do you feel full of energy?		
*22.	Do you feel that your situation is hopeless?		
*23.	Do you think that most people are better off than you are?		
24.	Do you frequently get upset over little things?		
25.	Do you frequently feel like crying?		
26.	Do you have trouble concentrating?		
27.	Do you enjoy getting up in the morning?		
28.	Do you prefer to avoid social gatherings?		
29.	Is it easy for you to make decisions?		
30.	Is your mind as clear as it used to be?		

Yesavage, J., et al. (1983). Development and validation of a geriatric depression screening scale: A preliminary report. *Journal of Psychiatric Research, 17,* 37–49, with permission.
* Items included in the 15-item Geriatric Depression Scale
# Items included in the 5-item Geriatric Depression Scale

BOX 18.6. Signs and Symptoms of Depression

Typical
- Changes in appetite
- Changes in sleep patterns
- Social withdrawal
- Loss of motivation
- Constipation
- Pessimism
- Guilt
- Decreased self-esteem
- Feelings of helplessness
- Hostility
- Agitation
- Aggression
- Anxiety

Atypical
- Vague somatic complaints—such as constipation, joint pain, fatigue, and memory changes—that seem to be out of proportion to the actual problem
- Client may become obsessed with the problems and feel that if problems are relieved, he or she will be fine

BOX 18.7. Mini-Mental Status Examination

Have the client answer the following questions or follow these instructions:

1. What is the season, month, day, and year?	5 points (subtract 1 point for each item left out)
2. Where are you (state, county, town, hospital floor)?	5 points (subtract 1 point for each item left out)
3. I will say the names of three objects. Repeat the names.	3 points (subtract 1 point for each word client forgets)
4. Counting backward from 100, subtract 7 five times (serial 7s) Or spell "world" backward	5 points
5. Recall the same three objects from a few minutes ago (question 3)	3 points (subtract 1 point for each word client forgets)

(continued)

BOX 18.7. Mini-Mental Status Examination (*Continued*)

6. I will show you two common objects. Tell me what they are.	2 points
7. Repeat the phrase "no ifs, ands, or buts."	1 point
8. I am going to give you a blank piece of paper. Take this paper, put it in your right hand, fold it in half, and put it on the floor.	3 points
9. I am going to print on a piece of paper. (Print "Close your eyes.") Read it and do it.	1 point
10. Write a sentence of your own.	1 point
11. Copy a pair of intersecting pentagons on a piece of paper.	1 point

Scoring:
24–30: No cognitive impairment
8–23: Mild cognitive impairment
0–7: Severe impairment

Adapted from Folstein, M., et al. (1975). Mini-mental state: A practical method for grading the cognitive state of clients for the clinician. *Journal of Psychiatric Research, 12,* 196–198.

BOX 18.8. Clock Scoring

Give the client a paper and ask him or her to draw a circle. Instruct him or her to draw the face of a clock inside the circle, putting the numbers in the correct positions. Then ask him or her to draw the hands to indicate 10 minutes after 11 or 20 minutes after 8.

Scoring:

Assign 1 point for each of the following:
• Draws closed circle
• Places numbers in correct positions
• Includes all 12 numbers in correct positions
• Places clock hands in correct positions

There are no specific cutoff scores. If performance on clock drawing is impaired, consider a complete diagnostic evaluation for dementia.

CHAPTER 19

ASSESSING THE HOMELESS PERSON

The components of the health history and physical examination are the same as for other patients. However, when dealing with homeless clients, your approach and focus will differ.

Approach and Focus

- Provide unconditional positive regard for the homeless client.
- Be accepting and nonjudgmental.
- Listen.
- Be sensitive to the reality of the homeless situation.
- Be direct in your communication with the client.
- Ask permission to touch the client. (Physical privacy may be one of the few prerogatives the client has left.)
- Focus more on addressing an immediate problem than on getting a complete history and physical examination.
- Use event markers for time periods; days, months, and years may not be meaningful to the homeless person.
- Schedule healthcare appointments early in the day because shelter management requires a person be present in the afternoon to secure a bed for the night. "Claiming a bed" may take priority over healthcare.
- Respond accurately and simply if the homeless person expresses concern about how his or her personal revelations are recorded and how the information will be used.
- Realize that the homeless person may be homeless by choice, be impatient, refuse to make eye contact, take a long time to respond, express minor complaints such as headache, have a mailing address or contact person, and see healthcare needs and priorities differently from you.

Health History

AREA/TYPES OF QUESTIONS	SIGNIFICANCE
Biographical Data	
Ask where patient is staying.	Less threatening to ask than "What is your address?" Questions about family members, telephone numbers, or additional demographic data may not be appropriate and may be met with silence. May also be reluctant to identify government agencies.
Current Health Survey	
Ask about injuries first.	Client may synthesize life and environmental factors to explain symptoms in ways that may not have occurred to you. Begin with questions about injuries; this may be a marker for time in an unstructured life.
Ask about symptoms of communicable diseases that may not have been reported.	Increased risk for communicable diseases as a result of crowded living quarters.
Ask about respiratory diseases, such as tuberculosis (TB).	Risk is high for those who sleep in close quarters in shelters or crowded spaces.
Ask about dermatological problems such as lesions, infestation.	No change of socks, no clean clothes, exposure to extremes, poor hygiene, living in close quarters increase risk.
Past Health History	
Ask about past injuries, infections, communicable diseases, hospitalizations, substance abuse, and psychiatric problems.	Determines compliance or completion of treatment and follow-up.
Family History	May not want to discuss family.
Review of Systems	
Ask about problems in the following systems that you may have missed in the current health survey.	Homeless patients are at increased risk for the problems identified by system below.

(continued)

AREA/TYPES OF QUESTIONS	SIGNIFICANCE
Integumentary	
	Skin problems: Scabies, lice.
HEENT	
	Ear and eye problems with children; dental problems with all ages.
Respiratory	
	Upper respiratory infection (URI), TB.
Cardiovascular	
	Hypertension (HTN).
Gastrointestinal	
	Alcohol abuse increases risk for GI disorders and poor nutrition.
Genitourinary	
	Women: Pregnancy, lack of prenatal care. *All:* Poor nutrition, complications, sexually transmitted diseases (STDs).
Musculoskeletal/Neurological	
	Neurological and psychiatric disorders.
Hematological/Immune/Endocrine	
	Anemia related to dietary deficiency, HIV/AIDS; diabetes.
Psychosocial Profile **Health Practices and Beliefs**	
	Gives client opportunity to present positive aspects of life. Acknowledging positive behaviors may help establish bond between you and client. Barriers to healthcare and limited resources limit preventive behaviors. Client's healthcare practices are often crisis or problem oriented and treated symptomatically. Follow-up is difficult.
Typical Day	
	May consist of being on feet all day, looking for food and a place to sleep.

(continued)

AREA/TYPES OF QUESTIONS	SIGNIFICANCE
Psychosocial Profile *Nutritional Patterns*	
	Nutrition is a problem. Tell client about available resources (e.g., food stamps, soup kitchens).
Activity and Exercise Patterns	
	Center on survival and meeting basic needs.
Sleep/Rest Patterns	
	Finding a safe place to sleep is a problem.
Personal Habits	
	Substance abuse and associated health problems are common among homeless people, but do not assume this is the case with your patient. Ask, "Do you smoke, drink alcohol, or use drugs?" If the answer is yes, ask "How much?"
Occupational Health Patterns	
	Patient may be working, but income may not be sufficient to maintain housing.
Socioeconomic Status	
	Homelessness denotes low socioeconomic status, poverty. Ask if client is a veteran. Identify available resources and make appropriate referrals.
Environmental Health Patterns	
	Thermoregulatory problems (hypothermia or hyperthermia) resulting from exposure. Alcohol increases risk for hypothermia. Using fire to keep warm increases risk for burns. Because the homeless person often wears everything he or she owns, risk for heat exhaustion, heat stroke, and dehydration increases in warm weather. Increased risk for being a victim of crime, robbery, assault, and rape. *(continued)*

AREA/TYPES OF QUESTIONS	SIGNIFICANCE
Psychosocial Profile *Roles/Relationships/Self-Concept*	
Cultural Influences	Low self-esteem, anxiety, and depression are common.
Religious Influences	Can be seen in both legal and illegal immigrants. Many groups have high poverty rates (e.g., 30% of Hispanics live in poverty). In homeless, language barriers can also add to problem of accessing health care.
Sexuality Patterns	Faith-based organizations are often major service providers for basic needs. Spiritual support may be integrated.
	Homeless client may still be sexually active and in a committed relationship. Ask, "Are you sexually active? With men, women, or both? Do you have genital itching, burning, or other symptoms?" Ask if client is a victim of abuse—50% of homeless women with children have been victims of domestic abuse.

HEENT =head, eyes, ears, nose, and throat

Physical Assessment

Conduct the physical assessment using tools and techniques appropriate for the age and gender of the client. Use gloves if risk for exposure to bodily fluids exists; otherwise, direct touch can convey trust. With the homeless client, the customary head-to-toe approach may not be practical. Close, face-to-face contact at the beginning of the exam may be seen as invasive or threatening by the client. Simply reverse the order, working from toe to head. This also minimizes the power position of the nurse standing over the client, giving directions while performing the exam.

Pay special attention to the client's feet. The homeless are at risk for foot problems because they are often on their feet most of the day, wearing poorly fitting shoes with no change of socks. Regardless of your findings, the act of touching and examining the feet demonstrates a thoroughness of approach and simple caring.

Also keep in mind that the homeless person may have all of his or her possessions on his or her person and may be reluctant to remove clothes. Assure the person that his or her clothing and belongings will be safe, and allow him or her to keep personal items.

The table below outlines a thorough physical assessment of a homeless client. Instead of performing a total assessment, you will usually focus on a specific area identified as a problem from the history data. Be as thorough as necessary to meet your client's health needs and as thorough as your client permits.

AREA	SIGNIFICANCE
General Health Survey	
Inspect general appearance, signs of injury, dress and grooming.	May have signs of injury—homeless people are more vulnerable to crime.
	Poor hygiene resulting from lack of resources may warrant referral.
Note any odors.	Body odors may be caused by poor hygiene or alcohol abuse.
Take vital signs: temperature, respirations, blood pressure (BP).	Hypothermia or hyperthermia from exposure often present.
	Upper respiratory problems common.
	HTN is chronic health problem.
Integumentary	
Inspect skin for lesions, color changes; inspect hair for infestation.	Lice or scabies caused by crowded living conditions.
Inspect feet for lesions and edema.	High incidence of hepatitis related to intravenous (IV) drug use.
	Cirrhosis related to alcohol abuse.
	Minor skin problems common.
	Poor wound healing because of poor nutrition.
	Being on feet most of day increases risk for peripheral vascular disease (PVD).
	Diabetes is also a chronic problem.

(continued)

AREA	SIGNIFICANCE
HEENT	
Inspect mouth and throat.	Dental problems and URI common among homeless.
Respiratory	
Auscultate lungs.	Respiratory problems and TB common.
Cardiovascular	
Palpate peripheral pulses.	PVD common.
Auscultate heart for normal and extra sounds.	HTN common.
Gastrointestinal	
Auscultate bowel sounds.	Gastrointestinal (GI) problems common.
Palpate abdomen.	Cirrhosis, pancreatitis associated with alcohol abuse common.
Genitourinary	
Inspect genitalia.	Homeless people, especially women, are susceptible to rape, increasing risk for STDs and pregnancy.
Musculoskeletal	
Inspect and palpate muscles.	Homeless people are susceptible to trauma from beatings.
Neurological	
Assess mental status.	Head trauma may result from beatings. Substance abuse (drugs and alcohol) can affect neurological status. Seizures can result from trauma and substance abuse. Psychiatric problems common, including depression, schizophrenia, and organic brain syndrome.

HEENT = head, eyes, ears, nose, and throat

CHAPTER 20

ASSESSING NUTRITION

Nutrition is the relative state of balance between nutrient intake and physiological requirements for growth and physical activity.

Malnutrition can represent a nutrient deficit or excess. Assessing nutritional status achieves the following:

- Identifies actual nutritional deficiencies.
- Illuminates dietary patterns that may contribute to health problems.
- Provides a basis for planning for more optimal nutrition.
- Establishes baseline data for evaluation.

Performing the Nutritional Assessment

Nutritional assessment is recommended for people with any of the following nutritional risks:

- Weight less than 80% or more than 120% of ideal body weight
- History of unintentional weight loss (greater than 10 lb or 10% of usual weight)
- Serum albumin concentration lower than 3.5 g/dL
- Total lymphocyte count lower than 1500 cells/mm^3
- History of illness, surgery, trauma, or stress
- Symptoms associated with nutritional deficiency or depletion
- Factors associated with inadequate nutritional intake or absorption

Health History

- Biographical data
- Current health status
- Past health history
- Family history
- Review of systems
  - Have you had unexplained weight loss, fatigue, activity intolerance, or inability to concentrate?

- Have you noticed changes in skin texture, skin discolorations, poor wound healing, or bruising?
- Do you have poor night vision or eye dryness?
- Do you have nosebleeds or bleeding gums? Cavities or lost teeth?
- Do you have chest pain or pressure?
- Are you constipated?
- Do you have diarrhea?
- *Women:* Have you had frequent miscarriages or irregular menses? How much caffeine do you consume a day?
- *Men:* Do you suffer from impotence?
- Do you have muscle weakness?
- Are you nervous or irritable? Do you have headaches, numbness or tingling, or muscle tics?
- Do you have frequent infections? Allergies?

- Psychosocial profile
  - Who shops and prepares meals in your family?
  - Are you able to plan and cook meals yourself, or do you depend on others to do this?
  - When was your last dental examination?
  - Do you go for routine physical examinations?
  - How do you usually spend your days? Do you go to restaurants frequently, and if so, where do you go and what types of foods do you eat? How much time do you spend shopping, preparing, and eating food?
  - What is your typical daily diet? How much water do you drink daily?
  - Do you actively try to maintain good nutrition and healthy weight? How?
  - Have your eating habits and appetite changed recently?
  - What is your usual activity and exercise level?
  - Do you feel that you have adequate energy? What activities do you not pursue because of lack of energy?
  - How many hours of sleep do you get a night? Do you wake up during the night? Are you taking more naps than usual? Do you feel rested? Do you use sleep aids? If so, what kinds?
  - Do you smoke?
  - Do you drink alcohol? If so, how much per day? Do you drink coffee, tea, or soft drinks every day? If so, how much?
  - Do you use over-the-counter drugs?
  - Do you use illegal drugs?
  - What do you do for a living?
  - How does your job affect daily meal routines?
  - Is your income adequate to meet your food needs?
  - Where do you buy your food? How do you store it? How do you prepare it?

- Do you have regular social interaction? Do you usually eat with other people or alone?
- Do you have any cultural influences that may affect your dietary practices? If so, what are they?
- Do you have any religious influences that may affect your dietary practices? If so, what are they?
- Are your social relationships satisfying or stressful? How much stress do you have in your life? How do you cope with it?

FOCUSED NUTRITIONAL HISTORY
- Have you lost or gained weight unintentionally in the past 6 months?
- What is the most you have ever weighed?
- How much did you weigh 6 months ago, and how much do you weigh now?
- What do you normally eat every day? Has your diet changed significantly? If so, how?
- Do you have any stomach or bowel symptoms (e.g., nausea, vomiting, diarrhea, or anorexia) that have lasted more than 2 weeks?
- Has anything happened in your life that has affected your ability to obtain or prepare food? If so, what?

COMPREHENSIVE NUTRITIONAL HISTORY
Two dietary analysis techniques are discussed below—24-hour recall and food intake records. You can use either technique as part of your comprehensive history.

24-Hour Recall
- Ask the client to write down what he or she ate and drank during the previous 24 hours.
- Use the Food Guide Pyramid to sort and categorize the foods and determine the general quality of his or her diet.
- Ask the client to record between-meal drinks and snacks, desserts, bedtime snacks, condiments, and food preparation items.
- Ask the client to record water intake.
- Be sure to have the client record the amount of each food or liquid he or she consumed, and translate these into standard servings according to the Food Pyramid.

Food Intake Records
- Food intake records are typically done on people who are debilitated, have severe burns, or are on chemotherapy.
- A food intake record is a quantitative listing of all food and fluid consumed within a designated time frame—usually 3 to 5 days.
- To analyze the data, reduce the recorded food items into their constituent nutrients, using United States Department of Agriculture food composition tables.

- A less specific but more practical approach involves analyzing the client's food intake record using food labels on packages.

Physical Assessment

APPROACH: You will mainly use the techniques of inspection and palpation. Evaluate the client's hydration status simultaneously.

TOOLBOX: Weight scale, flexible measuring tape, calipers, stethoscope, growth charts, weight and height tables, anthropometric tables, laboratory values, and a variety of containers.

PERFORMING A HEAD-TO-TOE PHYSICAL ASSESSMENT
- Look for changes in every system that might signal a nutritional problem.
- Anthropometry
- Growth charts
- Body mass index
- Arm measurements
  - Triceps skin fatfold
  - Midarm circumference
  - Midarm muscle circumference
  - Waist-to-hip ratio

AREA/SYSTEM AND NORMAL FINDINGS	ABNORMAL FINDINGS
General Health Survey	
No unexplained weight changes	Weight changes in short time: Fluid loss or gain
Vital signs within normal limits for person's age	Elevated BP: Fluid overload, high sodium intake, obesity
	Low BP: Dehydration
Integumentary *Skin*	
Skin intact, warm, and dry	Scaling: Low or high vitamin A, zinc, essential fatty acids
Texture smooth, no lesions	Transparent, cellophane appearance: Protein deficit
Color consistent with ethnicity	Cracking (cracked-pavement appearance): Protein deficit
	Follicular hyperkeratosis: Vitamins A, C deficits
	Petechiae (especially perifollicular): Vitamin C deficit
	Purpura: Vitamins C, K deficits
	Pigmentation/desquamation of sun-exposed areas: niacin deficit
	Edema: Protein and thiamin deficits
	Skin lesions, ulcers, nonhealing wounds: Protein, vitamin C, zinc deficits
	Yellow pigmentation (except sclerae): Excess carotene (benign)
	Poor skin turgor: Dehydration

(continued)

AREA/SYSTEM AND NORMAL FINDINGS	ABNORMAL FINDINGS
Integumentary *Hair*	
Even hair distribution, no alopecia	Transverse pigmentation of hair shaft; hair easy to pluck, breaks easily: Protein deficit Sparse hair distribution: Protein, biotin, zinc deficits; excess vitamin A Corkscrew hairs, unemerged hair coils: Vitamin C deficit
Nails	
Nails smooth and pink	Transverse ridges in nails: Protein deficit Concave "spoon" nails: Iron deficit
HEENT *Eyes*	
Eyes clear and bright, vision intact	Papilledema : Vitamin A excess Night blindness: Vitamin A deficit Sunken eyeballs, dark circles, decreased tears: Dehydration Sunken fontanels: Dehydration
Mouth and Throat	
Oral mucosa pink, moist, and intact without lesions	Angular stomatitis, cheilosis (dry, cracked, ulcerated lips): Riboflavin, niacin, pyridoxine deficits
Tonsils pink; gums pink and intact with no bleeding	Swollen, retracted, bleeding gums (if teeth present): Vitamin C deficit Atrophic lingual papillae (coated tongue): Riboflavin, niacin, folic acid, vitamin B_{12}, protein, iron deficits Glossitis (raw, red tongue): Riboflavin, niacin, pyridoxine, folic acid, vitamin B_{12} deficits
Parotid glands of normal size	Parotid gland enlargement: Protein deficit (consider bulimia)
Taste sensation intact	Hypogeusia (blunting of sense of taste): Zinc deficit
Swallow and gag reflex intact. Full mobility of tongue	Absent swallow and gag reflexes may impair eating Impaired tongue mobility may cause dysphagia.
Nose	
Sense of smell intact Nasal mucosa pink, moist, and intact without lesions	Hyposmia (defect in sense of smell): Zinc deficit Anosmia can affect taste. Dry mucous membranes: Dehydration
Respiratory Lungs clear, respirations normal	Increased respiratory rate: Iron-deficiency anemia

(continued)

AREA/SYSTEM AND NORMAL FINDINGS	ABNORMAL FINDINGS
Cardiovascular Regular heart rate/rhythm. PMI 1 cm at apex. No extra sounds	Heart failure, S_3: Thiamin, phosphorus, iron deficits Sudden heart failure, death: Vitamin C deficit Tachycardia and systolic murmur: Iron-deficiency anemia
Gastrointestinal Abdomen soft, nontender; no organomegaly	Hepatomegaly, ascites: Protein deficits, vitamin A excess Hyperactive bowel sounds: Hyperperistalsis with absorption problem
Musculoskeletal No deformities, tenderness, or swelling	Beading of ribs, epiphyseal swelling, bowlegs: Vitamin D deficit Tenderness, superperiosteal bleeding: Vitamin C deficit
Neurological No headache AAO × 3 DTR + 2/4 Senses intact	Headache: Vitamin A excess Drowsiness, lethargy, vomiting: Vitamin A, D excess Dementia: Niacin, vitamin B_{12} deficit Confusion, irritability: Dehydration Disorientation: Thiamin (Korsakoff's psychosis) deficit Ophthalmoplegia: Thiamin, phosphorus deficit Peripheral neuropathy (weakness, paresthesia, ataxia, decreased DTRs; diminished tactile, vibratory, and position sensation): Niacin, pyridoxine, vitamin B_{12} deficits Tetany, increased DTRs: Calcium, magnesium deficits

CHAPTER 21

ASSESSING SPIRITUALITY

Brief Review of Spiritual Health

- Does the client identify with any organized religion? If so, what religion?
- If the client does not identify with a particular religion, does he or she have a belief system that provides comfort and strength?
- Is the client an agnostic or an atheist? If so, does any belief system give meaning to his or her life?
- Bear in mind what is the primary nature of the client's religion.
- Are people of the client's religion monotheistic or pantheistic?

Developmental Considerations

Infants

- What concerns do the parents have about their child's illness?
- How can you help support your client's use of religious practices (e.g., by referral to the hospital chaplain or hospital meditation room)?
- Do parents ask why their child is ill?
- Do the parents see the infant's illness as a religious punishment?
- Are the parents practicing religious rituals?

Toddlers, Preschoolers, and School-Age Children

- How does the child feel about what is happening to him or her?
- To whom does the child talk when he or she is in trouble, sad, lonely, or scared?
- What makes the child feel better when he or she is scared, sad, or lonely?
- Does the child express concerns or show anxiety about illness and dying?
- Does he or she speak of being punished by a deity for "being bad?"
- Is he or she practicing religious rituals, such as saying bedtime prayers?

Adolescents and Young Adults

- How does the adolescent feel about what is happening to him or her?
- To whom does the adolescent usually go for support?
- What gives meaning to the adolescent's life? Has this changed since he or she got sick?
- Does the adolescent express concerns about dying or the seriousness of his or her illness?
- Does he or she practice any religious rituals?
- Does he or she verbalize his or her own beliefs and values?

Older Adults

- Ask the same questions as you would of an adolescent or young adult.
- Older clients often suffer many losses and therefore have fewer support systems, so you may need to make referrals to community services.

Cultural Considerations

- Familiarize yourself with your client's cultural domain.
- Learn about the use of prayer, meditation, and other activities or symbols that help people of your client's cultural or ethnic group reach fulfillment.
- Know what gives meaning to life for the client's cultural group. Identify the client's individual sources of strength.

- Become familiar with the way in which spiritual beliefs affect this cultural group's healthcare practices.

Health History

- Biographical data
  - Review the client's admission sheet for basic religious information, and be sure to ask questions to clarify this information.
  - Inquire about marital status and contact person.
  - Ask the client's age.
  - Be aware that the absence of religious identification does not mean that the client has no spiritual needs.
- Current health status
  - Your client's current physical health and spiritual health are intertwined.
  - Clients with chronic or terminal diseases are especially prone to spiritual distress.
- Past health history
  - Explore the connection between your client's health and spiritual needs.
- Family history
  - The family history is invaluable in identifying familial problems that pose a threat to your client's health, which may affect his or her spiritual needs.
- Psychosocial profile
  - Examine your client's typical day for activities that reflect spirituality.
  - Determine whether dietary preferences may also be influenced by religious practices.

Spiritual Assessment

Assessing Behavior

Is the client:

- Praying or meditating?
- Shutting others out?
- Constantly complaining?
- Having sleep difficulties?
- Pacing?

- Requesting frequent pain or sleep medication without apparent need?

Assessing Verbal Communication

Is the client talking about:

- God or another deity?
- Church, temple, mosque, or other place of worship?
- Prayer, hope, faith, or the meaning of life?
- The effect of the diagnosis on his or her quality of life?

Assessing Relationships

Does the client:

- Have many visitors? Who are his or her visitors (family, friends, clergy or other spiritual support people)?
- Interact with them well?

Assessing Environment

Does the client have:

- A Bible, Koran (Qur'an), or other religious reading material?
- Religious jewelry or symbols, such as a cross, Star of David, prayer cap or shawl, flowers from a church altar, or religious greeting cards?

Additional Questions for the Client

- Who are your support people?
- What provides you with strength and hope?
- What gives your life meaning and purpose?
- How has your life changed since you became ill?
- What is important to you?
- How is your religion, deity, or faith important to you?
- Is prayer important?
- What accommodations can be made to assist you in continuing any spiritual practices (e.g., religious symbols and/or dietary needs)?

CHAPTER 22

ASSESSING CULTURE

Because cultural background encompasses every aspect of a person's life, you need to be aware of how it influences your client's health and wellness. Consider the following areas—as adapted from Purnell, L.D., and Paulanka, B.J. (2003): *Transcultural Healthcare: A Culturally Competent Approach* (2nd ed.). Philadelphia: F. A. Davis Company—when determining the influence of culture on your client's health.

Overview

- Inhabited localities and topography
  - In what part of the world does this person's cultural or ethnic group originate?
  - What is the climate and topography there?
- Heritage and residence
  - Where does this person's cultural or ethnic group reside now?
- Reason for migration and associated economic factors
  - What were the major factors that motivated this person's cultural or ethnic group to emigrate?
- Educational status and occupations
  - What value does the person's cultural group place on education?
  - What are the predominant occupations of the group's members?

Communication

- Dominant language and dialects
  - What is the dominant language of the group?
  - Does the person use that language or a dialect that may interfere with communication?
  - Are there specific contextual speech patterns for this group? If so, what are they?
  - What is the usual volume and tone of speech?
- Cultural communication patterns
  - Is the person willing to share thoughts, feelings, and ideas?
  - What is the practice and meaning of touch in the person's society? With family, friends, strangers, same sex, opposite sex, and healthcare providers?
  - What are the personal spatial and distancing characteristics when communicating one-to-one? With friends vs. strangers?
  - Does this group use eye contact? Does avoidance of eye contact have special meaning? Is eye contact influenced by socioeconomic status?
  - Do various facial expressions have specific meanings? Are facial expressions used to express emotions?
  - Are there acceptable ways of standing and greeting outsiders? If so, what are they?
- Temporal relationships
  - Are people primarily past, present, or future oriented? How do they see the context of past, present, and future?
  - Are there differences in interpretation of social time versus clock time? If so, what are they?
  - Are people expected to be punctual in terms of jobs, appointments, and social engagements?
- Format and names
  - What is the format for a person's name?
  - How does the person expect to be greeted by strangers and healthcare practitioners?

Family Roles and Organization

- Head of household and gender roles
  - Who is the perceived head of household?

- How does this role change during different developmental aspects of life?
- What are the gender-related roles of men and women in the family system?
- Prescriptive, restrictive, and taboo behaviors
  - What are the prescriptive, restrictive, and taboo behaviors for children?
  - What are the prescriptive, restrictive, and taboo behaviors for adults?
- Family roles and priorities
  - What family goals and priorities are emphasized by this culture?
  - What are the developmental tasks of this group?
  - What is the status and role of older people in the family?
  - What are the roles and importance of extended family members?
  - How does one gain social status in this cultural system? Is there a caste system?
- How are alternative lifestyles and nontraditional families viewed by the society?

Workforce Issues

- Culture in the workplace
  - Are workforce issues, such as education, affected by immigration? If so, how?
  - What are the specific multicultural considerations when working with this culturally diverse person or group?
  - What factors influence patterns of acculturation in this cultural group?
  - How do the person's or group's healthcare practices influence the workforce?
- Issues related to autonomy
  - What are the cultural issues related to professional autonomy, superior or subordinate control, religion, and gender in the workforce?
  - Are there language barriers? For example, do people sometimes misunderstand English expressions by interpreting them concretely?

Biocultural Ecology

- Skin color and biological variations
  - Are there skin color and physical variations for this group? If so, what are they?
  - What special problems or concerns might the skin color pose for healthcare practitioners?
  - What are the biological variations in body habitus or structure?
- Diseases and health conditions
  - What are the risk factors for people related to topography or climate?
  - Are there any hereditary or genetic diseases or conditions that are common with this group? If so, what are they?
  - Are there any endemic diseases specific to this cultural or ethnic group? If so, what are they?
  - Are there any diseases or health conditions for which this group has increased susceptibility? If so, what are they?
- Does this group have any specific variations in drug metabolism, drug interactions, and related side effects? If so, what are they?

High-Risk Behaviors

- Are any high-risk behaviors common in this group? If so, what are they?
- What are the patterns of use of alcohol, tobacco, recreational drugs, and other substances in this group?

Healthcare Practices

- What are typical health-seeking behaviors for this group?
- What is this group's usual level of physical activity?
- Do people in this group use safety measures, such as seat belts?

Nutrition

- What does food mean to this group?
- Common foods and food rituals

- What specific foods, preparation practices, and major ingredients are commonly used by this group?
- Are there any specific food rituals for this group? If so, what are they?
- Dietary practices for health promotion
- Are enzyme deficiencies or food intolerances commonly experienced by this group? If so, what are they?
- Are large-scale or significant nutritional deficiencies experienced by this group? If so, what are they?
- Are there native food limitations in America that may cause special health difficulties? If so, what are they?

Pregnancy and Childbearing Practices

- Fertility practices and views regarding pregnancy
  - What are the cultural views and practices related to fertility control?
  - What are the cultural views and practices regarding pregnancy?
- Prescriptive, restrictive, and taboo practices in the childbearing family
  - What are the prescriptive, restrictive, and taboo practices related to pregnancy, such as food, exercise, intercourse, and avoidance of weather-related conditions?
  - What are the prescriptive, restrictive, and taboo practices related to the birthing process, such as reactions during labor, presence of men, position of mother for delivery, preferred types of health practitioners, or place of delivery?
  - What are the prescriptive, restrictive, and taboo practices related to the postpartum period, such as bathing, cord care, exercise, food, and roles of men?

Death Rituals

- Death rituals and expectations
  - Are there culturally specific death rituals and expectations? If so, what are they?
  - What is the purpose of the death rituals and mourning practices?

- What specific practices (e.g., cremation) are used for disposal of the body?
- Responses to death and grief
  - How are people expected to show grief and respond to the death of a family member?
  - What is the meaning of death, dying, and afterlife?

Spirituality

- Religious practices and use of prayer
  - How does the dominant religion of this group influence healthcare practices?
  - Are there activities such as prayer, meditation, or symbols that help people reach fulfillment? If so, what are they?
- Meaning of life and individual sources of strength
  - What gives meaning to people's lives?
  - What is the person's source of strength?
- What is the relationship between spiritual beliefs and healthcare practices?

Healthcare Practices

- Health-seeking beliefs and behaviors
  - What predominant beliefs influence healthcare practices?
  - What is the influence of health promotion and prevention practices?
- Responsibility for health care
  - Is the focus of acute-care practice curative or fatalistic?
  - Who assumes responsibility for health care in this culture?
  - What is the role of health insurance in this culture?
  - What are the behaviors associated with the use of over-the-counter medications?
- How do magicoreligious beliefs, folklore, and traditional beliefs influence healthcare behaviors?
- Are there barriers to health care such as language, economics, and geography for this group? If so, what are they?

- Cultural responses to health and illness
  - Are there cultural beliefs and responses to pain that influence interventions? If so, what are they?
  - Does pain have special meaning?
  - What are the beliefs and views about mental and physical illness in this culture?
  - Does this culture view mental handicaps differently from physical handicaps?
  - What are the cultural beliefs and practices related to chronicity and rehabilitation?
  - Are there any restrictions to the acceptance of blood transfusions, organ donation, and organ transplantation for this group? If so, what are they?

Healthcare Practitioners

- Traditional versus biomedical care
  - What are the roles of traditional, folklore, and magicoreligious practitioners, and how do they influence health practitioners?
  - How does this culture feel about healthcare practitioners providing care to patients of the opposite sex?
  - Does the age of the practitioner make a difference? If so, what?
- Status of healthcare providers
  - How does this culture feel about healthcare providers?
  - What is the status of healthcare providers in this culture?
  - How do different healthcare practitioners in this culture view each other?

CHAPTER 23

ASSESSING THE CLIENT'S ENVIRONMENT

Shorter stays in acute-care settings have increased the need for nursing care at home. Home care nursing can occur at both the primary and tertiary levels. At the primary care level, you will make postpartum visits to new mothers and babies. At the tertiary level, you will make follow-up visits to patients discharged from the hospital.

Assessing the Home

In the home, your assessment is based on the health history and physical examination findings. You need to assess your patient's response to the treatment plan and also identify any risk factors in his or her environment that may affect his or her health and well-being. Remember, the treatment plan established in the hospital will be effective only if your patient is able to follow it at home.

Begin by determining if your patient is able to perform activities of daily living (ADLs); then assess basic needs and environmental safety hazards. Also assess support systems and self-esteem or self-actualization. Keep in mind that financial status and religious and cultural beliefs influence health beliefs and practices.

AREAS/ QUESTIONS TO ASK	FACTORS IDENTIFIED BY QUESTIONS
Physical Needs *Food*	
What does the patient eat and drink? Who prepares food? Who buys food? Is food being stored properly? Is kitchen accessible? Clean? Are appliances in good operating condition? If you detect a nutritional deficit, does patient's illness have an effect on appetite? Is there an unexplained weight loss or gain? Does the patient drink alcohol? Does he or she have a dental problem? Are financial hardships limiting purchase of foods? Is the patient taking multiple medicines? Does he or she eat alone? Does he or she need assistance in eating?	Need for referrals for assistance, such as financial support, Meals on Wheels, home health aides Self-care deficits Teaching needs Nutritional deficits or problems affecting nutritional status
Elimination	
Is the bathroom accessible? Does patient need a commode? Does he or she need a raised toilet seat? Grab bars?	Need for assistive devices Self-care deficits Risk for falls Risk for incontinence problems
Bathing	
Does patient take baths, showers, or sponge baths? Does he or she care for his or her hair and teeth? Does he or she need assistance in bathing? Does he or she have a shower chair? Does the bathtub have grab bars? Rubber mats? Nonskid tiles?	Need for assistive devices Self-care deficits Risk for falls
Dressing	
Does patient have clean clothes? Do clothes fit? Des he or she need assistance with dressing?	Self-care deficits Risks for falls or skin breakdown Need for home health aide *(continued)*

AREAS/ QUESTIONS TO ASK	FACTORS IDENTIFIED BY QUESTIONS
Physical Needs *Dressing (Continued)*	
Do shoes fit properly? Who does the laundry? *Sleep*	
Where does the patient sleep? How much time does he or she spend in bed? Does the patient need a special mattress or bed? Are bedrails needed? How far is the bed from the bathroom? From other family members? Is there privacy for members in household?	Risk for skin breakdown Need for special equipment Safety issues
Medications Is patient able to take own medications as prescribed? Is he or she taking any over-the-counter medications, vitamins, or herbal supplements? Does he or she need medications pre-poured? Does he or she have any impairments that would prevent him or her from self-administering medications safely (e.g., cognitive or visual impairments)? Are medications safely stored? Can patient open medication containers? If using syringes, how does patient dispose of them? Obtain supplies? What is the name of patient's pharmacy? His or her medication insurance plan? Does patient have the finances to pay for medications and treatment? Does patient understand what medications he or she is taking and their purpose?	Compliance with medical treatment plan and reasons for noncompliance Problems associated with polypharmacy (e.g., side effects, drug interactions) Safety issues surrounding medication preparation and administration Need for assistive devices Need for referral or visiting nurse Teaching needs Financial needs for obtaining prescriptions
Shelter Is home maintained and clean? Who is responsible for managing and cleaning it?	Safety issues Need for referrals Need for assistance with

(continued)

AREAS/ QUESTIONS TO ASK	FACTORS IDENTIFIED BY QUESTIONS
Shelter (*Continued*)	
Are plumbing and sewage systems working properly?	home management and maintenance
What type of heating is there (gas, electric, oil, wood)? Central heating or space heating? Is heating system working properly?	
Is there air conditioning? Fans?	
Is ventilation adequate? Do windows open and close easily and completely?	
What type of insulation is there?	
Is home in need of repair (e.g., peeling paint or cracks in foundation or windows)?	
Is there evidence of insect or rodent infestation?	
Has home been tested for radon?	
Assessing Environmental Safety *Mobility/Fall Prevention*	
Is patient able to walk? Is his or her gait steady? Does patient use assistive devices correctly?	Risk for fall/injury Need for assistive devices
Do devices fit through pathways and doorways?	Need for referrals Need for teaching
Is house one level or more? Are there elevators or stairs?	
Can patient enter and exit home without difficulty?	
Are pathways and stairs clear?	
Are there throw rugs?	
Are there sturdy handrails on the stairs? Are first and last steps clearly marked?	
Are floors slippery or uneven?	
Is there adequate lighting in hallways, stairs, and path to bathroom?	
Is there need for restraints? If yes, what type and when?	
Are carpets in good repair without tears?	
Can patient walk on carpet? Does he or she have to hold onto furniture to maintain balance? If yes, is furniture sturdy and stable enough to provide support?	

(continued)

AREAS/ QUESTIONS TO ASK	FACTORS IDENTIFIED BY QUESTIONS
Assessing Environmental Safety *Mobility/Fall Prevention (Continued)*	
Are chairs sturdy and stable? Are there any cords or wires that may present a tripping hazard? *Fire/Burn Prevention*	
Are there working smoke detectors on each floor? Carbon monoxide detectors? Fire extinguisher? Is there an escape plan in case of fire? Are wires, plugs, and electrical equipment in good working condition? Is client using a heating pad or portable heaters safely? Does he or she smoke? If yes, does he or she smoke safely? Are there signs of cigarette burns? Are there signs of burns in the kitchen? Is stove free of grease? Does patient use oxygen? If yes, is tank stored safely away from heat or flame? *Crime/Injury*	Risk for injury Safety issues Teaching needs Referrals (e.g., local fire company for free smoke detectors)
Are there working locks on doors and windows? Is client able to make emergency calls? Are emergency numbers readily available? Is phone readily accessible? Are there firearms in home? If yes, are they safely secured with ammunition stored separately? Is there any evidence of criminal activity? Are poisonous or toxic substances properly stored?	Safety issues Need for referral to local police Teaching needs
Assessing Support Systems, Self-Esteem, and Self-Actualization *Roles*	
What roles does person play because of illness? How has this affected other family members?	Source of stress, depression, and anxiety Need for referrals

(continued)

AREAS/ QUESTIONS TO ASK	FACTORS IDENTIFIED BY QUESTIONS
Assessing Support Systems, Self-Esteem, and Self-Actualization *Caregivers*	
Is there a caregiver? Is caregiver competent, willing, and supportive? Does caregiver need support? Can caregiver hear client? Is there a need for an intercom, "baby monitor," or bell?	Supports Need for referrals (e.g., caregiver may need support, respite care, or home health aide) Need for assistive devices Teaching needs
Communication	
Is phone in easy reach? Can client dial phone and see numbers? Does he or she need oversized numbers, audio enhancer, or a memory feature? Is there a daily safety check system? Should there be an alert system like Lifeline? Are emergency numbers for police, fire, ambulance, nurse, doctor, relative, or neighbor clearly marked? How does patient get mail?	Emergency supports Teaching needs Need for assistive devices Safety issues
Family/Friends/Pets	
Who visits patient? Family, friends, church members? Who can drive patient to doctor appointments, church, and other places? Are there any pets? Is patient able to take care of them properly? Are pets well behaved?	Supports Need for referrals Ability to maintain follow-up care Teaching needs
Self-Esteem and Self-Actualization	
What does client like to do? Are there creative ways to enable him or her to do activities he or she enjoys? Are there meaningful solitary activities patient can do, such as reading or listening to music? Interactive activities?	Sources of meaning in patient's life Need for referral to community resources (e.g., library, senior citizen groups)

Adapted with permission from Narayan, M. (1997). Environmental assessment. *Home Healthcare Nurse, 15*(11):798. Philadelphia, Lippincott-Raven.

Assessing the Community

Assessment involves assessing the people within the community, the environment of the community, and the interaction between the two to identify any actual or potential health problems.

QUESTIONS TO ASK YOURSELF	SIGNIFICANCE
Boundaries	
What is the geographic description of the community (e.g., a town) or the criteria for membership in the community (e.g., a school)?	Boundaries can be real, concrete or conceptual. Identifies who and what is included in the community.
What are the neighboring areas (e.g., a city if the community is a suburb)?	Allows you to focus assessment on the community.
Are boundaries open or closed?	Some boundaries may exclude certain groups (e.g., communities with only high-priced housing may exclude lower socioeconomic groups).
What is the purpose or goals of the community (e.g., a school's mission statement)?	Identifies purpose of community (e.g., goal of a Catholic school is to educate children in Christian values).
Physical Characteristics	
How old is the community?	Older, well-established community may have more resources available than new, developing community. Or, older community's resources may be outdated, not meeting current needs.
What are community's demographics (e.g., age, race, sex, ethnicity, housing, density of population)?	You can identify healthcare needs of community by identifying health problems associated with age, gender, or race.
What are community's physical features?	Physical features can influence community's behavior and health (e.g., exposure to toxic substances).

(continued)

QUESTIONS TO ASK YOURSELF	SIGNIFICANCE
Psychosocial Characteristics	
What is the community's predominant religion, socioeconomic class, educational level, type of occupation, and marital status?	Religion influences what and how health issues are addressed (e.g., abortion/birth control contradicts Catholic beliefs).
	Socioeconomic class reflects affordability and accessibility of healthcare services. People in low socioeconomic areas may not have financial resources for health care or be able to practice preventive health care. Limited financial access to health care raises community's morbidity and mortality rates.
	Educational level identifies health teaching needs and approaches. The higher their educational level, the more likely people are to practice preventive health behaviors.
	Occupation can identify specific health issues for the group (e.g., blue collar workers may have a higher incidence of musculoskeletal problems; white collar workers may have a higher incidence of stress-related diseases).
	Marital status may identify stability and support sources within community.
External Influences	
Does the community receive any external funding?	Federal or state funding and grants may be available for health services.
Are there facilities outside community that are available to community members? Is there access or transportation to these facilities?	Identifies healthcare facilities needed (e.g., rural areas may need to go outside community for health services).
Are adequate healthcare providers available to community?	

(continued)

QUESTIONS TO ASK YOURSELF	SIGNIFICANCE
External Influences (*Continued*)	
Are volunteer groups available to the community?	Volunteer groups can be a valuable resource, especially if healthcare providers are limited.
How is health information communicated to community?	Determines if there is a need for further and better means of communication.
What laws affect the community?	Laws, such as zoning or pollution laws, can influence healthcare issues. Federal and state programs also can affect the health and well-being of some members of the community, such as senior citizens.
Are values of external influences consistent with those of community?	Inconsistent values can affect healthcare issues.
Internal Functions *Human Services*	
What human services are available within community? Nurses, doctors, volunteers? Is access to services adequate?	Determines if services meet community's needs.
What is community's budget? How much is allocated for healthcare services?	Identifies value of health care services and need for external funding sources.
What and how many healthcare facilities (hospitals, nursing homes, daycare centers) are available in community? Are there enough to meet people's needs? Are they well equipped? Accessible?	Determines availability and accessibility of healthcare facilities.
Does facility have goods and supplies to produce its goods? What is the product? What is the facility's contribution to the community?	Identifies both positive and negative effects to community (e.g., if facility is drug treatment center, drug dealers and abusers, as a community in itself, exert a negative effect on community at large).
Is education appropriate, accessible, and adequate for community? What types of schools are there? How much money is budgeted for education?	Identifies adequacy and availability of schools.

(continued)

QUESTIONS TO ASK YOURSELF	SIGNIFICANCE
Internal Functions *Politics*	
What is the organizational structure of the community? Elected vs. appointed positions? Terms? Formal vs. informal leaders?	Helps identify how decisions are made and who has power.
How are decisions made? Majority rule or consensus? Is community independent or dependent?	Identifies approaches needed to bring about change. Identifies role of nurse within community (e.g., if community is dependent, nurse may need to take more active role).
What are rules and laws of community? Formal and informal?	Identifies laws that regulate behaviors. Identifies expectations, peer pressures.
Communication	
Nonverbal: What is personality of community? How do people respond to outsiders?	Identifies approaches toward community.
Verbal: Who communicates with whom? What are means of communication? Is communication vertical or horizontal?	
Values	
What does the community value? What is important?	Identifies what is important to community.
Does the community have any traditions?	Can influence healthcare practices.
Are there subgroups within the community?	Can have own values and norms that affect community and influence healthcare practices.
What is the condition of the physical environment? Clean, dirty, in disrepair?	Condition of environment reflects value placed on it by community.
How is health defined by the community?	Identifies value community places on health.
How much does community value health?	
What type of healthcare facilities are there? How frequently are they used?	
Is the community homogeneous or heterogeneous?	Identifies approaches toward community.

(continued)

QUESTIONS TO ASK YOURSELF	SIGNIFICANCE
Health Behavior/Health Status *People*	
What is the growth rate of the community? Relationship between birth and death rates? Relationship between immigration and emigration? Is population young or old? Is it mobile?	Identifies health status and needs of community (e.g., health needs for retirement community are different from those of a community with mostly young couples). Indirectly identifies teaching needs. Identifies factors within community that affect health.
What are morbidity and mortality rates? The prevalence and incidence of disease?	Identifies focus and direction of health care needed by community. Identifies health teaching needs for community.
What types of risky behavior occur in the community? Are there at-risk groups?	Identifies at-risk groups. Identifies need for intervention and teaching.
What is the incidence of presymptomatic illnesses, such as HIV, hypertension (HTN), or high cholesterol?	Identifies need for screening programs. Determines effectiveness of existing screening programs. Identifies health teaching needs.
What is the level of functioning of community (e.g., dependent vs. independent)?	Identifies type and direction of intervention needed to maintain and promote health.
Are there people with disabilities? How many people and what types of disabilities?	Identifies resources required to meet need of community members with disabilities.
Environment	
What is the quality of the air?	Identifies possible exposure to pollutants.
What is the quality of the food supply?	Identifies possible contamination causing GI diseases.
What is the quality of the water supply? Is the water public or well? Is it fluoridated?	Identifies possible contamination causing GI problems.
What is the quality of the soil?	Identifies possible contamination with radioactive material, human or animal excreta, *Ascaris* worm.
Is there adequate housing?	Identifies possible crowding, radon and lead exposure.

(continued)

QUESTIONS TO ASK YOURSELF	SIGNIFICANCE
Health Behavior/Health Status *Environment (Continued)*	
What is the quality of home and work site?	Identifies possible occupational health risks.
What is the quality of solid waste disposal?	Identifies possible source of contamination.
What is the quality of hazardous waste disposal?	Identifies possible contamination from toxic substances.
Is there infestation by insects, rodents, and animals? Use of pesticides?	Identifies disease carriers. Pesticide use increases risk for exposure to toxic chemicals.
Are there natural disasters in the community? Incidences of violence or terrorism?	Identifies sources of stress.

Data from Smith, C., and Maurer, F. (2000). *Community Health Nursing Theory and Practice* (2nd ed.). Philadelphia: W. B. Saunders.

CHAPTER 24

ASSESSING ABUSE

Abuse can take many forms, can affect any age group, and knows no socioeconomic boundaries. It can be physical, sexual, emotional, or a combination of two or all of these. It may also be directed at property. As a nurse, you need to be alert for signs and symptoms of abuse at all levels of health care for all of your patients. This chapter covers child abuse, spousal or partner (domestic) abuse, and elder abuse.

Types of Abuse

- *Physical Abuse:* Physical contact with intent to harm, ranging from slapping, hitting, and biting to murder. Physical abuse includes neglect—depriving a person of basic needs such as food, water, or sleep.
- *Sexual Abuse:* Sexually oriented behavior without the consent of the other person or persons involved, ranging from sexually degrading remarks to rape.
- *Psychological (Emotional) Abuse:* Verbal abuse or actions that can be considered degrading, belittling, or threatening, used for control, often by evoking fear in the victim. This type of abuse is difficult to assess.
- *Property Abuse:* Deliberate destruction of a person's belongings.

Assessing Child Abuse

Child abuse and neglect are the leading cause of death in children younger than 3 years of age.

More than 2 million cases are reported every year. Child abuse can take the following forms:

- *Physical Abuse:* Includes actual physical trauma, such as bruising, breaking bones, intentional burns, and shaken-baby syndrome. It also includes Munchausen's syndrome by proxy (MSBP), in which the parent or caretaker intentionally causes a child to be ill to gain sympathy and recognition.
- *Neglect:* Failure to meet the child's basic needs.
- *Sexual Abuse:* Includes actual intercourse with either vaginal or anal penetration, genital fondling and other inappropriate touching, or pornographic photography of the child.
- *Psychological Abuse:* Includes emotional detachment from the child, constant belittling, fostering and enabling substance abuse and delinquency, and failing to provide adequate supervision.

Assessing for Physical Abuse

As you go through the assessment, ask yourself: Are the injuries inconsistent with the child's age or developmental stage (e.g., 1-month-old baby falling out of crib)? Is evidence of old fractures or trauma seen on current x rays?

TAKING THE HEALTH HISTORY
- Obtain separate statements from parents or caregivers. Be alert for inconsistencies (e.g., parent saying that hand-mark bruising on the child was inflicted by another child).
- Ask yourself: What is your perception of the child (e.g., difficult or quiet)?
- Ask the parent or caregiver:
    - Does the child have a history of past health problems? Where was the child treated? (Frequent emergency room [ER]) visits signal abuse. Parents may use different health care centers to avoid suspicion.)
    - What is the child's feeding history? (Compare the history given to the child's physical growth and development.)

- Ask the child (if old enough): What types of stress do you have in your life? Who are your supports?
- Suspect MSBP if:
  - Child does not respond to usual treatment.
  - Laboratory results are inconsistent with history or physically impossible.
  - Parent seems very knowledgeable about medical treatment.
  - Signs and symptoms of illness do not occur when parent is not present.
  - Similar findings or unexplained deaths have occurred in siblings.
  - Parent craves adulation for his or her care of child.

PERFORMING THE PHYSICAL EXAMINATION

- Obtain growth measurements and compare them with previous measurements. Nutritional neglect can cause failure to thrive.
- Look for distended abdomen, a sign of malnutrition.
- Observe child's grooming, dress, and hygiene.
- Examine all body surfaces for bruises, burns, and skin lesions, looking especially for the following signs of physical abuse:
  - Bruises that form the outline of a hand (from parent grabbing child)
  - Linear bruises (from belts)
  - Bruises on head, face, ears, buttocks, and lower back (consistent with abuse)
  - Obviously nonaccidental burns (e.g., burns on both lower legs)
  - Burn outline of an entire object, such as multiple cigarette burns on various parts of body
  - Detached retina and hemorrhages and subdural hematoma (shaken-baby syndrome)

Assessing for Sexual Abuse

TAKING THE HEALTH HISTORY

Be nonjudgmental when questioning caregivers about possible sexual abuse. Obtain the following information from patients or their caregivers:

- Ask children over 2½ years directly about being touched in "private parts." With older children, use an approach such as: "Sometimes people you know may touch or kiss you in a way that you feel is wrong. Has this ever happened to you?" With adolescents, use an approach such as: "Sometimes people touch you in ways you feel are wrong. This can be frightening, and it is wrong for people to do that to you. Has this ever happened to you?"
- Determine whether there has been a sudden onset of bedwetting in a child who was previously not a bedwetter.
- Determine whether the child masturbates or sexually acts out with other children.
- Determine whether the child has genitourinary symptoms, such as burning, itching, or vaginal discharge.
- Determine whether the child has a history of running away from home, especially to unsafe situations as opposed to a friend's home.

PERFORMING THE PHYSICAL ASSESSMENT
- Look for genital and anal irritation, discharge, swelling, redness, and bruising. In girls, carefully evaluate the vaginal introitus for evidence of penetration.
- During the examination, observe the child's behavior:
  - Is the child overly solicitous in a sexual manner?
  - Does he or she dress or act provocatively?
  - Is he or she overly fearful of the exam, especially the genital exam?

Assessing for Psychological Abuse

TAKING THE HEALTH HISTORY
Ask the parent or caregiver the following questions:

- Was this child the result of a planned pregnancy? What were the birth and postpartum period like? Were there many stressors at home at the time of your child's birth?
- How would you describe your child now?
- How is this child compared to others in your family?
- Is there a history of physical or developmental problems? If so, what kinds of supports do you receive?
- Has the child had many illnesses? If so, what are they? How has this affected your life?

- What are your expectations of the child?
- What form of discipline works best for the child?

PERFORMING THE PSYCHOLOGICAL ASSESSMENT
During the examination, observe the following:

- Compare parental description of the child with what you actually observe.
- Observe child-parent interaction. Is it distant or engaging? How does the parent comfort the child?
- If other siblings are present, does the parent respond to them differently from the child in question?
- Does the parent openly and repeatedly belittle the child (e.g., saying: "You're so dumb")?
- Does the child have developmental delays, poor social skills, speech problems, or regression?

Assessing Spousal or Partner Abuse (Domestic Violence)

Domestic violence is the leading cause of injury to women. One in every three women has been abused by a spouse or partner at least one time during the relationship. Here are more facts about domestic violence:

- Fifty percent of homeless women and children have been victims of abuse.
- The battering cycle consists of the tension-building phase, the battering phase, and the apologetic phase.
- Abuse occurs in same-sex relationships as well as heterosexual relationships.
- Abusers are usually emotionally dependent and egocentric.
- The battered partner is usually unsure, economically and emotionally dependent, and exhibiting learned helplessness.
- Spousal or partner abuse can take the form of physical, sexual, or psychological abuse (or a combination of two or all of these), or property abuse.
- Emotional abuse is difficult to assess because the effects are not as visible as those of physical abuse.
- To gain power and control, the abuser may:

- Use coercion and threats, such as threatening to leave the partner or commit suicide.
- Use intimidation to evoke fear by destroying personal belongings or hurting pets.
- Degrade and belittle, making the partner feel that it is his or her fault; make him or her feel guilty or blame abuse on him or her.
- Isolate the partner by limiting contacts with family and friends.
- Control or limit finances.
- Put children in the middle of the situation or threaten to take them away.
- If male, use male privilege by enforcing dominant role.

Assessing for Physical Abuse

TAKING THE HEALTH HISTORY
Ask the client:

- What is your chief complaint? Complaints are often vague and nonspecific; for example, headaches, gastrointestinal (GI) complaints, asthma, fatigue, and chronic vague pain.
- Do you have trouble sleeping? Do you have nightmares?
- Have you ever been hospitalized? Frequent ER visits are common, with injuries becoming progressively more severe. Current radiographs may reveal old fractures.
- How did the injury happen? Injury may not match the explanation (e.g., black eye from walking into door).
- Do you have a history of depression or attempted suicide? Abuse victim with a sense of hopelessness and powerlessness may be depressed and attempt suicide.
- Are you taking any prescribed or over-the-counter medications? Do you drink alcohol? If so, how much? Substance abuse may be used as an attempt to deal with physical abuse.
- Have you had any weight or appetite changes? Anorexia and bulimia are not uncommon.
- Have you ever been sexually assaulted? Are you satisfied with your sexual relationship with spouse or partner? Domestic violence can take the form of sexual abuse.

PERFORMING THE PHYSICAL EXAMINATION

- Assess for injuries suggesting abuse, such as cigarette burns; black eyes; facial injuries; injuries to the chest, back, breast, or abdomen; bruising on genitalia; or bruises in the shape of a hand or belt.
- During the examination, observe for the following:
  - Patient's lethargic, passive behavior
  - Patient's poor eye contact and anxious or fearful behavior
  - Patient' s visible fear when partner is in room; looking to partner before responding to questions
  - Partner answering for patient and being overly condescending

Assessing Elder Abuse and Neglect

More than 800,000 cases of elder mistreatment are reported annually. Elder abuse can be physical, sexual, or psychological. It can also take the form of neglect or financial or property abuse. During your assessment, be alert if the caregiver speaks for the patient, refuses to let the patient be examined alone, or underreacts when confronted with findings suggesting abuse.

Assessing for Physical Abuse

TAKING THE HEALTH HISTORY
Ask the following questions of the patient and caregiver:

- How did the injury happen? Suspect abuse if injury does not match explanation (e.g., caregiver says injury is from fall, but patient has no difficulty with balance or walking).
- When did the injury occur? Lengthy interval between injury and treatment suggests abuse.
- Who is the primary healthcare provider? "Doctor shopping" (using different healthcare providers) suggests abuse.
- To patient: Do you feel safe in your home?
- To patient: Are there any situations in which you feel afraid?
- To patient or caregiver: Have you ever given/taken the wrong dose of medication? Repeated medication errors by caregiver (e.g., oversedating patient) suggest abuse.

PERFORMING THE PHYSICAL EXAMINATION

During the examination, observe for the following:

- Whiplash burns from rope or cord
- Cigarette burns on palms and soles of feet
- Injuries with a pattern, such as that of a belt buckle or electrical cord
- Oral ecchymosis or injury from forced oral sex
- Whiplash injuries from shaking
- Hyphema, subconjunctival hemorrhage, detached retina, ruptured tympanic membrane
- Bruises on trunk, breast, abdomen, genitalia, and buttocks (bathing suit zone)
- Bleeding or bruising of genitalia, poor sphincter tone, and bruises on inner thighs
- Bruising on wrists and ankles from being bound or restrained
- Immersion burns (may follow a stocking-glove pattern)
- Evidence of old injuries
- Anxiety and depression

Assessing for Neglect

The following are signs of neglect in a patient:

- Never changing clothes, or wearing clothes that are dirty or inappropriate for the weather
- Poor hygiene or body odor
- Ingrown nails
- Decayed or missing teeth
- Untreated sores or pressure sores
- Matted hair
- Hypo/hyperthermia
- Untreated medical problems
- Dehydration
- Malnutrition, failure-to-thrive syndrome
- Weight loss
- Abnormal blood chemistry
- If you are making a home visit: Clutter, disconnected utilities, neglected pets, animal or human excrement, spoiled food

Assessing for Financial Abuse

The following are signs of financial abuse:

- Unusual activity in patient's bank account
- Bank statements diverted from patient's home
- Sudden disappearance of caregiver
- Patient asked to sign documents such as power of attorney
- Large withdrawals from patient's account
- Family that is reluctant to spend money on patient
- Disappearance of personal belongings
- Isolation of patient by caregiver
- Forged signatures on checks and documents
- Caregiver who is evasive about sources of income
- Lack of solid, legal financial arrangements in place for older person

Documentation

Physical, sexual, and financial abuse are crimes in all states. In most states, suspicion of abuse is grounds for reporting. Make sure that you document your findings clearly and objectively. Be specific and thorough because your assessment findings are crucial in early detection and prompt intervention.

INDEX □

Note: Page numbers followed by f indicate figures; page numbers followed by t indicate tables; and page numbers followed by b indicate boxed material.